Household Safety Sourcebook

Hypertension Sourcebook

Immune System Disorders Sourcebook

Infant & Toddler Health Sourcebook

Infectious Diseases Sourcebook

Injury & Trauma Sourcebook

Kidney & Urinary Tract Diseases & Disorders Sourcebook

Learning Disabilities Sourcebook, 2nd Edition

Leukemia Sourcebook

Liver Disorders Sourcebook

Lung Disorders Sourcebook

Medical Tests Sourcebook, 2nd Edition

Men's Health Concerns Sourcebook, 2nd Edition

Mental Health Disorders Sourcebook, 3rd Edition

Mental Retardation Sourcebook

Movement Disorders Sourcebook

Muscular Dystrophy Sourcebook

Obesity Sourcebook

Osteoporosis Sourcebook

Pain Sourcebook, 2nd Edition

Pediatric Cancer Sourcebook

Physical & Mental Issues in Aging Sourcebook

Podiatry Sourcebook

Pregnancy & Birth Sourcebook, 2nd Edition

Prostate Cancer

Public Health Sourcebook

Reconstructive & Cosmetic Surgery Sourcebook

Rehabilitation Sourcebook

Respiratory Diseases & Disorders Sourcebook

Sexually Transmitted Diseases Sourcebook, 2nd Edition

Skin Disorders Sourcebook

Sleep Disorders Sourcebook, 2nd Edition

Smoking Co...

Sports Injuries Sourcebook, 2nd Edition

Stress-Related Disorders Sourcebook

Stroke Sourcebook

Substance Abuse Sourcebook

Surgery Sourcebook

Thyroid Sourcebook

Transplantation Sourcebook

Traveler's Health Sourcebook

Vegetarian Sourcebook

Women's Health Concerns Sourcebook, 2nd Edition

Workplace Health & Safety Sourcebook

Worldwide Health Sourcebook

Teen Health Series

Alcohol Information for Teens

Asthma Information for Teens

Cancer Information for Teens

Diet Information for Teens

Drug Information for Teens

Eating Disorders Information for Teens

Fitness Information for Teens

Mental Health Information for Teens

Sexual Health Information for Teens

Skin Health Information for Teens

Sports Injuries Information for Teens

Suicide Information for Teens

Thyroid
Disorders
SOURCEBOOK

First Edition

Thyroid Disorders SOURCEBOOK

Basic Consumer Health Information about Disorders of the Thyroid and Parathyroid Glands, Including Hypothyroidism, Hyperthyroidism, Graves Disease, Hashimoto Thyroiditis, Thyroid Cancer, and Parathyroid Disorders, Featuring Facts about Symptoms, Risk Factors, Tests, and Treatments

Along with Information about the Effects of Thyroid Imbalance on Other Body Systems, Environmental Factors That Affect the Thyroid Gland, a Glossary, and a Directory of Additional Resources

Edited by
Joyce Brennfleck Shannon

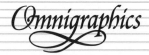

615 Griswold Street • Detroit, MI 48226

Bibliographic Note

Because this page cannot legibly accommodate all the copyright notices, the Bibliographic Note portion of the Preface constitutes an extension of the copyright notice.

Edited by Joyce Brennfleck Shannon

Health Reference Series

Karen Bellenir, *Managing Editor*
David A. Cooke, M.D., *Medical Consultant*
Elizabeth Barbour, *Research and Permissions Coordinator*
Cherry Stockdale, *Permissions Assistant*
Dawn Matthews, *Verification Assistant*
Laura Pleva Nielsen, *Index Editor*
EdIndex, Services for Publishers, *Indexers*

* * *

Omnigraphics, Inc.

Matthew P. Barbour, *Senior Vice President*
Kay Gill, *Vice President—Directories*
Kevin Hayes, *Operations Manager*
Leif Gruenberg, *Development Manager*
David P. Bianco, *Marketing Director*

* * *

Peter E. Ruffner, *Publisher*

Frederick G. Ruffner, Jr., *Chairman*

Copyright © 2005 Omnigraphics, Inc.

ISBN 0-7808-0745-6

Library of Congress Cataloging-in-Publication Data

Thyroid disorders sourcebook : basic consumer health information about disorders of the thyroid and parathyroid glands, including hypothyroidism, hyperthyroidism, Graves disease, Hashimoto thyroiditis, thyroid cancer, and parathyroid disorders, featuring facts about symptoms, risk factors, tests, and treatments, along with information about the effects of thyroid imbalance on other body systems, environmental factors that affect the thyroid gland, a glossary, and a directory of additional resources / edited by Joyce Brennfleck Shannon.-- 1st ed.
    p. cm. -- (Health reference series)
  Includes bibliographical references and index.
  ISBN 0-7808-0745-6 (hardcover : alk. paper)
  1. Thyroid gland--Diseases--Popular works. I. Shannon, Joyce Brennfleck.
II. Series.
  RC655.T4835 2005
  616.4'4--dc22
                                                                  2005003879

This book is printed on acid-free paper meeting the ANSI Z39.48 Standard. The infinity symbol that appears above indicates that the paper in this book meets that standard.

Printed in the United States

Table of Contents

Visit www.healthreferenceseries.com to view *A Contents Guide to the Health Reference Series*, a listing of more than 10,000 topics and the volumes in which they are covered.

Part III: Thyroid Tests

Part VII: Thyroid and Parathyroid Cancer

Part VIII: Thyroid and Parathyroid Disorder Treatments

Part IX: Thyroid Disorder Effects on Other Body Systems

Part X: Additional Help and Information

Preface

About This Book

The thyroid gland is central to the proper functioning of the body, regulating its metabolism and organ function. Thyroid imbalances can lead to symptoms such as fatigue, weight gain or loss, intolerance to cold or heat, sleep disturbances, and changes in bowel patterns. These symptoms can be subtle and develop slowly. According to the Colorado Thyroid Disease Prevalence Study, as many as 13 million Americans may have thyroid disease and not know it. Untreated, thyroid disease can cause elevated cholesterol levels, osteoporosis, depression, miscarriage, birth defects, anemia, and in extreme cases, death.

Thyroid Disorders Sourcebook provides essential information about thyroid and parathyroid function, related diseases, and treatments. Readers will learn about hypothyroidism, hyperthyroidism, Hashimoto thyroiditis, Graves disease, thyroid cancer, and diseases of the parathyroid glands. Facts about risk factors, symptoms, diagnostic tests, and treatments are included, along with information about how thyroid affects the body and how thyroid function can be impacted by environmental hazards. A glossary and a directory of resources provide additional help and information.

How to Use This Book

This book is divided into parts and chapters. Parts focus on broad areas of interest. Chapters are devoted to single topics within a part.

Part I: Thyroid Overview provides general information about the thyroid and parathyroid glands, the endocrine system, and the role of autoimmunity in thyroid disease. It describes thyroid screening guidelines and explains the various roles of physicians who specialize in treating thyroid disorders, including endocrinologists and thyroidologists.

Part II: Thyroid Disorder Symptoms and Risk Factors identifies the impact of genetics, chemical effects, environmental factors, radiation, and the use of iodine on the thyroid. It also discusses specific symptoms including goiter, depression, and prematurely gray hair.

Part III: Thyroid Tests describes tests used to identify thyroid disorders, including blood tests such as TSH, T3, and T4. It also gives detailed information about ultrasound, fine needle aspiration biopsy, and thyroid and parathyroid scans.

Part IV: Underactive Thyroid Gland Disorders contains detailed information about hypothyroidism, including common causes, diagnostic measures, treatments, and how low thyroid levels affect women who are pregnant. Individual chapters discuss disorders characterized by hypothyroidism.

Part V: Overactive Thyroid Gland Disorders contains detailed information about hyperthyroidism, including its causes and treatments, how high thyroid levels affect pregnant women, and special concerns related to high thyroid levels in older patients. Individual chapters discuss disorders characterized by hyperthyroidism.

Part VI: Parathyroid Gland Disorders explains the symptoms, diagnosis, and treatment of parathyroid disorders, including those characterized by hyperparathyroidism (overactive parathyroid gland disorders) and hypoparathyroidism (underactive parathyroid gland disorders).

Part VII: Thyroid and Parathyroid Cancer describes papillary, follicular, medullary, and anaplastic thyroid and parathyroid cancers, including facts about their diagnosis, staging, treatment options, and follow-up care. Information about thyroid cancer-related risks associated with nuclear testing in the U.S. between 1951 and 1963 is also included.

Part VIII: Thyroid and Parathyroid Disorder Treatments contains information about drugs used to increase or suppress thyroid hormone and radiation and radioiodine therapies. Surgical treatment options, such as removal of the thyroid or parathyroid glands, and clinical trials that provide access to innovative treatments are also described.

Part IX: Thyroid Disorder Effects on Other Body Systems includes information about the connection between thyroid dysfunction and disorders of the heart, eyes, blood, bones, and brain.

Part X: Additional Help and Information offers a glossary of important terms and a directory of thyroid-related government agencies and private organizations.

Bibliographic Note

This volume contains documents and excerpts from publications issued by the following U.S. government agencies: Agency for Toxic Substances and Disease Registry; Agency for Healthcare Research and Quality (AHRQ); Centers for Disease Control and Prevention (CDC); National Cancer Institute (NCI); National Cancer Institute–Surveillance, Epidemiology, and End Results (SEER) Program; National Institute of Arthritis and Musculoskeletal and Skin Diseases (NIAMS); National Institute of Child Health and Human Development (NICHD); National Institute of Diabetes and Digestive and Kidney Diseases (NIDDK); National Institute of Environmental Health Sciences (NIEHS); National Institutes of Health (NIH); National Institute of Neurological Disorders and Stroke (NINDS); National Library of Medicine (NLM); National Women's Health Information Center (NWHIC); Osteoporosis and Related Bone Diseases–National Resource Center (ORBD–NRC); U.S. Environmental Protection Agency (EPA); and the U.S. Food and Drug Administration (FDA).

In addition, this volume contains copyrighted documents from the following organizations and individuals: A.D.A.M., Inc.; American Academy of Family Physicians (AAFP); American Association of Clinical Endocrinologists (AACE); American Society of Health-System Pharmacists; American Thyroid Association (ATA); British Thyroid Foundation; Hormone Foundation; La Leche League International; Magic Foundation for Children's Growth; Memorial Sloan-Kettering Cancer Center; National Graves' Disease Foundation (NGDF); Nemours Center for Children's Health Media; James Norman, M.D. and Norman Endocrine Surgery Clinic; Paget Foundation; Santa Monica Thyroid Diagnostic Center; Thomson Micromedex, Inc.; Thyroid Federation International; Thyroid Foundation of America (TFA); UpToDate, Inc.; University of Wisconsin Department of Surgery; and Washington University School of Medicine in St. Louis–Office of Medical Public Affairs

Full citation information is provided on the first page of each chapter. Every effort has been made to secure all necessary rights to reprint the copyrighted material. If any omissions have been made, please contact Omnigraphics to make corrections for future editions.

Acknowledgements

In addition to the listed organizations, agencies, and individuals who have contributed to this *Sourcebook*, special thanks go to managing editor Karen Bellenir, permissions associate Liz Barbour, medical consultant Dr. David Cooke, verification assistant Dawn Matthews, and document engineer Bruce Bellenir for their help and support.

About the Health Reference Series

The *Health Reference Series* is designed to provide basic medical information for patients, families, caregivers, and the general public. Each volume takes a particular topic and provides comprehensive coverage. This is especially important for people who may be dealing with a newly diagnosed disease or a chronic disorder in themselves or in a family member. People looking for preventive guidance, information about disease warning signs, medical statistics, and risk factors for health problems will also find answers to their questions in the *Health Reference Series*. The *Series*, however, is not intended to serve as a tool for diagnosing illness, in prescribing treatments, or as a substitute for the physician/patient relationship. All people concerned about medical symptoms or the possibility of disease are encouraged to seek professional care from an appropriate health care provider.

Locating Information within the Health Reference Series

The *Health Reference Series* contains a wealth of information about a wide variety of medical topics. Ensuring easy access to all the fact sheets, research reports, in-depth discussions, and other material contained within the individual books of the *Series* remains one of our highest priorities. As the *Series* continues to grow in size and scope, however, locating the precise information needed by a reader may become more challenging.

A *Contents Guide to the Health Reference Series* was developed to direct readers to the specific volumes that address their concerns. It presents an extensive list of diseases, treatments, and other topics of general interest compiled from the Tables of Contents and major index headings. To access *A Contents Guide to the Health Reference Series*, visit www.healthreferenceseries.com.

Medical Consultant

Medical consultation services are provided to the *Health Reference Series* editors by David A. Cooke, M.D. Dr. Cooke is a graduate of Brandeis University, and he received his M.D. degree from the University of Michigan. He completed residency training at the University of Wisconsin Hospital and Clinics. He is board-certified in Internal Medicine. Dr. Cooke currently works as part of the University of Michigan Health System and practices in Brighton, MI. In his free time, he enjoys writing, science fiction, and spending time with his family.

Our Advisory Board

We would like to thank the following board members for providing guidance to the development of this *Series*:

- Dr. Lynda Baker,
  Associate Professor of Library and Information Science,
  Wayne State University, Detroit, MI

- Nancy Bulgarelli,
  William Beaumont Hospital Library, Royal Oak, MI

- Karen Imarisio,
  Bloomfield Township Public Library, Bloomfield Township, MI

- Karen Morgan,
  Mardigian Library, University of Michigan-Dearborn,
  Dearborn, MI

- Rosemary Orlando,
  St. Clair Shores Public Library, St. Clair Shores, MI

Health Reference Series *Update Policy*

The inaugural book in the *Health Reference Series* was the first edition of *Cancer Sourcebook* published in 1989. Since then, the *Series* has been enthusiastically received by librarians and in the medical community. In order to maintain the standard of providing high-quality health information for the layperson the editorial staff at Omnigraphics felt it was necessary to implement a policy of updating volumes when warranted.

Medical researchers have been making tremendous strides, and it is the purpose of the *Health Reference Series* to stay current with the most recent advances. Each decision to update a volume is made on an individual basis. Some of the considerations include how much new information is available and the feedback we receive from people who use the books. If there is a topic you would like to see added to the update list, or an area of medical concern you feel has not been adequately addressed, please write to:

Editor
Health Reference Series
Omnigraphics, Inc.
615 Griswold Street
Detroit, MI 48226
E-mail: editorial@omnigraphics.com

Part One

Thyroid Overview

Chapter 1

Your Thyroid Gland

Chapter Contents

Section 1.1

What Is the Thyroid Gland?

The thyroid gland is an endocrine gland. This means that it is a gland that manufactures certain hormones which are chemical substances secreted into the bloodstream that act as messengers to affect cells and tissues in distant parts of your body.

Where Is the Thyroid Gland?

The thyroid gland lies in the front of your neck in a position just below your Adam's apple. It is made up of two lobes—the right and the left lobes, each about the size of a plum cut in half—and these two lobes are joined by a small bridge of thyroid tissue called the isthmus. The two lobes lie on either side of your windpipe.

What Does the Thyroid Gland Do?

The thyroid makes two hormones that it secretes into the bloodstream. One is called thyroxine; this hormone contains four atoms of iodine and for short is often called T4. The other is called triiodothyronine, which contains three atoms of iodine and is often called T3. In the cells and tissues of the body, the T4 is converted to T3. It is the T3, derived from T4 or secreted as T3 from the thyroid gland, which is biologically active and influences the activity of all the cells and tissues of your body.

What Do the Thyroid Hormones Do?

The T4, or rather the T3 derived from it, and the T3 secreted direct by the thyroid gland influence the metabolism of your body cells. In other words it regulates the speed with which your body cells work. If too much of the thyroid hormones are secreted, the body cells work faster than normal, and you have hyperthyroidism. If you become hyperthyroid because of too much secretion of the hormones from the thyroid gland, the increased activity of your body cells or body organs may lead, for example, to a quickening of your heart rate or increased activity of your intestine so that you have frequent bowel movements or even diarrhea. On the other hand if too little of the thyroid hormones are produced (known as hypothyroidism), the cells and organs of your body slow down. Thus if you become hypothyroid, your heart rate, for example, may be slower than normal and your intestines work sluggishly so you become constipated.

How Is the Thyroid Gland Controlled?

There has to be some sort of mechanism that regulates very carefully the amount of T4 and T3 secreted by your thyroid gland so that just the right—the normal—amounts are manufactured and delivered into the bloodstream. The mechanism is very similar to that which regulates the central heating in a house where there is a thermostat in, say, the living room which is set to a particular temperature and

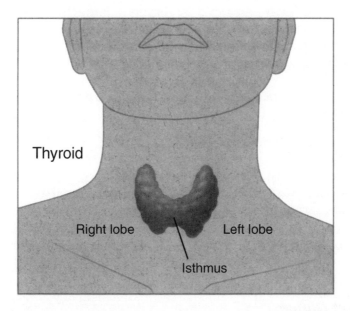

Figure 1.1. Thyroid Gland (Source: "What You Need to Know about Thyroid Cancer," National Cancer Institute, NIH Publication No. 01-4994, September 2001.)

which activates the gas- or oil-fired furnace or boiler that heats the hot water. In the case of the thyroid the thermostat consists of a little gland, called the pituitary gland that lies underneath your brain in your skull. The pituitary senses the level of thyroid hormones in your bloodstream, just as the thermostat in your living room senses the temperature. Under normal circumstances if the level drops just a little below normal, the pituitary reacts by secreting a hormone called the thyroid-stimulating hormone, also known as TSH, and this hormone activates the thyroid gland to put out more T4 and T3. Conversely, when the thyroid hormone levels rise above normal, the thermostat senses this and the pituitary stops secreting TSH so that the thyroid gland makes less T4 and T3.

How Is the Activity of Your Thyroid Gland Measured?

Your doctor will be able to get a good idea about the activity of your thyroid gland by listening to your symptoms, asking you some questions, and by examining you. By taking a small sample of blood, the levels of the hormones involved can be measured in the laboratory. By this means, it is possible to find out whether too much or too little T4 and/or T3 is being secreted by measuring the T4, T3, and TSH. These blood tests are essential in obtaining a diagnosis of a thyroid disturbance. Thyroid antibodies can also be measured to alert your doctor to the fact that you may be developing an autoimmune disorder, which may eventually lead to a thyroid disorder.

Treatment of Underactive and Overactive Thyroid Disorders

Hypothyroidism: Thyroxine is available as a synthetic hormone and is taken daily.

Hyperthyroidism: The available treatment consists of drugs to reduce the formation of thyroid hormones (anti-thyroid drugs), surgical removal of part of the gland (partial thyroidectomy), or reducing the gland's activity by giving radioiodine. You should ask your doctor to fully discuss management and treatment of your thyroid disorder with you.

Thyroid Cancer

Cancer of the thyroid gland is rare. Most lumps (nodules) in the thyroid turn out to be benign (non-cancerous). With modern treatments now available the outlook for people with cancer of the thyroid is very good and many people are completely cured.

Usually a person will begin by seeing their family doctor about a lump they have discovered in their neck or because of rapid growth of a goiter which they may have had for many years.

Related Thyroid Conditions

There are many related conditions that can accompany a thyroid disorder such as:

- thyroid eye disease
- some heart conditions
- altered cholesterol levels
- osteoporosis
- psychological symptoms
- infertility
- nodules and goiters
- rheumatism

Autoimmune disorders tend to run in families. The following conditions may be associated with autoimmune thyroid disease:

- Addison's disease
- diabetes mellitus
- vitiligo
- pernicious anemia
- polymyalgia rheumatica and giant-cell arteritis
- alopecia
- myasthenia gravis
- premature ovarian failure
- rheumatoid arthritis

It is very important for you and your doctor to be aware of your thyroid condition and understand all the related signs and symptoms in order to obtain the best possible means of treatment to manage the thyroid levels within a normal functioning range.

Section 1.2

Importance of Thyroid Health

Take Control of Your Health: Keep Your Thyroid in Balance

Every time you look in the mirror, a key to your well-being is staring you in the face: your thyroid gland. The thyroid gland is a small, butterfly-shaped gland located at the base of your neck just below your Adam's apple. Your thyroid gland helps control the function of many of your body's most important organs, including your heart, brain, liver, kidneys, and skin. Making sure that your thyroid gland is healthy and functioning properly is important to your body's overall well-being.

This section contains answers to commonly asked questions about thyroid health and will help you understand the role your thyroid gland plays in your health. The questions and answers will illustrate how you and your doctor can partner to identify your risk for thyroid disease, how to best treat your condition if you are diagnosed, and how to live an active and fulfilling life by keeping your thyroid in balance.

Be sure to speak to your doctor or nurse if you think you are at risk for thyroid disease, or if you are being treated for thyroid disease and are experiencing symptoms. If you are currently being treated for thyroid disease, make sure you follow your doctor's instructions—take the exact medicine your doctor prescribed every day. Your thyroid gland is more important than you might think.

Identifying the Symptoms and Risks of Thyroid Disease

What follows are commonly asked questions and answers about the importance of your thyroid health and the prevalence of thyroid disease to help you identify if you are at risk.

How common is thyroid disease?

Thyroid disease is more common than diabetes or heart disease. Thyroid disease is a fact of life for 27 million Americans—and more than half of those people remain undiagnosed. Women are 5 times more likely than men to suffer from hypothyroidism (when the thyroid gland is not producing enough thyroid hormone). Aging is just one risk factor that can contribute to hypothyroidism.

How important is my thyroid in my overall well-being?

The thyroid gland produces thyroid hormone, which controls virtually every cell, tissue, and organ in the body. If your thyroid is not functioning properly, it can produce too much thyroid hormone, which causes the body's systems to speed up—this is called hyperthyroidism; or it can create too little thyroid hormone, which causes the body's systems to slow down—this is called hypothyroidism. If your thyroid gland isn't working properly, neither will you. Untreated thyroid disease may lead to elevated cholesterol levels and subsequent heart disease, as well as infertility and osteoporosis. Research also shows that there is a strong genetic link between thyroid disease and other autoimmune diseases, including types of diabetes, arthritis, and anemia.

How do you know if you have a thyroid problem?

First, understand how to recognize the symptoms and risk factors of thyroid disease. Included in this section is a listing of specific symptoms and risk factors, including those for patients currently undergoing treatment for thyroid disorders to determine if their thyroid hormone levels are being maintained. Since many symptoms may be hidden, the best way to know for sure is to ask your doctor for a TSH (thyroid-stimulating hormone) test—a simple blood test to verify your thyroid gland's condition. Because thyroid disease often runs in families, examinations of your family members may reveal other individuals with thyroid problems.

Who should have a TSH test?

Individuals over the age of 35 and those who have any symptoms or risk factors associated with thyroid disease should talk to their doctor about undergoing a TSH test.

Treating Thyroid Disease

The first step toward taking control of your thyroid health is identifying whether your thyroid hormone levels are in balance. The second step is to recognize that there are effective treatments to manage thyroid disease, as long as you follow your doctor's instructions.

How is hypothyroidism usually treated?

Hypothyroidism is treated by replacing the body's thyroid hormone with a single daily dose of levothyroxine sodium (LT4). In order to ensure consistent treatment, your doctor may prescribe a specific brand of LT4 to treat your thyroid disease, and will prescribe the correct dose to keep your thyroid in balance. Since most cases of thyroid disease are permanent and often progressive, it is necessary to treat the disorder throughout one's lifetime. Periodic monitoring of TSH levels is necessary to ensure that the proper LT4 dose is being given, since medicine doses may have to be adjusted from time to time to ensure proper treatment. Precise dosing is critical since the body is sensitive to even small changes in thyroid hormone levels.

What causes hypothyroidism?

Hypothyroidism occurs when the thyroid gland does not produce enough thyroid hormone. The most common cause of hypothyroidism is an autoimmune disease called Hashimoto thyroiditis, in which the body's immune system attacks the thyroid. Hypothyroidism can also be caused by some treatments of hyperthyroidism because the remaining active thyroid cells cannot produce enough thyroid hormone. In addition, hypothyroidism can be caused by certain medicines such as lithium, iodine, and amiodarone. Hypothyroidism can temporarily arise after pregnancy or if the thyroid is inflamed due to a viral infection. This disease can also be present at birth, and tends to run in families.

What can affect my thyroid disease treatment results?

To reach optimal treatment results, it is important to take your medicine as instructed by your doctor. Do not stop taking your thyroid medicine, even if you feel better, without talking to your doctor first. It is important to stay on the exact dose and brand of medicine your doctor prescribes to help avoid any variations in your thyroid hormone levels. Thyroid hormone imbalance can result from untreated

10

thyroid disease, or from over- or under-treatment. In addition, various medicines and supplements may affect the absorption of thyroid hormone; therefore, you should talk to your doctor about any medicines and supplements you are taking and about the best time of day to take your thyroid medicine if you are taking other medicines.

Living with Thyroid Disease

The fact is, millions of people with thyroid disease are living active, healthy lives because they have taken control of their health and keep their thyroid in balance.

Can thyroid disease be cured?

No. Unfortunately, the majority of people with thyroid disease will not be cured of their condition. The good news is that both hypothyroidism and hyperthyroidism can be controlled. Patients with these conditions often remark that with therapy, they feel like they've rediscovered the life they lost. Hypothyroid patients on therapy can expect to lead a full and normal life.

Is it difficult to keep my thyroid in balance?

No, but it does require effort by the patient. If you are diagnosed with thyroid disease, be sure to take your thyroid medicine as instructed by your doctor, and refill your prescription on time so that you do not miss any doses. Your doctor may want to run TSH tests every 6 to 12 months to monitor your thyroid levels. Your body is sensitive to small changes in your TSH level and your thyroid medicine. In fact, thyroid medicines are measured in 1 one-millionth of a gram. Taking your medicine daily or as prescribed by your doctor, staying on the brand of thyroid medicine your doctor prescribed, and visiting your doctor every 6 to 12 months or as symptoms arise are the best ways to keep your thyroid in balance.

Once I'm taking a thyroid medicine, can I switch brands of thyroid medicine without my doctor's advice?

No, and there's an important reason why. Thyroid medicines are precisely dosed to meet your individual thyroid needs. Not all thyroid medicines deliver the same amount of thyroid hormone; therefore, switching medicines should only be done under the guidance of a doctor, and additional testing and dosage adjustment may be required to ensure you are receiving the amount of thyroid hormone your body needs. Even though two thyroid hormone replacement pills from different companies look the same and are the same dose, they may not perform in exactly the same way in your body. Therefore, it is important for you to know your medicine brand and dose, and ensure when you pick up your prescription at the pharmacy you are getting exactly what your doctor prescribed. This is especially important for elderly patients, patients with cardiovascular conditions or thyroid cancer, and pregnant patients. Changing brands of thyroid medicine without your doctor's supervision could cause you to receive too much or too little thyroid hormone, which may lead to a return of symptoms and other potential health problems.

What can I do to keep my thyroid in balance?

Speak candidly with your doctor about your family history, symptoms, and how you are feeling. If you have already been diagnosed, your priorities are to stay on therapy and stay on your brand of thyroid medicine, take it as your doctor has prescribed, and visit with your doctor regularly.

Symptoms and Risks

The first step in taking control of your thyroid health is to check your symptoms and risks. Take a moment to review the symptoms and risk-factor checklists. Share the results with your doctor.

Is your thyroid disease under control?

If you are currently being treated for thyroid disease, do you have any of the following symptoms? If you do, discuss them with your doctor.

Possible symptoms of over-treated hypothyroidism:

- Nervousness/irritability
- Irregular heart beat
- Heat intolerance
- Increased sweating
- Unexplained weight loss
- Diarrhea
- Sleeplessness
- Thyroid enlargement

- Decreased menstrual flow
- Impaired fertility

Possible symptoms of under-treated hypothyroidism:

- Fatigue
- Unexplained weight gain
- Dry skin and hair
- Difficulty concentrating
- Increased cholesterol
- Depression
- Cold intolerance
- Constipation
- Vague aches and pains
- Increased menstrual flow

Over- or under-treatment risk factors:

- You changed to a different thyroid medicine and have not had a new TSH test.
- You received a different thyroid medicine at the pharmacy than your doctor prescribed and you have not had a new TSH test.
- You recently started taking new medicines prescribed by another doctor.
- You recently started taking vitamins or herbal remedies and your doctor is not aware of them.
- Your thyroid medicine looks different from your previous medicine.

If you checked any of these risk factors or symptoms, you may need a new TSH test or dose adjustment to ensure your thyroid is in balance. To avoid over- or under-treatment, take your medicine every day and stay on the brand and dose of thyroid medicine your doctor prescribed.

Are you at risk for thyroid disease?

Do you have any of the following signs and symptoms? If you do, discuss them with your doctor.

Hypothyroidism risk factors:

- Fatigue
- Unexplained weight gain
- Dry skin and hair
- Difficulty concentrating
- Increased cholesterol
- Depression
- Always feeling cold
- Constipation
- Vague aches and pains
- Heavy menstrual flow

Hyperthyroidism risk factors:

- Nervousness/irritability
- Irregular heart beat
- Heat intolerance
- Increased sweating
- Unexplained weight loss
- Diarrhea
- Sleeplessness
- Thyroid enlargement
- Decreased menstrual flow
- Impaired fertility

Thyroid Disease Risk Factors

Do you have any of the following risk factors?

- Previous thyroid dysfunction
- Goiter
- Surgery or radiotherapy affecting the thyroid gland
- Diabetes mellitus
- Pernicious anemia
- Coarse or thinning hair

- Use of medicines such as lithium carbonate or iodine-containing compounds
- History of head or neck irradiations
- Family history of thyroid disease

If you have any of these signs and symptoms or risk factors, you may have undiagnosed thyroid disease. If you think you are at risk, ask your doctor for a TSH test. Now is the time to take control of your health.

References

AACE medical guidelines for clinical practice for the evaluation and treatment of hyperthyroidism and hypothyroidism. *Endocr Pract.* 2002; 8:457-469.

Canaris GJ, Manowitz NR, Mayor GM, Ridgway EC. The Colorado thyroid disease prevalence study. *Arch Intern Med.* 2000; 160:526-534.

Ayala AR, Wartofsky L. The case for more aggressive screening and treatment of mild thyroid failure. *Cleve Clin J Med.* 2002; 69:313-320.

Mechanick JL, et al. AACE medical guidelines for the clinical use of dietary supplements and nutraceuticals. *Endocr Pract.* 2003; 9:417-460.

Additional Information

American Association of Clinical Endocrinologists (AACE)
1000 Riverside Ave., Suite 205
Jacksonville, FL 32204
Phone: 904-353-7878
Fax: 904-353-8185
Website: http://www.aace.com
E-mail: info@aace.com

Chapter 2

Normal Parathyroid Function

Introduction to Normal Parathyroid Function

The sole purpose of the parathyroid glands is to control calcium within the blood in a very tight range between 8.5 and 10.2 mg/dl. In doing so, parathyroids also control how much calcium is in the bones, and therefore, how strong and dense the bones are. Although the parathyroid glands are located next to (and sometimes inside) the thyroid gland, they have no related function. The thyroid gland regulates the body's metabolism and has no effect on calcium levels while parathyroid glands regulate calcium levels and have no effect on metabolism. Calcium is the element that allows the normal conduction of electrical currents along nerves—its how our nervous system works and how one nerve talks to the next. Our entire brain works by fluxes of calcium into and out of the nerve cells. Calcium is also the primary element which causes muscles to contract.

Knowing these two major functions of calcium helps explain why people can get a tingling sensation in their fingers or cramps in the muscles of their hands when calcium levels drop below normal. A sudden drop in the calcium level (i.e., after a successful parathyroid operation where the patient doesn't take their calcium pills for the first few days after the surgery) can cause patients to feel foggy, weird, or confused like their brain isn't working correctly.

"Normal Parathyroid Function," by James Norman, M.D., Norman Endocrine Surgery Clinic, Tampa, Florida. © 2004 Norman Endocrine Surgery Clinic. Reprinted with permission.

The brain demands a normal steady-state calcium level, so any change in the amount of calcium can cause the brain to feel unloved and the patient to feel bad. Likewise, too much parathyroid hormone causes too high a calcium level—and this can make a person feel run down, cause them to sleep poorly, make them more irritable than usual, and even cause a decrease in memory. In fact, the most common symptoms for patients with parathyroid disease are related to the brain, and include depression and lack of energy. Even though one-fourth of patients with this disease will state that they feel just fine, after an operation more than 85 percent of these patients will claim to feel much better. Some say it's like someone turned the lights on. Even though you may think you have no symptoms from your calcium level being too high, nearly everybody feels better after the operation.

Normal Parathyroid Activity

Although the four parathyroid glands are quite small, they have a very rich blood supply. This suits them well since they are required to monitor the calcium level in the blood 24 hours a day. As the blood filters through the parathyroid glands, they detect the amount of calcium present in the blood and react by making more or less parathyroid hormone (PTH). When the calcium level in the blood is too low, the cells of the parathyroids sense it and make more parathyroid hormone. Once the parathyroid hormone is released into the blood, it circulates to act in a number of places to increase the amount of calcium in the blood (i.e., removing calcium from bones). When the calcium level in the blood is too high, the cells of the parathyroids make less parathyroid hormone—or stop making it altogether—thereby allowing calcium levels to decrease. This feedback mechanism runs constantly, thereby maintaining calcium (and parathyroid hormone) in a very narrow normal range. In a normal person with normal parathyroid glands, their parathyroid glands will turn on and off dozens of times per day in an attempt to keep the calcium level in the normal range so the brain and muscles function properly.

How Does Parathyroid Hormone Increase Blood Calcium?

Like all endocrine glands, parathyroids make a hormone (a small protein capable of causing distant cells in the body to react in a specific manner). Parathyroid hormone (PTH) has a very powerful influence on the cells of the bones which causes them to release their calcium into the bloodstream. Calcium is the main structural component of bones which give them their rigidity—but remember, the principle purpose of the bones is to provide a storage system for calcium—so the brain will never be without calcium. Under the presence of parathyroid hormone, bones will give up their calcium in an attempt to increase the blood level of calcium. Under normal conditions, this process is very highly tuned and the amount of calcium in our bones remains at a normal high level. Under the presence of too much parathyroid hormone, however, the bones will continue to release their calcium into the blood at a rate which is too high resulting in bones which have too little calcium. This condition is called osteopenia and osteoporosis.

When bones are exposed to high levels of parathyroid hormone for several years they become brittle and much more prone to fractures. Another way in which the parathyroid hormone acts to increase blood levels of calcium is through its influence on the intestines. Under the presence of parathyroid hormone the lining of the intestine becomes more efficient at absorbing calcium normally found in our diet.

Parathyroid Function Quick Facts

- The parathyroid glands monitor the calcium in the blood 24 hours per day.
- The four parathyroid glands make more or less parathyroid hormone (PTH) in response to the level of calcium in the blood.
- When the calcium in our blood goes too low, the parathyroid glands make more PTH.
- Increased PTH causes the body to put more calcium into the blood.
- Increased PTH causes the bones to release their calcium into the blood.
- When the calcium in our blood goes too high, the parathyroid glands stop making PTH—they shut down.
- Calcium is the most important element for the nervous system, the muscular system, and the skeletal system. This is why parathyroid disease (over-production of PTH) causes symptoms of the brain, muscles, and bones.

Chapter 3

Thyroid and Parathyroid Glands Are Part of the Endocrine System

Although we rarely think about them, the glands of the endocrine system and the hormones they release influence almost every cell, organ, and function of our bodies. The endocrine system is instrumental in regulating mood, growth and development, tissue function, and metabolism, as well as sexual function and reproductive processes.

In general, the endocrine system is in charge of body processes that happen slowly, such as cell growth. Faster processes like breathing and body movement are monitored by the nervous system. But even though the nervous system and endocrine system are separate systems, they often work together to help the body function properly.

What Is the Endocrine System?

The foundations of the endocrine system are the hormones and glands. As the body's chemical messengers, hormones (pronounced: hor-moanz) transfer information and instructions from one set of cells to another. Although many different hormones circulate throughout the bloodstream, each one affects only the cells that are genetically programmed to receive and respond to its message. Hormone levels

"Endocrine System," this information was provided by KidsHealth, one of the largest resources online for medically reviewed health information written for parents, kids, and teens. For more articles like this one, visit www.KidsHealth.org, or www.TeensHealth.org. © 2004 The Nemours Center for Children's Health Media, a division of The Nemours Foundation.

21

can be influenced by factors such as stress, infection, and changes in the balance of fluid and minerals in blood.

A gland is a group of cells that produces and secretes, or gives off, chemicals. A gland selects and removes materials from the blood, processes them, and secretes the finished chemical product for use somewhere in the body. Some types of glands release their secretions in specific areas. For instance, exocrine (pronounced: ek-suh-krin) glands, such as the sweat and salivary glands, release secretions in the skin or inside of the mouth. Endocrine glands, on the other hand, release more than 20 major hormones directly into the bloodstream where they can be transported to cells in other parts of the body.

The major glands that make up the human endocrine system are the hypothalamus, pituitary, thyroid, parathyroids, adrenals, pineal body, and the reproductive glands, which include the ovaries and testes. The pancreas is also part of this hormone-secreting system, even though it is also associated with the digestive system because it also produces and secretes digestive enzymes. Although the endocrine glands are the body's main hormone producers, some non-endocrine organs—such as the brain, heart, lungs, kidneys, liver, thymus, skin, and placenta—also produce and release hormones.

The hypothalamus (pronounced: hi-po-tha-luh-mus), a collection of specialized cells that is located in the lower central part of the brain, is the primary link between the endocrine and nervous systems. Nerve cells in the hypothalamus control the pituitary gland by producing chemicals that either stimulate or suppress hormone secretions from the pituitary.

Although it is no bigger than a pea, the pituitary (pronounced: puh-too-uh-ter-ee) gland, located at the base of the brain just beneath the hypothalamus, is considered the most important part of the endocrine system. It s often called the master gland because it makes hormones that control several other endocrine glands. The production and secretion of pituitary hormones can be influenced by factors such as emotions and seasonal changes. To accomplish this, the hypothalamus relays information sensed by the brain (such as environmental temperature, light exposure patterns, and feelings) to the pituitary.

The tiny pituitary is divided into two parts: the anterior lobe and the posterior lobe. The anterior lobe regulates the activity of the thyroid, adrenals, and reproductive glands. Among the hormones it produces are:

- **growth hormone**, which stimulates the growth of bone and other body tissues and plays a role in the body's handling of nutrients and minerals

- **prolactin** (pronounced: pro-lak-tin), which activates milk production in women who are breastfeeding

- **thyrotropin** (pronounced: thigh-ruh-tro-pin), which stimulates the thyroid gland to produce thyroid hormones

- **corticotropin** (pronounced: kor-tih-ko-tro-pin), which stimulates the adrenal gland to produce certain hormones

The pituitary also secretes endorphins (pronounced: en-dor-finz), chemicals that act on the nervous system to reduce sensitivity to pain. In addition, the pituitary secretes hormones that signal the ovaries and testes to make sex hormones. The pituitary gland also controls ovulation and the menstrual cycle in women.

The posterior lobe of the pituitary releases antidiuretic (pronounced: an-ty-dy-uh-reh-tik) hormone, which helps control body water balance through its effect on the kidneys and urine output; and oxytocin (pronounced: ahk-see-toe-sin), which triggers the contractions of the uterus that occur during labor.

The thyroid (pronounced: thigh-royd), located in the front part of the lower neck, is shaped like a bowtie or butterfly and produces the thyroid hormones thyroxine (pronounced: thigh-rahk-seen) and triiodothyronine (pronounced: try-eye-uh-doe-thigh-ruh-neen). These hormones control the rate at which cells burn fuels from food to produce energy. As the level of thyroid hormones increases in the bloodstream, so does the speed at which chemical reactions occur in the body. Thyroid hormones also play a key role in bone growth and the development of the brain and nervous system in children. The production and release of thyroid hormones is controlled by thyrotropin (pronounced: thigh-ruh-tro-pin), which is secreted by the pituitary gland.

Attached to the thyroid are four tiny glands that function together called the parathyroids (pronounced: par-uh-thigh-roydz). They release parathyroid hormone, which regulates the level of calcium in the blood with the help of calcitonin (pronounced: kal-suh-toe-nin), which is produced in the thyroid.

The body has two triangular adrenal (pronounced: uh-dree-nul) glands, one on top of each kidney. The adrenal glands have two parts, each of which produces a set of hormones and has a different function. The outer part, the adrenal cortex, produces hormones called corticosteroids (pronounced: kor-tih-ko-ster-oydz) that influence or regulate salt and water balance in the body, the body's response to stress, metabolism, the immune system, and sexual development and function.

The inner part, the adrenal medulla (pronounced: muh-duh-luh), produces catecholamines (pronounced: kah-tuh-ko-luh-meenz), such as epinephrine (pronounced: eh-puh-neh-frun). Also called adrenaline, epinephrine increases blood pressure and heart rate when the body experiences stress. (Epinephrine injections are often used to counteract a severe allergic reaction.)

The pineal (pronounced: pih-nee-ul) body, also called the pineal gland, is located in the middle of the brain. It secretes melatonin (pronounced: meh-luh-toe-nin), a hormone that may help regulate the wake-sleep cycle.

The gonads are the main source of sex hormones. In males, they are located in the scrotum. Male gonads, or testes (pronounced: testeez), secrete hormones called androgens (pronounced: an-druh-junz), the most important of which is testosterone (pronounced: teh-stass-tuh-rone). These hormones regulate body changes associated with sexual development, including enlargement of the penis, the growth spurt that occurs during puberty, and the appearance of other male secondary sex characteristics such as deepening of the voice, growth of facial and pubic hair, and the increase in muscle growth and strength. Working with hormones from the pituitary gland, testosterone also supports the production of sperm by the testes.

The female gonads, the ovaries (pronounced: o-vuh-reez), are located in the pelvis. They produce eggs and secrete the female hormones estrogen (pronounced: es-truh-jen) and progesterone (pronounced: projes-tuh-rone). Estrogen is involved in the development of female sexual features such as breast growth, the accumulation of body fat around the hips and thighs, and the growth spurt that occurs during puberty. Both estrogen and progesterone are also involved in pregnancy and the regulation of the menstrual cycle.

The pancreas (pronounced: pan-kree-us) produces (in addition to others) two important hormones, insulin (pronounced: in-suh-lin) and glucagon (pronounced: gloo-kuh-gawn). They work together to maintain a steady level of glucose, or sugar, in the blood and to keep the body supplied with fuel to produce and maintain stores of energy.

What Does the Endocrine System Do?

Once a hormone is secreted, it travels from the endocrine gland through the bloodstream to the cells designed to receive its message. These cells are called target cells. Along the way to the target cells, special proteins bind to some of the hormones. The special proteins act as carriers that control the amount of hormone that is available to interact with and affect the target cells. Also, the target cells have receptors that latch onto only specific hormones, and each hormone has its own receptor, so that each hormone will communicate only with specific target cells that possess receptors for that hormone. When the hormone reaches its target cell, it locks onto the cell's specific receptors and these hormone-receptor combinations transmit chemical instructions to the inner workings of the cell.

When hormone levels reach a certain normal or necessary amount, further secretion is controlled by important body mechanisms to maintain that level of hormone in the blood. This regulation of hormone secretion may involve the hormone itself or another substance in the blood related to the hormone. For example, if the thyroid gland has secreted adequate amounts of thyroid hormones into the blood, the pituitary gland senses the normal levels of thyroid hormone in the bloodstream and adjusts its release of thyrotropin, the pituitary hormone that stimulates the thyroid gland to produce thyroid hormones. Another example is parathyroid hormone, which increases the level of calcium in the blood. When the blood calcium level rises, the parathyroid glands sense the change and decrease their secretion of parathyroid hormone. This turnoff process is called a negative feedback system.

Things That Can Go Wrong with the Endocrine System

Too much or too little of any hormone can be harmful to the body. For example, if the pituitary gland produces too much growth hormone, a child may grow excessively tall. If it produces too little, a child may be abnormally short. Controlling the production of or replacing specific hormones can treat many endocrine disorders in children and adolescents, some of which include:

- **Adrenal insufficiency.** This condition is characterized by decreased function of the adrenal cortex and the consequent underproduction of adrenal corticosteroid hormones. The symptoms of adrenal insufficiency may include weakness, fatigue, abdominal pain, nausea, dehydration, and skin changes. Doctors treat adrenal insufficiency by giving replacement corticosteroid hormones.

- **Cushing syndrome.** Excessive amounts of glucocorticoid hormones in the body can lead to Cushing syndrome. In children, it most often results when a child takes large doses of synthetic corticosteroid drugs (such as prednisone) to treat autoimmune diseases such as lupus. If the condition is due to a tumor in the pituitary gland that produces excessive amounts of corticotropin and stimulates the adrenals to overproduce corticosteroids, it's known as Cushing disease. Symptoms may take years to develop and include obesity, growth failure, muscle weakness, easy bruising of the skin, acne, high blood pressure, and psychological changes. Depending on the specific cause, doctors may treat this condition with surgery, radiation therapy, chemotherapy, or drugs that block the production of hormones.

- **Type 1 diabetes.** When the pancreas fails to produce enough insulin, type 1 diabetes (pronounced: dy-uh-be-teez and previously known as juvenile diabetes) occurs. Symptoms include excessive thirst, hunger, urination, and weight loss. In children and teens, the condition is usually an autoimmune disorder in which specific immune system cells and antibodies produced by the child's immune system attack and destroy the cells of the pancreas that produce insulin. The disease can cause long-term complications including kidney problems, nerve damage, blindness, and early coronary heart disease and stroke. To control their blood sugar levels and reduce the risk of developing diabetes complications, children with this condition need regular injections of insulin.

- **Type 2 diabetes.** Unlike type 1 diabetes, in which the body can't produce normal amounts of insulin, in type 2 diabetes the body is unable to respond to insulin normally. Children and teens with the condition tend to be overweight, and it is believed that excess body fat plays a role in the insulin resistance that characterizes the disease. In fact, the rising prevalence of this type of diabetes in children has paralleled the dramatically increasing rates of obesity among children and teens in recent years. The symptoms and possible complications of type 2 diabetes are basically the same as those of type 1. Some kids and teens can control their blood sugar level with dietary changes, exercise, and oral medications, but many will need to take insulin injections like patients with type 1 diabetes.

- **Growth hormone problems.** Too much growth hormone in children who are still growing will make their bones and other body parts grow excessively, resulting in gigantism. This rare condition is usually caused by a pituitary tumor and can be treated by removing the tumor. In contrast, when the pituitary gland fails to produce adequate amounts of growth hormone, a child's growth in height is impaired. Hypoglycemia (low blood sugar) may also occur in children with growth hormone deficiency, particularly in infants and young children with the condition.

- **Hyperthyroidism.** Hyperthyroidism (pronounced: hi-per-thigh-roy-dih-zum) is a condition in which the levels of thyroid hormones in the blood are excessively high. Symptoms may include weight loss, nervousness, tremors, excessive sweating, increased heart rate and blood pressure, protruding eyes, and a swelling in the neck from an enlarged thyroid gland (goiter). In children and teens the condition is usually caused by Graves disease, an autoimmune disorder in which specific antibodies produced by the child's immune system stimulate the thyroid gland to become overactive. The disease may be controlled with medications or by removal or destruction of the thyroid gland through surgery or radiation treatments.

- **Hypothyroidism.** Hypothyroidism (pronounced: hi-po-thigh-roy-dih-zum) is a condition in which the levels of thyroid hormones in the blood are abnormally low. Thyroid hormone deficiency slows body processes and may lead to fatigue, a slow heart rate, dry skin, weight gain, constipation, and, in children, slowing of growth and delayed puberty. Hashimoto thyroiditis, which results from an autoimmune process that damages the thyroid and blocks thyroid hormone production, is the most common cause of hypothyroidism in children. Infants can also be born with an absent or underdeveloped thyroid gland, resulting in hypothyroidism. The condition can be treated with oral thyroid hormone replacement.

- **Precocious puberty.** Body changes associated with puberty may occur at an abnormally young age in some children if the pituitary hormones that stimulate the gonads to produce sex hormones rise prematurely. An injectable medication is available that can suppress the secretion of these pituitary hormones (known as gonadotropins) and arrest the progression of sexual development in most of these children.

Chapter 4

Autoimmunity and Thyroid Disease

What is autoimmunity?

When your body is attacked—perhaps by a virus or germs on a nail you stepped on—your immune system defends you. It sees and kills the germs that might hurt you.

But when the system doesn't work right, this process can cause harm. Immune cells can mistake your body's own cells as invaders and attack them. This "friendly fire" can affect almost any part of the body. It can sometimes affect many parts of the body at once. This is called autoimmunity (meaning self-immunity).

What causes autoimmunity?

No one knows why the immune system treats some body parts like germs. We do know that you cannot catch autoimmune diseases from another person.

Most scientists think that our genes and things in the environment are involved. If you have a certain gene or combination of genes, you may be at higher risk for autoimmune disease. But you won't get the disease until something around you turns on your immune system. This may include the sun, infections, drugs, or, in some women, pregnancy.

"Questions and Answers about Autoimmunity," National Institute of Arthritis and Musculoskeletal and Skin Diseases (NIAMS), NIH Publication No. 02-4858, January 2002.

What kinds of problems are caused by autoimmunity?

Autoimmunity can affect almost any organ or body system. The exact problem one has with autoimmunity (or its diseases) depends on which tissues are targeted.

If the skin is the target, you may have skin rashes, blisters, or color changes. If it's the thyroid gland, you may be tired, gain weight, be more sensitive to cold, and have muscle aches. If it's the joints, you may have joint pain, stiffness, and loss of function.

You may know which organ or system is affected from the start. But you may not know the site of the attack. In many people, the first symptoms are fatigue, muscle aches, and low fever.

How are autoimmune diseases diagnosed?

Autoimmune diseases often do not show a clear pattern of symptoms at first. So diagnosing them can be hard. But with time, a diagnosis can usually be made by using:

- **Medical history:** The doctor will ask about your symptoms and how long you have had them. Your symptoms may not point to one disease. But they can be a starting point for your doctor. You should tell your doctor if you have a family member with autoimmune disease. You may not have the same disease as your family member. But having a family history of any autoimmune disease makes you more likely to have one.

- **Physical exam:** During the exam, the doctor will check for any signs. Inflamed joints, swollen lymph nodes, or discolored skin might give clues.

- **Medical tests:** No one test will show that you have an autoimmune disease, but doctors may find clues in a blood sample. For example, people with lupus or rheumatoid arthritis often have certain autoantibodies in their blood. Autoantibodies are blood proteins formed against the body's own parts. Not all people with these diseases have these autoantibodies, and some people without autoimmune disease do have them. So blood tests alone may not always help. But if a person has disease symptoms and autoantibodies, the doctor can be more sure of a diagnosis.

The key is patience. Your doctor may be able to diagnose your condition quickly based on your history, exam, and test results. But the process often takes time. It may take several visits to find out exactly what's wrong and the best way to treat it.

How are autoimmune diseases treated?

Autoimmunity takes many forms. There are also many treatments for it. Treatment depends on the type of disease, how severe it is, and its symptoms. Generally, treatments have one of three goals:

- **Relieving symptoms:** If your symptoms bother you, your doctor may suggest treatments that give some relief. Relieving symptoms may be as simple as taking a drug for pain relief. It may also be as involved as having surgery.

- **Preserving organ function:** When autoimmune diseases threaten organs, treatment may be needed to prevent damage. Such treatments may include drugs to control an inflamed kidney in people with lupus. Insulin injections can regulate blood sugar in people with diabetes. These treatments don't stop the disease, but they can save organ function. They can also help people live with disease complications.

- **Targeting disease mechanisms:** Some drugs may also be used to target how the disease works. In other words, they can suppress the immune system. These drugs include cyclophosphamide (Cytoxan*) and cyclosporine (Neoral and Sandimmune). The same immune-suppressing drug may be used for many diseases.

Your doctor may not prescribe a treatment. If your symptoms are mild, the risks of treatment may be worse than the symptoms. You may choose to put off treatment for now, but you should watch for signs that your disease is progressing. Visit your doctor regularly. You need to catch changes before they lead to serious damage.

*Brand names included in this chapter are provided as examples only, and their inclusion does not mean that these products are endorsed by the National Institutes of Health or any other Government agency. Also, if a particular brand name is not mentioned, this does not mean or imply that the product is unsatisfactory.

What types of doctors treat autoimmune diseases?

Treatments for autoimmune diseases vary. So do the types of doctors who provide them. For some people, one doctor will be enough to manage their disease. Others may require a team approach. One doctor might coordinate and give care, and others would treat specific organ problems. For example, a person with lupus might be seen by a rheumatologist. But that person might also see a nephrologist for related kidney problems and a dermatologist for skin problems.

Specialists you may need to see include:

- A rheumatologist, who treats arthritis and other rheumatic diseases. These include scleroderma and systemic lupus erythematosus (lupus or SLE).

- An endocrinologist, who treats gland and hormone problems. These include diabetes and thyroid disease.

- A neurologist, who treats nerve problems. These include multiple sclerosis and myasthenia gravis.

- A hematologist, who treats diseases that affect the blood. These include pernicious anemia and autoimmune hemolytic anemia.

- A gastroenterologist, who treats problems with the digestive system. These include Crohn disease and ulcerative colitis.

- A dermatologist, who treats problems of the skin, hair, and nails. These include psoriasis, pemphigus/pemphigoid, and alopecia areata.

- A nephrologist, who treats kidney problems. These include glomerulonephritis—inflamed kidneys associated with lupus.

What are some other problems related to autoimmune diseases?

Having a chronic disease can affect almost every part of your life. The problems you might have with an autoimmune disease vary. They may include:

- **How you look and your self-esteem:** Depending on your disease, you may have discolored or damaged skin or hair loss. Your joints may look different. These can all affect how you look and your self-esteem. Such problems can't always be prevented, but their effects can be reduced with treatment. Cosmetics, for example, can hide a skin rash. Surgery can correct a malformed joint.

- **Caring for yourself:** Painful joints or weak muscles can make it hard to do simple tasks. You may have trouble climbing stairs, making your bed, or brushing your hair. If doing daily tasks is hard, talk with a physical therapist. The therapist can teach you exercises to improve strength and function. An occupational therapist can show you new ways to do things or tools to make tasks easier. Sometimes regular exercise or simple devices can help you do more things on your own.

- **Family relationships:** Family members may not understand why you don't have energy to do things you used to do. They may even think you are just being lazy. But they may also be overly concerned and eager to help you. They may not let you do the things you can do. They may even give up their own interests to be with you. Learn as much as you can about your disease. Share what you learn with your family. Involve them in counseling or a support group. It may help them better understand the disease and how they can help.

- **Sexual relations:** Sexual relationships can also be affected. For men, diseases that affect blood vessels can lead to problems with erection. In women, damage to glands that produce moisture can lead to vaginal dryness. This makes intercourse painful. In both men and women, pain, weakness, or stiff joints may make it hard for them to move the way they once did. They may not be sure about how they look. Or they may be afraid that their partner will no longer find them attractive. With communication, good medical care, and perhaps counseling, many of these issues can be overcome or at least worked around.

- **Pregnancy and childbearing:** In the past, women with some autoimmune diseases were told not to have children, but better treatments and understanding have changed that advice. Autoimmune diseases can affect pregnancy, and pregnancy can affect autoimmune diseases. But women with many such diseases can safely have children. How a pregnancy turns out can vary by disease and disease severity. If you have an autoimmune disease, you should consult your doctor about having children.

Glossary of Terms

Antibodies. Special proteins produced by the body's immune system that help fight and destroy viruses, bacteria, and other foreign substances that invade the body.

Antigen. A substance (usually foreign) that stimulates the immune response. In people with autoimmune disease, the body's own cells may be seen as antigens.

Autoantibodies. Abnormal antibodies that attack parts of the body, causing autoimmune disease.

Autoimmune disease. A disease that occurs when the immune system turns against parts of the body it is designed to protect.

Fever. A rise in body temperature caused by the immune system's response to infection or disease.

Immune response. The reaction of the immune system against foreign substances. When the reaction occurs against the body's own cells or tissues, it is called an autoimmune reaction.

Immune system. A complex system that normally protects the body from infections. The immune system consists of a group of cells, the chemicals that control those cells, and the chemicals that those cells release.

Immunosuppressive drugs. Drugs that suppress the immune response and can be used to treat autoimmune disease. Unfortunately, because normal immunity is also suppressed with these drugs, they leave the body at risk for infection.

Infection. Invasion of the body tissues by bacteria or other tiny organisms that cause illness.

Inflammation. A reaction of tissues to injury or disease, typically marked by four signs: swelling, redness, heat, and pain.

Trigger. Something that either sets off a disease in people who are genetically predisposed to developing the disease, or that causes a certain symptom to occur in a person who has a disease. For example, sunlight can trigger rashes in people with lupus.

Autoimmune Thyroid Diseases

Graves disease. An autoimmune disease of the thyroid gland that results in the overproduction of thyroid hormone. This causes such symptoms as nervousness, heat intolerance, heart palpitations, and unexplained weight loss.

Pernicious anemia. A deficiency of the oxygen-carrying red blood cells that often occurs in people with autoimmune diseases of the thyroid gland.

Thyroiditis. An inflammation of the thyroid gland that causes the gland to become underactive. This condition results in symptoms such as fatigue, weakness, weight gain, cold intolerance, and muscle aches.

Additional Information

National Health Information Center
P.O. Box 1133
Washington, DC 20013-1133
Toll-Free: 800-336-4797
Phone: 301-565-4167
Website: http://www.healthfinder.gov
E-mail: healthfinder@nhic.org

American Autoimmune Related Diseases Association
22100 Gratiot Avenue
East Detroit, MI 48201-2227
Toll-Free Literature Requests: 800-598-4668
Phone: 586-776-3900
Fax: 586-776-3903
Website: http://www.aarda.org
E-mail: aarda@aarda.org

Chapter 5

Screening Guidelines for Thyroid Disease

This chapter includes screening guidelines from the U.S. Preventive Services Task Force (USPSTF), the American Thyroid Association, the Canadian Task Force on the Periodic Health Examination, the American College of Physicians, the American Association of Clinical Endocrinologists, the American College of Obstetricians and Gynecologists, and the American Academy of Family Physicians.

U.S. Preventive Services Task Force Thyroid Disease Screening Guidelines

This statement summarizes the current U.S. Preventive Services Task Force (USPSTF) recommendations on screening for thyroid disease and the supporting scientific evidence, and updates the 1996 recommendations contained in the *Guide to Clinical Preventive Services, Second Edition: Periodic Updates.*[1]

The complete information on which this statement is based, including evidence tables and references, is available in the Systematic Evidence Review "Screening for Thyroid Disease,"[2] available through the USPSTF website (http://www .preventiveservices.ahrq.gov) and through the National Guideline Clearinghouse™ (http://www.guideline .gov).

Recommendations made by the USPSTF are independent of the U.S. Government. They should not be construed as an official position

"Screening for Thyroid Disease: Recommendation Statement," Agency for Healthcare Research and Quality (AHRQ), Pub. No. 04-0530A, January 2004.

of AHRQ or the U.S. Department of Health and Human Services. This article first appeared in *Ann Intern Med.* 2004;140:125–127.

U.S. Preventive Services Task Force—Recommendations and Ratings

The Task Force grades its recommendations according to one of 5 classifications (A, B, C, D, I) reflecting the strength of evidence and magnitude of net benefit (benefits minus harms):

A.   The USPSTF strongly recommends that clinicians provide [the service] to eligible patients. The USPSTF found good evidence that [the service] improves important health outcomes and concludes that benefits substantially outweigh harms.

B.   The USPSTF recommends that clinicians provide [the service] to eligible patients. The USPSTF found at least fair evidence that [the service] improves important health outcomes and concludes that benefits outweigh harms.

C.   The USPSTF makes no recommendation for or against routine provision of [the service]. The USPSTF found at least fair evidence that [the service] can improve health outcomes, but concludes that the balance of benefits and harms is too close to justify a general recommendation.

D.   The USPSTF recommends against routinely providing [the service] to asymptomatic patients. The USPSTF found at least fair evidence that [the service] is ineffective or that harms outweigh benefits.

I.   The USPSTF concludes that the evidence is insufficient to recommend for or against routinely providing [the service]. Evidence that [the service] is effective is lacking, of poor quality, or conflicting, and the balance of benefits and harms cannot be determined.

U.S. Preventive Services Task Force—Strength of Overall Evidence

The USPSTF grades the quality of the overall evidence for a service on a 3-point scale (good, fair, poor):

- **Good:** Evidence includes consistent results from well-designed, well-conducted studies in representative populations that directly assess effects on health outcomes.

- **Fair:** Evidence is sufficient to determine effects on health outcomes, but the strength of the evidence is limited by the number, quality, or consistency of the individual studies, generalization to routine practice, or indirect nature of the evidence on health outcomes.

- **Poor:** Evidence is insufficient to assess the effects on health outcomes because of limited number or power of studies, important flaws in their design or conduct, gaps in the chain of evidence, or lack of information on important health outcomes.

Summary of Recommendation

The U.S. Preventive Services Task Force (USPSTF) concludes the evidence is insufficient to recommend for or against routine screening for thyroid disease in adults. **I recommendation.** [See "U.S. Preventive Services Task Force—Recommendations and Ratings" for an explanation of what this rating means.]

The USPSTF found fair evidence that the thyroid stimulating hormone (TSH) test can detect subclinical thyroid disease in people without symptoms of thyroid dysfunction, but poor evidence that treatment improves clinically important outcomes in adults with screen-detected thyroid disease. Although the yield of screening is greater in certain high-risk groups (e.g., postpartum women, people with Down syndrome, and the elderly), the USPSTF found poor evidence that screening these groups leads to clinically important benefits. There is the potential for harm caused by false positive screening tests; however, the magnitude of harm is not known. There is good evidence that over-treatment with levothyroxine occurs in a substantial proportion of patients, but the long-term harmful effects of over-treatment are not known. As a result, the USPSTF could not determine the balance of benefits and harms of screening asymptomatic adults for thyroid disease.

Clinical Considerations

- Subclinical thyroid dysfunction is defined as an abnormal biochemical measurement of thyroid hormones without any specific clinical signs or symptoms of thyroid disease and no history of thyroid dysfunction or therapy. This includes individuals who have mildly elevated thyroid stimulating hormone (TSH) and normal thyroxine (T4) and triiodothyronine (T3) levels (subclinical hypothyroidism), or low TSH and normal T4 and T3 levels (subclinical hyperthyroidism). *Individuals with symptoms of thyroid dysfunction, or those with a history of thyroid disease or treatment, are excluded from this definition and are not the subject of these recommendations.*

• When used to confirm suspected thyroid disease in patients referred to a specialty endocrine clinic, TSH has a high sensitivity (98%) and specificity (92%). When used for screening primary care populations, the positive predictive value (PPV) of TSH in detecting thyroid disease is low; further, the interpretation of a positive test result is often complicated by an underlying illness or by frailty of the individual. In general, values for serum TSH below 0.1 milliunit/liter (mU/L) are considered low and values above 6.5 mU/L are considered elevated.

• Clinicians should be aware of subtle signs of thyroid dysfunction, particularly among those at high risk. People at higher risk for thyroid dysfunction include the elderly, postpartum women, those with high levels of radiation exposure (under 20 milligray [mGy]), and patients with Down syndrome. Evaluating for symptoms of hypothyroidism is difficult in patients with Down syndrome because some symptoms and signs (e.g., slow speech, thick tongue, and slow mentation) are typical findings in both conditions.

• Subclinical hyperthyroidism has been associated with atrial fibrillation, dementia, and, less clearly, with osteoporosis. However, progression from subclinical to clinical disease in patients without a history of thyroid disease is not clearly established.

• Subclinical hypothyroidism is associated with poor obstetric outcomes and poor cognitive development in children. Evidence for dyslipidemia, atherosclerosis, and decreased quality of life in adults with subclinical hypothyroidism in the general population is inconsistent and less convincing.

Discussion

Subclinical thyroid disease is much more common than overt disease in primary care populations. Up to 5% of women and 3% of men have subclinical hypothyroidism;[3] prevalence increases with age and is greater in whites than in blacks.[3, 4] Untreated hypothyroidism can lead to fatigue, weight gain, mental slowing, heart failure, and elevated lipid levels. Subclinical hyperthyroidism is less common, occurring in 1% of men over age 60 and 1.5% of women over age 60.[5] Untreated hyperthyroidism can lead to atrial fibrillation, congestive heart failure, osteoporosis, and neuropsychiatric problems.

The goal of screening for thyroid disease is to identify and treat patients at risk for the health consequences of thyroid dysfunction before they become clinically apparent. The USPSTF examined the evidence for screening people who have no known history of thyroid disease and no or few signs or symptoms. The USPSTF found no controlled studies that examined whether routine screening for thyroid disease in the primary care setting leads to improved symptoms or other health outcomes.

Screening for thyroid dysfunction can be performed using the medical history, physical examination, or any of several serum thyroid function tests. The TSH is usually recommended because it can detect abnormalities before other tests become abnormal. When used to confirm suspected disease in patients referred to an endocrine specialty clinic, the TSH test has a sensitivity above 98% and a specificity greater than 92% for the clinical and functional diagnosis.[6] The accuracy of TSH screening in primary care patients is difficult to evaluate, as TSH is often considered the gold standard for assessing thyroid function. A severe non-thyroid disease can lead to a false positive TSH test result; in a recent systematic review of TSH used to screen patients admitted to acute care and geriatric hospitals, the PPV of a low TSH was 0.24 for hyperthyroidism and 0.06 for hypothyroidism.[7] In screening programs, patients who have normal thyroxine levels, but have mild elevations of TSH or low TSH levels often revert to normal over time.[8–10]

In a review of observational studies conducted among groups of people who were exposed to radiation from nuclear fallout, high doses of I-131 (under 20 mGy) were associated with hypothyroidism (Helfand, unpublished data, 2003). There is fair evidence to suggest that exposure to I-131 increases the risk for developing thyroid antibodies, which may lead to autoimmune thyroid disease. The evidence for an increased risk for hypothyroidism from exposure to low doses of I-131 (under 20 mGy) is inconclusive, making it difficult to ascertain whether there is a threshold dose of I-131 exposure that confers no added risk for hypothyroidism. Thus, clinicians need to be extra vigilant in this high risk group for the possibility of thyroid dysfunction.

The USPSTF found no randomized trials of treatment for overt or subclinical hyperthyroidism. Limited evidence is available from observational studies regarding cardiac function parameters pre- and post-treatment, but no studies reported clinical outcomes. [3]

The USPSTF found 14 randomized trials of treatment using levothyroxine (LT4) therapy,[2] but few were relevant to the issue of treating screen-detected subclinical hypothyroidism in primary care clinical settings, and most of the potentially relevant studies suffered

41

from significant design flaws. Most studies were in groups of patients known to have thyroid disease (e.g., patients with Hashimoto thyroiditis or Graves disease). Results from 3 small studies of women with screen-detected subclinical hypothyroidism showed no improved clinical outcomes (in 2 of the studies) and some improved clinical outcome in the third.[11–13] Data from observational studies, most of which were judged to be of poor quality, showed that treatment of subclinical hypothyroidism leads to modestly improved serum lipid levels.[14] No trials of treatment of subclinical hypothyroidism in pregnant women were identified.

A potential benefit of treating subclinical hypothyroidism is to prevent the spontaneous development of overt hypothyroidism, but this potential benefit has not been studied in clinical trials. If the potential benefit suggested by data from a longitudinal survey is real, the USPSTF estimates that in a reference population of 1,000 women screened, 3 cases of overt hypothyroidism would be prevented in 5 years, but 40 people would have taken medication for 5 years without a clear benefit.[2]

The potential harms of screening and treatment are principally the adverse effects of antithyroid drugs, radioiodine, thyroid surgery, and thyroid replacement therapy if detection and early treatment for subclinical disease are unnecessary. People with a false positive TSH test result (more common in those with a severe underlying illness or those who are frail or elderly) may be subjected to unnecessary treatment or may have adverse psychological consequences (e.g., labeling). The USPSTF reviewed only the adverse effects of LT4 replacement therapy for mild thyroid failure and potential adverse effects of long-term treatment. These adverse effects were not carefully assessed in the randomized trials. Although some studies have suggested that women with a low TSH as a result of taking thyroid hormone replacement are at higher risk for developing osteoporosis,[15, 16] a recent systematic review did not support this finding.[17] Over-treatment with LT4 is a potential risk: about 1 in 4 patients receiving LT4 are maintained unintentionally on doses sufficient to fully suppress TSH.[18, 19] Data from the Framingham Study suggest that 1 excess case of atrial fibrillation might occur for every 114 patients treated with LT4 sufficient to suppress TSH.[19]

Recommendations of Other Groups

The American Thyroid Association recommends measuring thyroid function in all adults beginning at age 35 years and every 5 years thereafter, noting that more frequent screening may be appropriate in high-risk or symptomatic individuals.[20]

The Canadian Task Force on the Periodic Health Examination recommends maintaining a high index of clinical suspicion for nonspecific symptoms consistent with hypothyroidism when examining perimenopausal and postmenopausal women.[21]

The American College of Physicians recommends screening women older than age 50 with 1 or more general symptoms that could be caused by thyroid disease.[22]

The American Association of Clinical Endocrinologists recommends TSH measurement in women of childbearing age before pregnancy or during the first trimester.[23]

The American College of Obstetricians and Gynecologists recommends that physicians be aware of the symptoms and risk factors for postpartum thyroid dysfunction and evaluate patients when indicated.[24]

The American Academy of Family Physicians recommends against routine thyroid screening in asymptomatic patients younger than age 60.[25]

References

1. U.S. Preventive Services Task Force. *Guide to Clinical Preventive Services. 2nd ed.* Alexandria, Virginia: International Medical Publishing, Inc.; 1996:209–218.

2. Helfand, M. *Screening for Thyroid Disease. Systematic Evidence Review No. 23.* (Prepared by the Oregon Health & Science University Evidence-based Practice Center under Contract No. 290-97-0018). Rockville, MD: Agency for Healthcare Research and Quality. (Available on the AHRQ website at: http://www.ahrq.gov/clinic/serfiles.htm).

3. Hollowell JG, Staehling NW, Flanders WD, et al. Serum TSH, T(4), and thyroid antibodies in the United States population (1988 to 1994): National Health and Nutrition Examination Survey (NHANES III). *J Clin Endocrinol Metab.* 2002;87(2): 489–499.

4. Tunbridge WM, Vanderpump MP. Population screening for autoimmune thyroid disease. *Endocrinol Metab Clin North Am.* 2000;29(2):239–253.

5. Helfand M, Redfern CC. Clinical guideline, part 2. Screening for thyroid disease: an update. American College of Physicians [published erratum appears in *Ann Intern Med.* 1999 Feb 2;130(3):246]. *Ann Intern Med.* 1998;129(2):144–158.

6. Helfand M, Crapo LM. Testing for suspected thyroid disease. In: Sox HC, ed. *Common Diagnostic Tests.* Philadelphia: American College of Physicians; 1990.

7. Attia J, Margetts P, Guyatt G. Diagnosis of thyroid disease in hospitalized patients. A systematic review. *Arch Intern Med.* 1999;159:658–665.

8. Jaeschke R, Guyatt G, Gerstein H, et al. Does treatment with L-thyroxine influence health status in middle-aged and older adults with subclinical hypothyroidism? *J Gen Intern Med.* 1996;11(12):744–749.

9. Parle J, Franklyn J, Cross K, Jones S, Sheppard M. Prevalence and follow-up of abnormal thyrotropin (TSH) concentrations in the elderly in the United Kingdom. *Clin Endocrinol* (Oxf). 1991;34:77–83.

10. Sundbeck G, Jagenburg R, Johansson PM, Eden S, Lindstedt G. Clinical significance of a low serum thyrotropin concentration by chemiluminometric assay in 85-year-old women and men. *Arch Inten Med.* 1991;151:549–556.

11. Nystrom E, Caidahl K, Fager G, Wikkelso C, Lundberg PA, Lindstedt G. A double-blind cross-over 12-month study of L-thyroxine treatment of women with 'subclinical' hypothyroidism. *Clin Endocrinol.* 1988;29(1):63–75.

12. Ross DS. Bone density is not reduced during the short-term administration of levothyroxine to postmenopausal women with subclinical hypothyroidism: a randomized, prospective study. *Am J Med.* 1993;95(4):385–388.

13. Monzani F, Di Bello V, Caraccio N, et al. Effect of levothyroxine on cardiac function and structure in subclinical hypothyroidism: a double blind, placebo-controlled study. *J Clin Endocrinol Metab.* 2001;86(3):1110–1115.

14. Danese MD, Ladenson PW, Meinert CL, Powe NR. Clinical review 115: effect of thyroxine therapy on serum lipoproteins in patients with mild thyroid failure: a quantitative review of the literature. *J Clin Endocrinol Metab.* 2000;85(9):2993–3001.

15. Uzzan B, Campos J, Cucherat M, Nony P, Boissel JP, Perret GY. Effects on bone mass of long term treatment with thyroid hormones: a meta-analysis. *J Clin Endocrinol Metab.* 1996; 81:4278–4289.

16. Faber J, Galloe AM. Changes in bone mass during prolonged subclinical hyperthyroidism due to L-thyroxine treatment: a meta-analysis. *Eur J Endocrinol.* 1994;130(4):350–356.

17. Greenspan SL, Greenspan FS. The effect of thyroid hormone on skeletal integrity. *Ann Intern Med.* 1999;130(9):750–758.

18. Canaris GJ, Manowitz NR, Mayor G, Ridgway EC. The Colorado thyroid disease prevalence study. *Arch Intern Med.* 2000;160(4):526–534.

19. Sawin C, Geller A, Wolf P. Low serum thyrotropin concentrations as a risk factor for atrial fibrillation in older persons. *N Engl J Med.* 1994;331:1249–1252.

20. Ladenson PW, Singer PA, Ain KB, et al. American Thyroid Association guidelines for detection of thyroid dysfunction. [erratum appears in *Arch Intern Med.* 2001 Jan 22;161(2):284]. *Arch Intern Med.* 2000;160(11):1573–1575.

21. Canadian Task Force on the Periodic Health Examination. *Canadian Guide to Clinical Preventive Health Care.* Ottawa: Canada Communication Group; 1994:611–618.

22. American College of Physicians. Clinical guideline, part 1. Screening for thyroid disease. Ann Intern Med. 1998;129(2): 141–143.

23. AACE Thyroid Task Force. American Association of Clinical Endocrinologists medical guidelines for clinical practice for the evaluation and treatment of hyperthyroidism and hypothyroidism. *Endocrine Prac.* 2002;8:457–469.

24. American College of Obstetricians and Gynecologists. *Thyroid disease in pregnancy.* Technical Bulletin no. 37. Washington,

DC: American College of Obstetricians and Gynecologists, 2002.

25. American Academy of Family Physicians. *Summary of Policy Recommendations for Periodic Health Examinations.* Leawood, KS: American Academy of Family Physicians; 2002.

Additional Information

U.S. Preventive Services Task Force
Project Director, USPSTF
Agency for Healthcare Research and Quality
540 Gaither Road
Rockville, MD 20850
Toll-Free: 800-358-9295
Website: http://www.preventiveservices.ahrq.gov
E-mail: uspstf@ahrq.gov

Chapter 6

Doctors Who Specialize in Thyroid Disorders

What Is a Thyroidologist?

A clinical thyroidologist is the one who is best equipped to render the care needed to diagnose and plan treatment for a lifetime of thyroid disease care. A thyroidologist is trained in internal medicine, endocrinology, thyroid hormone analysis, nuclear medicine, cytopathology, oncology, and ultrasound. When you visit the thyroid clinics, they can do almost all the studies in house, and results are obtained immediately, or in a few days.

What Are the Usual Reasons That You Should See a Thyroidologist?

There are good studies showing that you will save yourself from all types of problems, if you see a thyroidologist at the first sign you might have a thyroid problem. It is sad to see patients handled improperly at first, requiring more extensive therapy later. There are many examples of this:

Reprinted with permission from "What is a Thyroidologist?" by Richard B. Guttler, M.D., Director, Santa Monica Thyroid Center, 1328 16th Street, Santa Monica, CA 90404, 310-393-8860, 800-408-4909 (outside California), Dr.Guttler@ thyroid.com. © 2003. For additional information about thyroid disorders, visit Dr. Guttler's educational website at http://www.thyroid.com. Text under the heading "What Is an Endocrinologist?" is reprinted with permission from "Your Endocrinologist: A Patient's Guide to Endocrinology." © 2004 The Hormone Foundation. All rights reserved. For additional information, visit http://www.hormone.org.

- The patient is told she has a high TSH, and needs thyroid hormone, but is not studied to find the underlying cause and structure of the thyroid until a nodule is noted a few years later.

- The patient who has surgery by an inexperienced surgeon and as a result experiences nerve damage or calcium problems, when the surgery was not indicated in the opinion of the thyroidologist. Even if the surgery is needed, a thyroidologist will refer the patient to the surgeons who do at least 50 thyroidectomies per year to cut down the risk of complications.

Signs That It Is Time to See a Thyroidologist

1. When you are told there is an abnormal thyroid blood result and your physician wants to treat you, request a consultation first. The most common mistake is failure to get a consultation when the TSH test is abnormal. Both hypothyroidism and hyperthyroidism have abnormal TSH testing, but this is not enough reason for treatment until the cause is known. Treatment by your family physician may be risky without a thyroid consultation.

2. When you are told there is a mass in the thyroid. It is best to stop there and get a referral to a thyroid expert before you allow a biopsy, or any further studies.

3. If you fail to see a specialist, allow a biopsy by other physicians, and are told you need surgery, you still have time to get an expert opinion. A complete thyroid evaluation may turn up reasons for the biopsy results, or after review of the biopsy, render a different diagnosis. The adequacy of the biopsy can be determined and if inadequate for proper diagnosis a repeat can be performed. The surgery may not be needed.

4. It is still not too late to see a thyroidologist, even when the surgery is set. The thyroidologist will frankly tell you if he/she thinks the surgery is needed, and if so, if the surgeon is qualified to offer low risk care. He/she can recommend a thyroid surgeon. Remember, thyroid surgery for nodules is not an emergency. You have time to make sure you are doing the right thing with the best qualified thyroid surgeon.

5. When you are told you have thyroid cancer. Most people think an oncologist is the right physician to see. However, since thyroid cancer is treated without the chemotherapy

drugs or radiation therapy typically used by an oncologist, a thyroidologist consultation would be beneficial. External radiation therapy is not useful in most cases. Thyroid cancer is a thyroid hormone cancer and is best treated by a thyroidologist. The nuclear medicine physician, unless he/she has special training in thyroidology, may not be the best physician to captain your thyroid cancer team. Radioiodine studies and treatment are not always necessary with other modern methods of cancer diagnosis and therapy that are not related to the use of radioiodine.

6. You are told to withdraw from thyroid medication for up to six weeks prior to radioiodine testing and treatment for your cancer. You know you were sick the last time, but feel you have no choice. Well, you do have a choice today. Request a second opinion. The thyroidologist will decide if you really need to have the treatment or study. Then, if it is needed, there are modern methods that do not make you sick from hypothyroidism, and allow you to keep on thyroid medication during the testing and treatment.

7. You have thyroid antibodies in your blood, but your physician, tells you other thyroid tests are normal. He/she wants you to do nothing and return in a year. These are great markers for disease, and a consult should not be put off for a year. Request a consultation, whether through your physician or on your own initiative.

8. Pregnancy and post-pregnancy are dangerous times for thyroid patients. This is when you need to see a thyroidologist, even if the OB/GYN physician thinks it isn't necessary. Possible problems include child I.Q. losses due to early pregnancy hypothyroidism in the mother, fetal hyperthyroidism passed to the baby by a mother treated for Graves disease in the past, changing thyroid hormone dose during pregnancy, improper instructions on neonatal vitamin use with thyroid hormone resulting in hypothyroidism, and hyperthyroid and hypothyroidism occurring postpartum.

There are many more examples of the value of early consultations with a thyroidologist, but anytime is better than never, as the thyroid gland diseases are long-term and intervention at any stage can be very helpful.

What Is an Endocrinologist?

An endocrinologist is a specially trained doctor. Endocrinologists diagnose diseases that affect your glands. They know how to treat these conditions, which are often complex and involve many systems and structures within your body. Your regular doctor refers you to an endocrinologist when you have a problem with your endocrine system.

What is the endocrine system?

Your endocrine system is a system of glands. Glands are organs that make hormones. These are substances that help to control activities in your body. Hormones control reproduction, metabolism (food burning and waste elimination), and growth and development. Hormones also control the way you respond to your surroundings. They help to provide the proper amount of energy and nutrition. The endocrine glands include the thyroid, parathyroid, pancreas, ovaries, testes, adrenal, pituitary, and hypothalamus.

What do endocrinologists do?

Endocrinologists are trained to recognize and uncover hormone problems. They help to restore the natural balance of hormones in your system. Endocrinologists also conduct basic research to learn the secrets of glands. Clinical research helps them learn the best ways to treat patients. Endocrinologists develop new drugs and treatments for hormone problems. They take care of many functions and problems:

- diabetes
- thyroid diseases
- metabolism
- hormonal imbalances
- menopause
- osteoporosis
- hypertension
- cholesterol (lipid) disorders
- infertility and birth control
- shortness (short stature)
- cancers of the glands

What type of medical training do endocrinologists receive?

Endocrinologists finish four years of medical school. They spend three or four years in an internship and residency program. These specialty programs cover internal medicine, pediatrics, or obstetrics and gynecology. They spend two or three more years learning how to diagnose and treat hormone conditions.

What are the most common endocrine diseases and disorders?

Endocrine diseases and disorders are grouped into several areas. Some endocrinologists focus on one or two areas, such as diabetes, pediatric disorders, thyroid, or reproductive and menstrual disorders. Others work in all areas of endocrinology. The major areas of endocrinology are:

Diabetes: Patients with diabetes have too much sugar in their blood. Recent studies have found that excellent blood sugar control helps prevent problems from diabetes. Problems in the eyes, kidneys, and nerves can be very serious. They can lead to blindness, dialysis, or amputation. Endocrinologists treat diabetes with diet and medications, including insulin. They also work closely with patients to control blood sugar and monitor them so they can prevent health problems.

Thyroid: Patients with thyroid disorders often have problems with their energy levels. They may also have trouble with muscle strength, emotions, weight control, and tolerating heat or cold. Endocrinologists treat patients with too much or too little of the thyroid hormones. They help patients reach a hormone balance by replacing thyroid hormone. Endocrinologists also receive special training to manage patients with thyroid growths or cancer, and swollen thyroid glands.

Bone: Osteomalacia (rickets, which causes bones to soften) and osteoporosis are bone diseases that endocrinologists diagnose and treat. Osteoporosis is a disease that weakens your skeleton. Certain hormones act to protect bone tissue. When these hormone levels drop, bones can lose tissue and weaken. Menopause, loss of testicle function, and aging may put you at risk for bone breaks. Endocrinologists treat other disorders that can affect bones, such as too much parathyroid hormone.

Reproduction/Infertility: About one in ten American couples are infertile. Endocrine research has helped thousands of couples to have children. Endocrinologists diagnose and treat the precise hormone imbalance that causes infertility. Endocrinologists also assess and treat patients with reproductive problems based in glands. They work with patients who need hormone replacement. Problems that they treat include menopause symptoms, irregular periods, endometriosis, polycystic ovary syndrome, premenstrual syndrome, and impotence.

Obesity and Overweight: Endocrinologists treat patients who are overweight or obese, often because of metabolic and hormonal problems. The sign of obesity is too much body fat. Thyroid, adrenal, ovarian, and pituitary disorders can cause obesity. Endocrinologists also identify factors linked with obesity. These factors include insulin resistance and genetic problems.

Pituitary Gland: The pituitary is often called the master gland of the body because it controls other glands. The pituitary makes several vital hormones. Over- or under- production of pituitary hormones can lead to infertility, menstrual disorders, growth disorders (acromegaly or short stature), and too much cortisol (Cushing's syndrome). Endocrinologists control these conditions with medications and refer patients who need surgery.

Growth: Pediatric endocrinologists treat children with endocrine problems that cause short stature and other growth problems. Thanks to endocrine research, safe and effective treatments are available for people whose growth is abnormal.

Hypertension: Hypertension is high blood pressure, and it is a risk factor for heart disease. Up to 10% of people have hypertension because of too much aldosterone, a hormone produced in the adrenal glands. About half of these cases are caused by growths that can be removed with surgery. Conditions such as the metabolic syndrome or a growth called a pheochromocytoma also may cause hypertension. These conditions also can be treated successfully.

Lipid Disorders: Patients with lipid disorders have trouble maintaining normal levels of body fats. One of the most common lipid disorders is hyperlipidemia—high levels of total cholesterol, low-density lipoprotein cholesterol (known as bad cholesterol), and/or triglycerides in the blood. High levels of these fats are linked to heart and blood vessel (coronary heart) disease, strokes, and other diseases. Hypertension is common in people with lipid disorders, and together these factors put patients at higher risk for coronary heart disease. Endocrinologists are trained to detect factors that may be related to lipid disorders, such as hypothyroidism, drug use (such as steroid use), or genetic or metabolic conditions. Lipid disorders can be found in several conditions that require special management, including the metabolic syndrome, polycystic ovary syndrome, and obesity. Special diets, exercise, and medications, including estrogen replacement therapy in some cases, may be prescribed to manage hyperlipidemia and other lipid disorders.

Additional Information

The Hormone Foundation
8401 Connecticut Ave., Suite 900
Chevy Chase, MD 20815-5817
Toll-Free: 800-HORMONE (467-6663)
Website: http://www.hormone.org

Dr. Richard Guttler
Santa Monica Thyroid Diagnostic Center
1328 16th Street
Santa Monica, CA 90404
Toll-Free: 800-408-4909 (outside California)
Phone: 310-393-8860
Fax: 310-395-8147
Website: http://www.thyroid.com
E-mail: Dr.Guttler@thyroid.com

Part Two

Thyroid Disorder
Symptoms and Risk Factors

Chapter 7

Possible Signs and Symptoms of Thyroid Disorders

Frequently Asked Questions about Thyroid Disorders

What is the thyroid and why should I worry about it?

The thyroid is a small gland in the neck, just under the Adam's apple. Shaped like a butterfly, the thyroid plays an important role in a person's health and affects every organ, tissue, and cell in the body. It makes hormones that help to regulate the body's metabolism (how the body uses and stores energy from foods eaten) and organ functions. When the thyroid is not working properly (called thyroid disorder), it can affect your body weight, energy level, muscle strength, skin health, menstrual cycle (periods), memory, heart rate, and cholesterol level. Thyroid disorders happen: when the thyroid gland is not as active as it should be (called underactive thyroid); when the thyroid is more active than it should be (called overactive thyroid); or when the thyroid is enlarged (called goiter or nodule). People with thyroid enlargement can have underactive, overactive, or normal thyroid function. Thyroid disorders are much more common in women than in men. About 1 out of every 8 American women will develop a thyroid disorder. Underactive or overactive thyroid can be found with a simple blood test (called a thyroid stimulating hormone or TSH test), and is

Excerpts from "Frequently Asked Questions about Thyroid Disorders," National Women's Health Information Center, October 2002. Also, "Important Information for Thyroid Patients," © Thyroid Federation International. Reprinted with permission. Reviewed in November 2004 by David A. Cooke, M.D., Diplomate, American Board of Internal Medicine.

most often treated with medication and sometimes surgery or radio-active iodine.

What are the different types of thyroid disorders?

- **Hypothyroidism (underactive thyroid).** This is the most common type of thyroid disorder, where the thyroid makes too little of the thyroid hormone that your body needs to function properly. It is most often caused by Hashimoto disease. With this disease, the body's immune system (which normally protects you from disease) thinks the thyroid is a foreign invader and tries to destroy the thyroid. When damage is done to the thyroid, it can become larger (called goiter). Not getting enough iodine in a person's diet can also cause hypothyroidism, but this is more common outside of the United States (in the U.S., many products such as salt and bread are supplemented with iodine, making iodine deficiency rare). Being female, over 40 years of age, having a close family member with thyroid disease, and recently having had a baby are things that can increase the chance of getting hypothyroidism.

- **Hyperthyroidism (overactive thyroid).** When the thyroid gland is overactive, it makes too much of the thyroid hormone that your body needs to be healthy. This condition affects women more than men. In young women, hyperthyroidism is most often caused by Graves disease. With this disease, the body's immune system tricks the thyroid into making too much thyroid hormone. The entire thyroid becomes enlarged and over-active. Older women may get another form of hyperthyroidism (toxic nodular goiter), where overactive thyroid cells group to-gether and form a lump in the neck (called a thyroid nodule) that makes more of the thyroid hormone than the body needs. Some thyroid disorders initially cause overactive thyroid, but at a later point in time cause underactive thyroid, due to damage done to the thyroid gland.

- **Postpartum thyroiditis.** After giving birth, a woman's thyroid can swell and become larger or inflamed. This can cause chang-ing levels of thyroid hormone in the body. Sometimes high levels can be followed by low levels of thyroid hormone. After 6 months or less, this condition usually goes away with no permanent damage to the thyroid. While common, thyroid disorders after pregnancy are often hard to detect since some of the symptoms, such as having trouble sleeping, fatigue, depression, or weight change are viewed as normal when a woman has a new baby. The symptoms can also be mild. Usually only short-term treatment is required until the thyroid recovers normal function. Sometimes after pregnancy, a woman can get hypothyroidism (underactive thyroid), which persists and needs long-term treatment with medication.

- **Thyroid cancer.** This type of cancer is most often found as a lump (or nodule) in the thyroid gland. It is not a common type of cancer and most thyroid nodules are benign (not cancer). Other signs of thyroid cancer include swelling in the lymph nodes of the neck and trouble swallowing or breathing. Although anyone can get thyroid cancer, people who as children had head or neck x-ray treatments for tonsillitis or other conditions (from about the 1920s to the 1960s) are more likely to get this cancer. It is treated with surgery, which removes the cancer, sometimes followed by radioactive iodine therapy, which kills the cancer.

What are the signs of a thyroid disorder?

It can be hard to tell if you have a thyroid disorder because these disorders can have signs that are common and often confused with other conditions. If you think you have a thyroid disorder, talk with your health care provider and ask if a blood test for a thyroid disorder is indicated. A simple blood test measures thyroid stimulating hormone, or TSH, to find overactive and underactive thyroid disorders.

Important Information for Thyroid Patients from Thyroid Federation International

Since thyroid hormones affect every cell in your body, an overactive or underactive thyroid can produce a wide variety of symptoms. Your thyroid gland is located in the front of your neck below your Adam's apple. It plays an important role in regulating your body's metabolism.

Hypothyroidism (Underactive Thyroid)

Hypothyroidism may occur at any age, but is especially common in older individuals. It affects 17% of women and 9% of men by age 60.

Skin, Hair, and Nails

- Is your skin: cold, thick, dry with little or no sweating, waxy, flaky, itchy, pale ivory, or jaundiced?
- Do you bruise easily, do wounds heal slowly?
- Are you always feeling cold?
- Is your body temperature below normal?
- Have you noticed puffiness of hands and face—especially of the eyelids and under the eyes?
- Do you get "pins and needles"?
- Do you have carpal tunnel syndrome?
- Have you noticed hair loss of scalp, groin, outer half of eyebrows?
- Are you constantly cleaning out the sink and tub drains after each shampoo?
- Is your scalp dry?
- Does your hair feel like straw? Is it starting to frizzle?
- Are your nails brittle and thick and always breaking, splitting, layering?

Digestive System

- Are you always constipated?
- Have you gained weight and feel bloated?
- Is your cholesterol high?

Reproductive System

- Do you have heavy menstruation (clotting is common)?
- Have you had low birth weight babies and early delivery?
- Did you have a miscarriage your last pregnancy?
- Have you recently given birth? Postpartum thyroiditis occurs in approximately 8% of women after delivery and involves a hypothyroid stage 12–14 weeks after delivery.

Cardiac System

- Is your pulse slower than normal?

- Do you experience skipped beats followed by a boom, chest pain, shortness of breath?
- Are you sleeping excessively yet still feel totally drained and lifeless?
- Is everything an extreme effort?
- Have you lost your get up and go?
- Do your family and co-workers (if you're still able to work) think of you as lazy?
- Do you feel 100 years old?
- Do you take iron medication for chronic anemia?
- Has your blood pressure changed—gone either up or down?

The Mind and Emotions

- Does your mind feel foggy?
- Does your mental process seem slower than usual making thinking and decision making more difficult?
- Is your memory poor?
- Do you feel depressed, sad, and cry easily for no reason?
- Do you see something in your peripheral vision when nothing is there?

Muscular System

- Is it hard to keep your arms up when curling your hair?
- Do you get muscle cramps, lose your balance, and have a sluggish tendon reflex?

Eyes, Ear, Nose, and Throat

Although thyroid eye disease is more commonly associated with Graves disease (hyperthyroidism), it can also be associated with hypothyroidism.

- Do you find you have to listen harder to hear conversations and need the radio or television turned up?
- Does your voice seem deeper and hoarse?
- Is your speech slurred at times?

- Do you notice swelling at the front of your neck and feel pressure on your throat which is making swallowing more difficult?

- Do you suffer from frequent chest colds and other infections?

- Have you been treated for hyperthyroidism? (hypothyroidism often develops after treatment).

- Do you have a family history of thyroid disease and/or diabetes?

A TSH test is the most important test for detecting primary hypothyroidism.

Note: If you have had x-ray therapy as a child for enlarged adenoids or tonsils, enlargements of the thymus gland as a newborn, birthmarks, whooping cough, acne, or ringworm of the scalp, your physician should palpate your neck carefully to check for thyroid nodules as in almost every instance the thyroid function test will be normal, even in patients who have a proven carcinoma. The T4 (a thyroid hormone) and TSH (thyroid stimulating hormone) value can be misleading in this case, as they reflect the state of the total thyroid function, rather than the presence or significance of a thyroid nodule.

Hyperthyroidism (Overactive Thyroid)

Hyperthyroidism is most common between the ages of 20–40 but may occur at any age. Possible signs and symptoms of hyperthyroidism include the following.

Skin, Hair, and Nails

- Do you always feel hot and can't stand the heat?
- Is your skin warm and velvety to touch?
- Is your face flushed?
- Do you have increased sweating and frequent hives/itching?
- Have you noticed increased pigmentation of palms/soles?
- Do you have orange skin like lumps on the skin of the shins?
- Is your hair very soft, hard to curl and diffusely thinning?
- Are your nails soft, grow quickly and lift allowing dirt to get trapped underneath which is hard to get out?
- Have you noticed your fingers taking on the shape of a club—fingertips widen at sides of nail (rare)?

Possible Signs and Symptoms of Thyroid Disorders

Digestive System

- Are you shoveling food into your system because of an excessive appetite, but losing weight?
- Do you have frequent bowel movements/diarrhea?

Reproductive System

- Is your period now scant or stopped altogether?
- Have you been told you are experiencing early menopause?
- Are you having difficulty to conceive?
- Decreased sex drive due to total exhaustion of constantly being driven is common.
- Have you recently given birth? Postpartum thyroiditis involves a hyperthyroid stage 6–12 weeks after delivery followed by a hypothyroid stage 12–14 weeks post partum.

Cardiac System

- Is your pulse faster than normal with times when it goes so fast (tachycardia) you become very weak?
- Are you short of breath?
- Do you have swelling of your ankles?
- Do you get chest pain and palpitations, but a cardiac checkup reveals nothing wrong?
- When your doctor checks your blood pressure is your systolic blood pressure reading (top number) elevated with diastolic reading (bottom number) normal? This is known as wide pulse pressure.

The Mind and Emotions

- Do you feel as if you are in overdrive and out of control?
- Are you restless, nervous, impatient, irritable, unable to stop cleaning house, etc.?
- Do you feel ready to explode, have mood swings, panic attacks, headaches, difficulty sleeping you're so wound up?

Muscular System

- Do you find yourself pulling on the bannister with your arms to help you climb stairs due to weak thigh muscles?

63

- Have you noticed a fine tremor (you can check this by placing a sheet of paper on the back of your hand) or obvious shakiness of your hands?
- Is your knee jerk response exaggerated?
- Are your ankles swollen?

Eye, Ear, Nose, and Throat

- Do you stare a lot without blinking?
- Have you noticed changes in your eyes such as eye lid elevation, a feeling of sand in eyes, pain, watering, redness, possible protrusion.

If you have thyroid eye disease symptoms, you should be seen by a specialist. Do not hesitate to ask for a second opinion on treatment options.

According to Dr. Robert Volpe, FRCP, FACP, Toronto, Canada, "the general view is that if patients do have eye signs to begin with and yet radioactive iodine is the treatment of choice, then prednisone given concurrently with the radioactive iodine and for 6–8 weeks tends to prevent the aggravation of the eye signs. There is some suggested evidence that patients should not be allowed to become hypothyroid after treatment and possibly thyroxine should be given after the radioactive iodine so as to prevent hypothyroidism. However, this is somewhat controversial and most endocrinologists would wait until the TSH begins to rise before prescribing thyroxine."

- Are you very sensitive to noise now?
- Have you noticed a lump or swelling on the front of your neck?
- Do you have a family history of thyroid disease and/or diabetes?

Please note the listed symptoms are extensive in order to present the whole picture. You probably won't have all of these symptoms. Seniors usually present atypically so TSH testing is very important. Early diagnosis with a simple TSH blood test followed by correct treatment will prevent serious complications.

It is extremely important for you to tell your doctor all of your symptoms—copy and highlight or circle them from this chapter and take it with you. Also write down any questions you may have and give a copy to your doctor.

We urge all doctors to take time to listen to your patients—do not isolate symptoms, but look at the whole spectrum. If a patient tells you she/he feels as if she/he's falling apart and nothing seems to be working properly, chances are she/he's right.

Additional Information

American Foundation of Thyroid Patients
4322 Douglas Ave.
Midland, TX 79703
Phone: 915-694-9966
Website: http://www.thyroidfoundation.org
E-mail: thyroid@flash.net

American Thyroid Association
6066 Leesburg Pike, Suite 550
Falls Church, VA 22041
Toll-Free: 800-THYROID (849-7643)
Phone: 703-998-8890
Fax: 703-998-8893
Website: http://www.thyroid.org
E-mail: admin@thyroid.org

Endocrine Society
8401 Connecticut Ave., Suite 900
Chevy Chase, MD 20815-5817
Phone: 301-941-0200
Website: http://www.endo-society.org
E-mail: societyservices@endo-society.org

National Institute of Diabetes and Digestive and Kidney Diseases (NIDDK)
NIH Building 31, Room 9A04
Center Drive, MSC 2560
Bethesda, MD 20892
Phone: 301-496-3583
Website: http://niddk.nih.gov

National Women's Health Information Center (NWHIC)
8550 Arlington Blvd., Suite 300
Fairfax, VA 22031
Toll-Free: 800-994-9662
Website: http://www.4woman.gov

Thyroid Federation International
797 Princess St., Suite 304
Kingston, ON K7L 1G1
Canada
Phone: 613-544-9731
Fax: 613-544-9731
Website: http://www.thyroid-fed.org
E-mail: tfi@on.aibn.com

Thyroid Foundation of America, Inc.
One Longfellow Place, Suite 1518
Boston, MA 02114
Toll-Free: 800-832-8321
Phone: 617-534-1500
Fax: 617-534-1515
Website: http://www.allthyroid.org
E-mail: info@allthyroid.org

Chapter 8

Goiter

Definition: A goiter is an enlargement of the thyroid gland that is not associated with inflammation or cancer.

Causes, Incidence, and Risk Factors

There are different kinds of goiters. A simple goiter usually occurs when the thyroid gland is not able to produce enough thyroid hormone to meet the body's requirements. The thyroid gland compensates by enlarging, which usually overcomes mild deficiencies of thyroid hormone.

A simple goiter may be classified as either an endemic (colloid) goiter or a sporadic (nontoxic) goiter.

Endemic goiters occur within groups of people living in geographical areas with iodine-depleted soil, usually regions away from the sea coast. People in these communities might not get enough iodine in their diet. (Iodine is vital to the formation of thyroid hormone.) The modern use of iodized table salt in the U.S. prevents this deficiency; however, it is still common in central Asia and central Africa.

In most cases of sporadic goiter the cause is unknown. Occasionally, certain medications such as lithium or aminoglutethimide can cause a nontoxic goiter.

Hereditary factors may cause goiters. Risk factors for the development of a goiter include female sex, age over 40 years, inadequate dietary intake of iodine, residence in an endemic area, and a family history of goiter.

Symptoms

- Thyroid enlargement varying from a single small nodule to massive enlargement (neck lump)
- Breathing difficulties, cough, or wheezing due to compression of the trachea
- Swallowing difficulties due to compression of the esophagus
- Neck vein distention and dizziness when the arms are raised above the head

Signs and Tests

- Measurement of thyroid stimulating hormone (TSH) and free thyroxine (T4) in the blood
- Thyroid scan and uptake
- Ultrasound of thyroid—if nodules are present, a biopsy should be done to evaluate for thyroid cancer

Treatment

A goiter only needs to be treated if it is causing symptoms. The enlarged thyroid can be treated with radioactive iodine to shrink the gland or with surgical removal of part or all of the gland (thyroidectomy). Small doses of iodine (Lugol's or potassium iodine solution) may help when the goiter is due to iodine deficiency.

Expectations (Prognosis)

A goiter is a benign (harmless) process. Simple goiters may disappear spontaneously, or may become large. Over time, hypothyroidism may develop due to destruction of the normal thyroid tissue. This can be treated with medications to replace the thyroid hormone.

Occasionally, a goiter may progress to a toxic nodular goiter when a nodule is making thyroid hormone on its own. This can cause hyperthyroidism and can be treated with radioactive iodine to destroy the nodule.

Complications

- Progressive thyroid enlargement and/or the development of hardened nodules may indicate thyroid malignancy. All thyroid nodules should be biopsied to evaluate for malignancy.

- A simple goiter may progress to a toxic nodular goiter.
- Hypothyroidism may occur after treatment of a large goiter with radioactive iodine or surgery.

Calling Your Health Care Provider

Call your health care provider if you experience any swelling or enlargement in the front of your neck, increased resting pulse rate, palpitations, diarrhea, nausea, vomiting, sweating without exercise or increased room temperature, tremors, agitation, shortness of breath, or signs of hypothyroidism such as fatigue, constipation, or dry skin.

Prevention

The use of iodized table salt prevents endemic goiter.

Chapter 9

Thyroid Nodules

Symptoms and Causes of Thyroid Nodules

What is a thyroid nodule?

The term thyroid nodule refers to any abnormal growth of thyroid cells into a lump within the thyroid. Although the vast majority of thyroid nodules are benign (noncancerous), a small proportion of thyroid nodules do contain thyroid cancer. Because of this possibility, the evaluation of a thyroid nodule is aimed at discovering a potential thyroid cancer.

What are the symptoms of a thyroid nodule?

Most thyroid nodules do not cause any symptoms. Your doctor usually discovers them during a routine physical examination, or you might notice a lump in your neck while looking in a mirror. If the nodule is made up of thyroid cells that actively produce thyroid hormone without regard to the body's need, a patient may complain of hyperthyroid symptoms. A few patients with thyroid nodules may complain of pain in the neck, jaw, or ear. If the nodule is large enough, it may cause difficulty swallowing or cause a tickle in the throat or shortness of breath if it is pressing on the windpipe. Rarely, hoarseness can be caused if the nodule irritates a nerve to the voice box.

What causes a thyroid nodule?

The thyroid nodule is the most common endocrine problem in the United States. The chances are 1 in 10 that you or someone you know will develop a thyroid nodule. Although thyroid cancer is the most important cause of the thyroid nodule, fortunately it occurs in less than 10% of nodules. This means that about 9 of 10 nodules are benign (noncancerous). The most common types of noncancerous thyroid nodules are known as colloid nodules and follicular neoplasms. If a nodule produces thyroid hormone without regard to the body's need, it is called an autonomous nodule, and it can occasionally lead to hyperthyroidism. If the nodule is filled with fluid or blood, it is called a thyroid cyst.

We do not know what causes most noncancerous thyroid nodules to form. A patient with hypothyroidism may also have a thyroid nodule, particularly if the cause is the inflammation known as Hashimoto thyroiditis. Sometimes a lack of iodine in the diet can cause a thyroid gland to produce nodules. Some autonomous nodules have a genetic defect that causes them to grow.

Diagnosis of Thyroid Nodules

Since most patients with thyroid nodules do not have symptoms, most nodules are discovered during an examination of the neck for another reason, such as during a routine physical examination or when you are sick with a cold or flu. Once the nodule is discovered, your doctor will try to determine whether the lump is the only problem with your thyroid or whether the entire thyroid gland has been affected by a more general condition such as hyperthyroidism or hypothyroidism. Your physician will feel the thyroid to see whether the entire gland is enlarged, whether there is a single nodule present, or whether there are many lumps or nodules in your thyroid. The initial laboratory tests may include blood tests to measure the amount of thyroid hormone (thyroxine, or T4) and thyroid-stimulating hormone (TSH) in your blood to determine whether your thyroid is functioning normally. Most patients with thyroid nodules will also have normal thyroid function tests.

Rarely is it possible to determine whether a thyroid nodule is cancerous by physical examination and blood tests alone, and so the evaluation of the thyroid nodule often includes specialized tests such as a thyroid fine needle biopsy, a thyroid scan, and/or a thyroid ultrasound.

Thyroid Fine Needle Biopsy

A fine needle biopsy of a thyroid nodule may sound frightening, but the needle used is very small and a local anesthetic can be used. This simple procedure is done in the doctor's office. It does not require any special preparation (no fasting), and patients usually return home or to work after the biopsy without any ill effects. For a fine needle biopsy, your doctor will use a very thin needle to withdraw cells from the thyroid nodule. Ordinarily, several samples will be taken from different parts of the nodule to give your doctor the best chance of finding cancerous cells if a tumor is present. The cells are then examined under a microscope by a pathologist.

The report of a thyroid fine needle biopsy will usually indicate one of the following findings:

1. **The nodule is benign (noncancerous).** This result is obtained in 50% to 60% of biopsies and often indicates a colloid nodule. The risk of overlooking a cancer when the biopsy is benign is generally under 3 in 100 and is even lower when the biopsy is reviewed by an experienced pathologist at a major medical center. Generally, these nodules need not be removed, but another biopsy may be required in the future, especially if they get bigger.

2. **The nodule is malignant (cancerous).** This result is obtained in about 5% of biopsies and often indicates papillary cancer, one of the most common thyroid cancers. All of these nodules should be removed surgically, preferably by an experienced thyroid surgeon.

3. **The nodule is suspicious.** This result is obtained in about 10% of biopsies and indicates either a follicular adenoma (noncancerous) or a follicular cancer. Often, your doctor may want to obtain a thyroid scan to determine which nodules should be removed surgically.

4. **The biopsy is nondiagnostic or inadequate.** This result is obtained in up to 20% of biopsies and indicates that not enough cells were obtained to make a diagnosis. This is a common result if the nodule is a cyst. These nodules may be removed surgically or be re-evaluated with second fine needle biopsy, depending on the clinical judgment of your doctor.

Thyroid Scan

The thyroid scan uses a small amount of a radioactive substance, usually radioactive iodine, to obtain a picture of the thyroid gland. Because thyroid cancer cells do not take up radioactive iodine as easily as normal thyroid cells do, this test is used to determine the likelihood that a thyroid nodule contains a cancer. If done as the first test, the thyroid scan is used to determine those patients who most need a biopsy. The scan usually gives the following results.

1. **The nodule is cold.** In other words, the nodule is not taking up radioactive iodine normally. This patient is referred for a fine needle biopsy of the nodule.

2. **The nodule is functioning.** The nodule's uptake of radioactive iodine is similar to that of normal cells. A biopsy is not needed right away since the likelihood of cancer is very low.

3. **The nodule is hot.** The nodule's uptake of radioactive iodine is greater than that of normal cells. The likelihood of cancer is extremely rare, and so biopsy is usually not necessary.

If the fine needle biopsy was done as the first test, then a scan is usually ordered to evaluate a suspicious biopsy result. In this case, patients with a cold nodule result should have their nodule removed. Patients with functioning or hot nodules on a scan and a suspicious biopsy can be watched, and surgery is not immediately necessary.

Thyroid Ultrasound

The thyroid ultrasound uses high frequency sound waves to obtain a picture of the thyroid. This very sensitive test can easily determine if a nodule is solid or cystic, and it can determine the precise size of the nodule. The thyroid ultrasound can be used to keep an eye on thyroid nodules that are not removed by surgery to determine if they are growing or shrinking. Some ultrasound characteristics of a nodule are more frequent in thyroid cancer than in noncancerous nodules. Even so, the thyroid ultrasound alone is rarely able to determine if a nodule is a thyroid cancer. The thyroid ultrasound also can be used to assist the placement of the needle within the nodule during a fine needle biopsy, especially if the nodule is hard to feel. Finally, the thyroid ultrasound can identify nodules that are very small and cannot be felt during a physical examination. The clinical importance of these very small nodules is uncertain; however, the ultrasound provides a means by which an accurate fine needle biopsy can be performed if your doctor thinks a biopsy is needed.

Treatment of Thyroid Nodules

All thyroid nodules that are found to contain a thyroid cancer, or that are highly suspicious of containing a cancer, should be removed surgically by an experienced thyroid surgeon. Most thyroid cancers are curable and rarely cause life threatening problems. Any thyroid nodule not removed needs to be watched closely, with an examination of the nodule every 6 to 12 months. This follow-up may involve a physical examination by a doctor or a thyroid ultrasound or both. Occasionally, your doctor may want to try to shrink your nodule by treating you with thyroid hormone at doses slightly higher that your body needs (called suppression therapy). Whether you are on thyroid hormone suppression therapy or not, a repeat fine needle biopsy may be indicated if the nodule gets bigger. Also, even if the biopsy is benign, surgery may be recommended for removal of a nodule that is getting bigger.

Additional Information

American Thyroid Association
6066 Leesburg Pike, Suite 550
Falls Church, VA 22041
Toll-Free: 800-THYROID (849-7643)
Phone: 703-998-8890
Fax: 703-998-8893
Website: http://www.thyroid.org
E-mail: admin@thyroid.org

Chapter 10

Prematurely Gray Hair and Thyroid Dysfunction

Years ago an association was made between prematurely gray hair and pernicious anemia. Pernicious anemia is an autoimmune disorder in which antibodies damage stomach cells. The damaged cells lose the ability to absorb vitamin B_{12} and the result is known as pernicious anemia.

Then doctors began to notice that prematurely gray hair was also associated with other autoimmune disorders, particularly hyperthyroidism due to Graves disease and hypothyroidism due to chronic thyroiditis (Hashimoto disease). Because of this, many physicians routinely ordered vitamin B_{12} levels, as well as thyroid hormone test in individuals whom they know were prematurely gray.

Now some physicians may not know whether their patient has gray hair because more and more women are coloring their hair. The doctor may not ask whether they were prematurely gray and therefore at risk for these autoimmune disorders.

The Risks of Hidden Thyroid Illness

There are some serious health risks for individuals who have untreated hidden thyroid illness.

- For young women there are risks in pregnancy. A women who is pregnant and has even mild thyroid deficiency manifested by an elevation of serum thyroid stimulating hormone (TSH) level could face serious problems. Her risks are increased for miscarriage, premature delivery, a low birth weight baby, and hypertension before delivery.

- Older individuals with unrecognized hypothyroidism could experience fatigue, depression, fluid retention, muscle cramps, and an elevation in cholesterol, increasing their risk for heart disease.

- Individuals with unrecognized hyperthyroidism may experience difficulty getting pregnant, miscarriage, osteoporosis, and serious heart complications, including atrial fibrillation (a rhythm disorder) and heart attacks.

A program being carried out by the hair stylists at Daryl Christopher Salons and the Thyroid Foundation of America (TFA) educates the public about these relationships.

"We are sincerely hoping to facilitate communication between patients and their physicians, so that individuals who should be screened for thyroid dysfunction are having the appropriate tests," says Dr. Lawrence C. Wood, TFA's Medical Director. "The tests are simple and accurate. A blood sample is taken and measured for thyroid stimulating hormone (TSH) and antithyroid peroxidase (anti-TPO) antibody. The TSH tells whether the patient needs treatment now (a low TSH indicates hyperthyroidism while an increased TSH indicates an underactive thyroid). The anti-TPO antibody test tells whether an individual is at increased risk for thyroid dysfunction. Most thyroid specialists would recommend that an individual who tests positive for this antibody should have repeat tests for TSH every three months if pregnant or once a year if not pregnant."

In this program, patients will take their knowledge about prematurely gray hair and thyroid dysfunction to their physician and ask the physician whether its appropriate for them to have a serum TSH and an anti-TPO antibody test to find out whether they have a thyroid problem now and are at risk for one in the future.

"Of course it is up to the patients' physicians to decide whether testing should be done," according to Dr. Wood. "The Thyroid Foundation of America recognizes that it is the responsibility of the physician to make these choices. Our program is designed to remind physicians of the significance of prematurely gray hair as a clue to hidden thyroid problems."

Other Health Problems May Also Be Found in These Families

The idea of family screening means that the individuals who are prematurely gray should consider their family's health as well. On the side of the family where the prematurely gray hair comes from there may be relatives who have thyroid dysfunction or other medical conditions that need treatment. For example physicians may want to measure vitamin B_{12} levels in older individuals to look for pernicious anemia which may present as anemia, peripheral neuropathy with numb hands and feet, or even as an emotional disorder.

Patient Privacy Preserved

Dr. Wood pointed out that the study is being done with great care to protect the privacy of the individuals involved. Patients are given a numbered document that they take to their physicians. When they and their relatives have completed thyroid testing they will return the results of their test in their numbered report rather than with their name. Information will then be complied anonymously to find out how many individuals were tested and how many new individuals were found who had hidden thyroid problems that needed treatment.

All participants will be sent a summary of the reports, which also will be made available to their physicians.

Additional Information

Thyroid Foundation of America, Inc.
One Longfellow Place, Suite 1518
Boston, MA 02114
Toll-Free: 800-832-8321
Phone: 617-534-1500
Fax: 617-534-1515
Website: http://www.allthyroid.org
E-mail: info@allthyroid.org

79

Chapter 11

Depression May Indicate Thyroid Imbalance

Depression and Thyroid Illness

Depression may be the first sign of an overactive or underactive thyroid. The nervousness, anxiety, and hyperactivity of hyperthyroidism often interfere with a person's ability to function in normal daily activities. Both anxiety and depression can be severe, but should improve once the hyperthyroidism is recognized and treated.

Depression is more commonly associated with hypothyroidism with its fatigue, mental dullness, and lethargy leading to depression which is often profound and severe enough that a physician may mistakenly treat the patient first for depression without testing for underlying hypothyroidism. Since most hypothyroidism begins after age fifty, the symptoms are often attributed to aging, menopause, and/or depression.

Postpartum Depression

Approximately one in twenty women experience a change in thyroid function following pregnancy. Since this is a time when the responsibilities of the young mother are considerable, she may attribute the fatigue and emotional symptoms as a natural result of her increased duties and lack of sleep. Some physicians have suggested, however, that every young mother who experiences depression should have a TSH test to be sure her thyroid function is normal.

Bipolar Mood Disorders and Thyroid Disease

Bipolar Disorder is a new term for an old illness, which was formerly called manic depression. People with bipolar disorder have periods of depression, which may last weeks or months. They may also have periods of a week or more of mania or hypomania. These are marked by varying degrees of hyperactivity, excessive happiness, unrealistic ambitions, and impaired judgment. A minority of patients with bipolar disorder experience rapid cycling, meaning that they have at least four major episodes of mood change per year. Studies of patients with rapid cycling bipolar disorder, (80% of whom are women) have shown that 25–50% have evidence of thyroid deficiency. Some feel well, and their only evidence of thyroid failure is an increased level of TSH in their blood. Others are clearly hypothyroid.

Lithium: A Problem for Some Patients

Physicians have prescribed lithium in the treatment of depression for years. It has a low incidence of side effects and a high success rate in treating depression, especially bipolar disorders including the rapid cycling.

Unfortunately, in individuals with an underlying tendency toward thyroid dysfunction, lithium may cause hypothyroidism. Since most physicians are aware of this relationship, it is now common for a physician to first check the serum TSH levels of a patient before prescribing lithium, repeating the thyroid test periodically while the patient is on the medication.

Are You at Risk?

Not all individuals with depression have a thyroid problem. Nevertheless, because thyroid dysfunction can be so difficult to recognize yet so responsive to treatment, most physicians will order an initial serum TSH test to evaluate thyroid function.

You are at increased risk if you or a close relative has had a thyroid problem. Your risk is also increased if you have a related autoimmune condition such as diabetes requiring insulin treatment, pernicious anemia, or the white skin spots of vitiligo. You are also more likely to develop thyroid dysfunction if you or a close relative have had prematurely gray hair (one gray hair before thirty) or any degree of ambidexterity or left-handedness.

Why risk missing a thyroid problem if you are depressed? Discuss these concerns with your physicians and be sure that your TSH has been checked before you are treated for depression.

Information about Depression

In any given 1-year period, 9.5 percent of the population, or about 18.8 million American adults, suffer from a depressive illness.[1] The economic cost for this disorder is high, but the cost in human suffering cannot be estimated. Depressive illnesses often interfere with normal functioning and cause pain and suffering not only to those who have a disorder, but also to those who care about them. Serious depression can destroy family life as well as the life of the ill person. But much of this suffering is unnecessary.

Most people with a depressive illness do not seek treatment, although the great majority—even those whose depression is extremely severe—can be helped. Thanks to years of fruitful research, there are now medications and psychosocial therapies such as cognitive/behavioral, talk, or interpersonal that ease the pain of depression.

Unfortunately, many people do not recognize that depression is a treatable illness. If you feel that you or someone you care about is one of the many undiagnosed depressed people in this country, the information presented here may help you take the steps that may save your own or someone else's life.

Depressive Disorders

A depressive disorder is an illness that involves the body, mood, and thoughts. It affects the way a person eats and sleeps, the way one feels about oneself, and the way one thinks about things. A depressive disorder is not the same as a passing blue mood. It is not a sign of personal weakness or a condition that can be willed or wished away. People with a depressive illness cannot merely pull themselves together and get better. Without treatment, symptoms can last for weeks, months, or years. Appropriate treatment, however, can help most people who suffer from depression.

Types of Depression

Depressive disorders come in different forms, just as is the case with other illnesses such as heart disease. This section briefly describes three of the most common types of depressive disorders. However, within these types there are variations in the number of symptoms, their severity, and persistence.

Major depression is manifested by a combination of symptoms that interfere with the ability to work, study, sleep, eat, and enjoy once pleasurable activities. Such a disabling episode of depression may occur only once but more commonly occurs several times in a lifetime.

Dysthymia, a less severe type of depression, involves long-term, chronic symptoms that do not disable, but keep one from functioning well or from feeling good. Many people with dysthymia also experience major depressive episodes at some time in their lives.

Bipolar disorder, another type of depression, is also called manic-depressive illness. Not nearly as prevalent as other forms of depressive disorders, bipolar disorder is characterized by cycling mood changes: severe highs (mania) and lows (depression). Sometimes the mood switches are dramatic and rapid, but most often they are gradual. When in the depressed cycle, an individual can have any or all of the symptoms of a depressive disorder. When in the manic cycle, the individual may be overactive, talkative, and have a great deal of energy. Mania often affects thinking, judgment, and social behavior in ways that cause serious problems and embarrassment. For example, the individual in a manic phase may feel elated, full of grand schemes that might range from unwise business decisions to romantic sprees. Mania, left untreated, may worsen to a psychotic state.

Symptoms of Depression and Mania

Not everyone who is depressed or manic experiences every symptom. Some people experience a few symptoms, some many. Severity of symptoms varies with individuals and also varies over time.

Depression

- Persistent sad, anxious, or empty mood
- Feelings of hopelessness, pessimism
- Feelings of guilt, worthlessness, helplessness
- Loss of interest or pleasure in hobbies and activities that were once enjoyed, including sex
- Decreased energy, fatigue, being slowed down

- Difficulty concentrating, remembering, making decisions
- Insomnia, early-morning awakening, or oversleeping
- Appetite and/or weight loss or overeating and weight gain
- Thoughts of death or suicide; suicide attempts
- Restlessness, irritability
- Persistent physical symptoms that do not respond to treatment, such as headaches, digestive disorders, and chronic pain

Mania

- Abnormal or excessive elation
- Unusual irritability
- Decreased need for sleep
- Grandiose notions
- Increased talking
- Racing thoughts
- Increased sexual desire
- Markedly increased energy
- Poor judgment
- Inappropriate social behavior

How to Help Yourself If You Are Depressed

Depressive disorders make one feel exhausted, worthless, helpless, and hopeless. Such negative thoughts and feelings make some people feel like giving up. It is important to realize that these negative views are part of the depression and typically do not accurately reflect the actual circumstances. Negative thinking fades as treatment begins to take effect. In the meantime:

- Set realistic goals in light of the depression and assume a reasonable amount of responsibility.
- Break large tasks into small ones, set some priorities, and do what you can as you can.
- Try to be with other people and to confide in someone; it is usually better than being alone and secretive.
- Participate in activities that may make you feel better.

- Mild exercise, going to a movie, a ball game, or participating in religious, social, or other activities may help.

- Expect your mood to improve gradually, not immediately.

- Feeling better takes time. It is advisable to postpone important decisions until the depression has lifted. Before deciding to make a significant transition—change jobs, get married, or divorced—discuss it with others who know you well and have a more objective view of your situation.

- People rarely snap out of a depression. But they can feel a little better day-by-day.

- Remember, positive thinking will replace the negative thinking that is part of the depression and will disappear as your depression responds to treatment.

- Let your family and friends help you.

How Family and Friends Can Help the Depressed Person

The most important thing anyone can do for the depressed person is to help him or her get an appropriate diagnosis and treatment. This may involve encouraging the individual to stay with treatment until symptoms begin to abate (several weeks), or to seek different treatment if no improvement occurs. On occasion, it may require making an appointment and accompanying the depressed person to the doctor. It may also mean monitoring whether the depressed person is taking medication. The depressed person should be encouraged to obey the doctor's orders about the use of alcoholic products while on medication. The second most important thing is to offer emotional support. This involves understanding, patience, affection, and encouragement. Engage the depressed person in conversation and listen carefully. Do not disparage feelings expressed, but point out realities and offer hope. Do not ignore remarks about suicide. Report them to the depressed person's therapist. Invite the depressed person for walks, outings, to the movies, and other activities. Be gently insistent if your invitation is refused. Encourage participation in some activities that once gave pleasure, such as hobbies, sports, religious or cultural activities, but do not push the depressed person to undertake too much too soon. The depressed person needs diversion and company, but too many demands can increase feelings of failure.

Do not accuse the depressed person of faking illness or of laziness, or expect him or her to snap out of it. Eventually, with treatment, most people do get better. Keep that in mind, and keep reassuring the depressed person that, with time and help, he or she will feel better.

Reference

[1] "The Numbers Count: Mental Disorders in America," National Institute of Mental Health, 2001. Available at http://www.nimh.nih.gov/publicat/numbers.cfm.

Additional Information

Thyroid Foundation of America
One Longfellow Place, Suite 1518
Boston, MA 02114
Toll-Free: 800-832-8321
Phone: 617-534-1500
Fax: 617-534-1515
Website: http://www.allthyroid.org
E-mail: info@allthyroid.org

Chapter 12

Genetic Links and Thyroid Disease

Understanding the Link between Genetics and Thyroid Disease

Most Americans are aware that heart disease and cancer patients may be genetically predisposed to these conditions, but according to a national survey released in January 2002 by the American Association of Clinical Endocrinologists (AACE), more than three-fourths (76%) of the population do not know that thyroid disease runs in families.[1]

To counteract this lack of awareness, and encourage Americans to uncover their family health history to discover their at-risk medical conditions, AACE is launching a new campaign, "The Neck's Generation: Thyroid Genealogy," to educate the public about the genetic links associated with thyroid disease. Research shows that there is a strong genetic link between thyroid disease and other autoimmune diseases including certain types of diabetes, anemia, and arthritis.[2] In fact, thyroid disease affects more than 13 million Americans, yet more than half remain undiagnosed.[3]

"AACE's call to action is for each American to educate themselves about their family health history and how it can affect their chances of developing a thyroid disorder. If thyroid disease or other autoimmune diseases run in their family, a conversation with their doctor and a simple blood test can rule out their risk for thyroid problems," says Rhoda Cobin, M.D., F.A.C.E., and president of AACE. Health issues have increasingly become a family concern. According to the Council on Family Health, consumers are playing an increasingly active role in managing their health and treating their ailments.[4] Because autoimmune disorders are hereditary, and some disorders run strongly in families, AACE encourages Americans to keep an open health dialogue between family members, including education on the risks of undiagnosed thyroid disease.

"Communication was the key that allowed both myself and my daughter to get early diagnoses of thyroid disease," said Wanda Rockwell of Waldwick, New Jersey, a patient with hypothyroidism. "If my mother, who also has an underactive thyroid, and I hadn't discussed her diagnosis as soon as she went on medication, I would not have known the symptoms to look for—nor would I have realized my daughter was also at risk."

The thyroid is a butterfly-shaped gland located in the neck, just below the Adam's apple and above the collarbone. Left untreated, thyroid disease causes serious long-term complications such as elevated cholesterol levels and subsequent heart disease, infertility, muscle weakness, and osteoporosis. "Fifty percent of thyroid disease patients' offspring will inherit the thyroid disease gene. Since the thyroid gland is critical to every cell, tissue, and organ in the body, it is very important for Americans to get tested for thyroid disease—especially if they are experiencing some of the most common symptoms like fatigue, forgetfulness, depression, and changes in weight and appetite," says Hossein Gharib, M.D., F.A.C.E, a Vice-President of AACE and Professor of Medicine at the Mayo Medical School.

According to the AACE survey, more than half (56%) of the American population has never been tested for thyroid disease.[5] The millions who remain undiagnosed reflect the widespread lack of awareness of this serious condition that is easily treatable by taking a levothyroxine sodium pill once a day to restore thyroid hormone to its normal level.

The Diabetes and Thyroid Connection

AACE's survey found that 79 percent of Americans did not know there is a connection between diabetes and thyroid disease.[6] In fact, fifteen to twenty percent of diabetics and their siblings or parents are at a greater risk of presenting with thyroid disease compared to 4.5 percent of the general population.[7] Patients with thyroid disease and their relatives are also at an increased risk of the type of diabetes that develops in children or young adults called type one diabetes.[8] These two disorders rarely occur in the same person, but frequently can occur among family members. For example, it would not be uncommon to have a grandmother who suffers from diabetes and a grandchild that develops thyroid disease because both of these diseases fall into the autoimmune disorder category.

The Arthritis and Thyroid Connection

Since 90 percent of AACE survey respondents did not know that people with arthritis may be at increased risk for thyroid disease,[9] it is not surprising that patients who suffer from certain types of joint and tendon inflammation rarely make the thyroid link. Painful tendonitis and bursitis of the shoulder was reported in 6.7 percent of thyroid disease patients, but occurs in only about 1.7 percent of the general population.[10] In some cases, the pain and stiffness improves in thyroid patients when their thyroid condition is diagnosed and stabilized on medication.

There is also a higher prevalence of thyroid disease among patients suffering from rheumatoid arthritis than in the general population. In a group of 383 patients with documented rheumatoid arthritis, 9.3 percent had thyroid antibodies.[11] Rheumatoid arthritis occurs when there is inflammation of many joints of the body, typically the knuckles, wrists, and elbows. This type of arthritis also can improve when a patient's thyroid condition is treated.

The Anemia and Thyroid Connection

According to the AACE survey, only 15 percent of Americans are aware of the link between anemia and thyroid disease, but research shows that thyroid antibodies are frequently found in patients with pernicious anemia and their relatives. Pernicious anemia is a vitamin B_{12} deficiency that usually develops in patients over the age of 60. This is an age group also at strong risk for thyroid disease. In fact, one in five women over the age of 65 have an increased thyroid stimulating hormone (TSH) blood level, indicating a failing thyroid gland.

In a large series of American patients with pernicious anemia, nearly half (48.3%) had laboratory test evidence of thyroid disease.[12] The overall prevalence of pernicious anemia among children, siblings, parents, and parents' siblings of patients with pernicious anemia is about 2.5 percent, or about 20 times the prevalence in the population at large.[13] This figure becomes even greater if age and closeness of the family relationship are considered.

Additional AACE Survey Findings[14]

* A majority of survey respondents correctly identified multiple sclerosis (75%) and epilepsy (73%) as non-genetic disorders; however, only 24% correctly identified thyroid disease as having genetic links.

* Forty-seven percent of Americans know that thyroid disease affects primarily women. In fact, women are five to eight times more likely than men to have thyroid disease.

* Most survey respondents correctly identified weight gain or loss (70%) and fatigue (62%) as symptoms of a possible under-lying thyroid condition. Fewer people knew that changes in hair, skin, and nails (40%), depression (37%), and intolerance to heat and/or cold (34%) are also symptoms associated with thyroid disorder.

* In the same vein, much of the public is not aware of other complications that can stem from thyroid disease. Only 28 percent of survey takers knew of the link between elevated cholesterol and thyroid disease. Twenty-four percent knew that thyroid disease puts patients at increased risk for infertility, while 22 percent understood the link between osteoporosis and thyroid conditions.

The American Association of Clinical Endocrinologists and the Neck Check™

While the TSH blood test is the most sensitive and accurate diagnostic tool for thyroid disease, AACE also recommends that patients perform a simple self-examination called the Neck Check™. This easy, quick self-exam unveiled by AACE in 1997, helps Americans detect if they have an enlarged thyroid gland and should speak with their doctor about further testing. For step-by-step instructions on how to perform the Neck Check™, refer to chapter 17 of this book, or visit the AACE website at http://www.aace.com.

References

1. ORC *International Omnitel Survey*, December 2001.

2. Dayan CM, Daniels GH Chronic Autoimmune Thyroiditis, *NEJM* 335: 2 99-107, 1996.

3. www.aace.com

4. Hayes, Jr. M.D., Arthur Hull "Did You Know...Focus: Preventing Drug Interactions," Council on Family Health, www.cfhinfo.org/educationResources/did_you.htm 12/11/01.

5. ORC *International Omnitel Survey*, December 2001.

6. ORC *International Omnitel Survey*, December 2001.

7. Adams A Walston J Silver K *Autoimmune Disease Risk in Families with Type 1 Diabetes*, www.genetichealth.com 10/27/01.

8. Wood M.D., Lawrence C *Your Thyroid: A Home Reference*, Ballantine Books, New York, 1995.

9. ORC *International Omnitel Survey*, December 2001.

10. Wood M.D., Lawrence C *Your Thyroid: A Home Reference* Ballantine Books, New York, 1995.

11. Wood M.D., Lawrence C *Your Thyroid: A Home Reference* Ballantine Books, New York, 1995.

12. Carmel R, Spencer CA. Clinical and subclinical thyroid disorders associated with pernicious anemia. *Arch Inter Med* 1982: 142: 1465.

13. Lee: Wintrobe's *Clinical Hematology, 10th ed.*, Lippincott Williams & Wilkins, 1999.

14. ORC *International Omnitel Survey*, December 2001.

Additional Information

American Association of Clinical Endocrinologists (AACE)
1000 Riverside Avenue, Suite 205
Jacksonville, FL 32204
Phone: 904-353-7878
Fax: 904-353-8185
Website: http://www.aace.com
E-mail: info@aace.com

As part of The Neck's Generation campaign, AACE's website also provides tools such as a chart to track your own family health history and testing reminder e-postcards to help the general public educate themselves and others about the genetic link in thyroid disease.

Chapter 13

Environmental Factors Affect the Thyroid Gland

Public and scientific unease about possible disruption of hormones by man-made substances in the environment has gathered steam steadily over the last decade, propelled significantly by two events of 1996: the publication of *Our Stolen Future*, by Theo Colborn, Dianne Dumanoski, and John Peterson Myers, and the passage by Congress of the Food Quality Protection Act and amendments to the Safe Drinking Water Act, directing the U.S. Environmental Protection Agency (EPA) to determine whether and to what extent industrial chemicals disrupt reproductive and thyroid hormones.

In response to its congressional mandate, the EPA formed the Endocrine Disruptor Screening and Testing Advisory Committee (EDSTAC). In its 1998 final report, EDSTAC recommended that the EPA address the effects of pesticides, commercial chemicals, and other environmental contaminants on the endocrine system, which comprises the body's hormones and glands—the pituitary gland, the adrenal gland, the ovaries, the testes, the pancreas, the hypothalamus, the parathyroid gland, and the thyroid gland.

Because the thyroid affects the adult body's major systems, and because it is crucial to fetal development, its disruption by exogenous chemicals is of intense interest. Moreover, the thyroid, along with breast tissue and bone marrow, is especially vulnerable to ionizing radiation. Taken

"Disrupting a Delicate Balance: Environmental Effects on the Thyroid," *Environmental Health Perspectives,* Volume 111, Number 12, September 2003, National Institute of Environmental Health Sciences.

together, these aspects of the thyroid make understanding environmental influences on it a fascinating puzzle requiring a multidisciplinary meld of endocrinology, toxicology, and nuclear medicine to untangle.

A Difficult Subject

The study of the thyroid and its products presents special challenges to researchers. Thyroid hormones differ markedly from reproductive hormones in several respects, and these differences have made it difficult to transfer the reproductive hormone model of chemical endocrine disruption to the thyroid system. For one thing, estrogens and androgens are released into the body in what endocrinologist R. Thomas Zoeller of the University of Massachusetts Amherst, who was a member of EDSTAC, calls a "regulatory pulse." In contrast, thyroid product levels "stay pretty much the same all the time," and if disturbed will attempt to return to normal levels. Further, the thyroid system affects bodily processes more globally and more subtly than reproductive hormones. Thyroid products are "necessary but not sufficient" to affect physiological processes, says Zoeller; they are likely to work in concert with other hormones or vitamins rather than independently.

Whereas much of the early endocrine disruption research started with the effects of chemicals on nuclear receptors, research into thyroid disruption initially concentrated on trying to determine whether chemicals affect circulating levels of TSH and T4. But measuring TSH and T4 is a relatively uncertain assay for detecting the effects of low-level or chronic chemical or radiation exposure. Assays for serum hormones including T3, T4, and TSH are fairly sophisticated, says Zoeller, "but measuring hormone levels as an assay of thyroid disruption does not tell us whether there are adverse effects of this disruption."

For example, he explains, scientists are finding that very subtle reductions in circulating T4—reductions so subtle that they can't be measured directly but can only be deduced from a small increase in TSH—can cause a change in specific developmental processes in the brain that are controlled by thyroid hormone. Thus, he says, the typical interpretation of this observation would be that the increase in TSH was compensatory because there were no end points incorporated into the experimental design to track the effects of these changes. This uncertainty has made it more difficult for researchers to identify possible changes in thyroid function and metabolism that may not be reflected in circulating hormone levels.

With regard to reproductive hormones, "It's [relatively] easy to pick out measurements that will provide some degree of specificity of effect—if you see the effect, you can be reasonably sure that the compound was an estrogen or androgen," says developmental toxicologist George Daston, a research fellow at Procter & Gamble in Cincinnati who served on EDSTAC. "With the thyroid, we're having a lot of difficulty pinning down that degree of specificity." For example, the markers of congenital hypothyroidism, such as small stature, low birth weight, and vision and motor problems, can be caused by factors other than developmental thyroid disruption.

Thyroid and Brain Development

Although it is important to understand how environmental exposures may affect adults, effects in adults may be less significant as the thyroid's self-correcting feedback system helps the adult body right itself, and if this fails, hormone supplementation usually reestablishes balance. However, the developing fetus depends upon maternal thyroid hormones until around the beginning of the second trimester, and at no time is thyroid hormone more crucial than during brain development. Thus, it is in fetal and childhood development that environmental factors may have their greatest impact.

Some neurodevelopmental problems, such as extreme mental retardation and deaf-mutism, can be prevented or at least mitigated with postnatal hormone treatment. But even with treatment, children of hypothyroidal mothers have a higher-than-normal incidence of difficulties with spatial, perception, memory, language, and other skills. In a review of thyroid and brain development in the June 1994 issue of *EHP Supplements*, Susan Porterfield, an endocrinologist at the Medical College of Georgia in Augusta, suggested that these problems probably stem more from the fetus's lack of available thyroid hormone than from inadequate hormone replacement for the newborn. Therefore, because most developmental deficits are irreversible, mechanisms by which environmental exposures disrupt the thyroid's role in development are currently the focus of much research interest.

Basic fetal brain development is under way in humans within the first few weeks of gestation. Spinal cord and hindbrain components grow at this point, and cerebral cortex structures begin to take shape about halfway through gestation. Neural synapses begin forming as early as the second month of gestation, peaking in the child's first year of life, and many parts of the brain continue to develop postnatally and even into adulthood. Thyroid hormone is essential for neuron formation, synapse development, formation of myelin (the sheath surrounding neurons that enhances nerve impulse transmission), and migration of neurons to their proper places in the brain.

Although the fetal thyroid begins to grow around the end of the first trimester, it does not begin producing its own products until the second trimester, and the hypothalamic-pituitary-thyroid axis is not mature until the last trimester. Thus, maternal thyroid hormone must be continuously available until birth because crucial brain development takes place before the fetus's thyroid system is up and running.

Extreme maternal hypothyroidism leads to neurological cretinism, which can include spastic diplegia (a form of cerebral palsy), deafness, and severe mental retardation. On the other hand, maternal hyperthyroidism can result in low birth weight, prematurity, and, in the case of maternal Graves disease (an autoimmune disorder marked by hyperthyroidism), an increased incidence of congenital malformations.

Even small changes in thyroid hormone availability during critical periods of brain development can have troubling results. Children born to mothers with hypothyroxinemia, or low circulating levels of T4, may have difficulty with motor coordination, balance, and other psychomotor problems. Some research also suggests that attention deficit/hyperactivity disorder may result in children of hypothyroidal mothers, and studies summarized by Gabriella Morreale de Escobar and colleagues from Madrid's Alberto Sols Biomedical Research Institute in the November 2000 issue of the *Journal of Clinical Endocrinology & Metabolism* demonstrate 5- to 6-point intelligence quotient (IQ) deficits in children of mothers with hypothyroxinemia.

For these reasons, elucidating the effects of low-level exposures to environmental toxicants during gestation is vital, says Ted Schettler, science director for the Science and Environmental Health Network, a non-governmental organization. Schettler, who served on EDSTAC, points out that even small changes in IQ resulting from fetal thyroid hormone disruption can have important ramifications, depending on where the person falls on the IQ spectrum. A drop in IQ from 75 to 70, for example, can make the difference between institutional care and independent living, which in turn translates to significant economic effects on society.

Answering the questions regarding environmental factors in fetal brain development involving the thyroid would be easier if there were only one or two mechanisms by which thyroid function can be disrupted. But in a comprehensive September 1998 review article in *Thyroid*, Françoise Brucker-Davis, now on the faculty at the Centre Hospitalier Universitaire in Nice, France, identified nearly 90 separate compounds having thyroid-disrupting properties. And in the June 2002 issue of *EHP Supplements*, Kembra L. Howdeshell, now a post-doctoral fellow working at the University of Michigan in Ann Arbor, noted 12 separate types of interference in thyroid mechanisms. This recent work builds on earlier research and analysis by scientists such as Charles Capen, a professor of veterinary bioscience at The Ohio State University in Columbus, and R. Michael McClain, formerly a research leader at Hoffman-La Roche, who in the 1980s first espoused the idea that there are multiple mechanisms by which environmental agents alter thyroid function.

The primary types of interference in thyroid mechanisms are inhibition of iodine uptake by the thyroid gland, binding of exogenous chemicals to the serum proteins normally intended to transport T4 to target cells, inhibition of hormone synthesis in the gland, and breakdown and elimination of thyroid products by the liver. There is also the possibility that some chemicals interfere with cellular utilization of thyroid hormone by attaching to the receptors and acting as agonists or antagonists of the hormone action itself, or by interacting with receptor cofactors. Research has not yet clearly established these processes, however.

Chemical Culprits?

In her 1998 review of both animal and human studies, Brucker-Davis found that, in general, there was abundant evidence from wildlife and laboratory animal research that environmental chemicals do disrupt thyroid function. Yet she could come to few firm conclusions with respect to humans, partly because many human studies indicate only mild effects, and, she wrote, because "the presence of multiple contaminants makes it difficult to sort out the respective role of individual chemicals."

Brucker-Davis argued in her review that the strongest evidence of thyroid disruption by chemicals is that iodine deficiency occurs in iodine-sufficient areas, implying that some unidentified influence interrupts what would otherwise be a fairly straightforward process. As a research agenda, she suggested concentrating on the chemicals having structures similar to thyroid hormone and those that alter liver metabolism of thyroid hormone. The former are candidates for action at cell receptor sites and binding to carrier proteins, and the latter could trigger the TSH feedback mechanism.

Many of the same chemicals thought to damage the reproductive hormone system are also suspected or known to affect the thyroid.

These include polychlorinated biphenyls (PCBs) and their relatives the polybrominated diphenyl ethers (PBDEs), ethylenebisdithio-carbamates (EBDCs), dioxins, and perchlorate. Each family of compounds may contain several different congeners that have similar but not identical actions—or very dissimilar actions, or no actions at all—further complicating the puzzle.

PCBs, once used widely in electrical equipment, were banned in the United States in 1979 because they were associated with cognitive impairments, immune disorders, and cancer in humans. PBDEs have come into widespread use over the last 20 years as flame retardants in products such as carpet and computer plastics. Both groups are persistent in the environment and bioaccumulation up the food web. Dioxins—by-products of organochlorine synthesis, waste combustion, and paper production—are structurally similar to PCBs and PBDEs. They, too, are persistent and are often mixed with PCBs in the environment.

PCBs probably affect thyroid function by displacing T4 from serum-binding proteins in blood and by increasing liver metabolism of thyroid hormones. A paradox of PCB effects, says Zoeller, is that they reduce circulating T4 without increasing TSH. PBDEs and dioxins have similar effects.

EBDCs are potent fungicides. They are used on many plants, including root and leafy vegetables, fruits, and cereals, both in the field and after harvest. They have been known since the 1960s to cause goiter and to inhibit iodine uptake. The body breaks them down to ethylenethiourea, which has been identified by the EPA as a thyroid carcinogen in rats and mice and a probable human carcinogen. EBDCs can lower levels of thyroid hormone in rats at low doses, and may affect TSH. Ethylenethiourea also inhibits thyroid peroxidase, an enzyme necessary for synthesis of T3 and T4.

Perchlorate, used as an oxygen source in missile and rocket fuel, is common in drinking water in the southwestern United States. It inhibits iodine uptake by the thyroid, which can result in hypothyroidism and thyroid tumors. The EPA is in the process of setting a reference dose for perchlorate exposure in humans.

But these toxicants aren't the only chemicals that affect the thyroid. Fluoride, an element common in U.S. drinking water either naturally or added as a dental caries preventive, also suppresses thyroid hormone, although the mechanism is not understood, according to Paul Connett, a professor of chemistry at St. Lawrence University in Canton, New York, and an activist opposing the addition of fluoride to water. But the U.S. Food and Drug Administration emphasizes that fluoride concentrations in drinking water are safe, and most thyroid researchers believe many other chemicals pose a greater threat.

Another culprit, cyanide, occurs naturally in more than 1,000 plants, including cassava, sorghum, and bamboo, all important food sources in many parts of the developing world. At chronic subacute levels of exposure, cyanide can produce goiter and hypothyroidism. According to the Cassava Cyanide Diseases Network, a collaborative group of government officials and academics in Mozambique and Australia, cyanide contributes to goiter when the diet is already iodine-deficient. Traditional methods of processing cassava effectively neutralize cyanide's health effects, but according to WHO regional surveys of iodine deficiency status in Africa, ongoing wars, famines, and resulting mass migrations of African peoples dependent on cassava have interrupted such processing methods in many places, increasing the exposure of these already-stressed populations.

Soy isoflavones, touted by many as a benign substitute for endogenous estrogens for postmenopausal women, can be goitrogenic, although the amounts usually consumed by adults are insufficient to have that effect. Findings by toxicologist Daniel Doerge of the National Center for Toxicological Research and colleague Daniel M. Sheehan, reported in the June 2002 issue of *EHP Supplements*, suggest that soy isoflavones' ability to disrupt the thyroid depends on other factors such as iodine deficiency, other dietary goitrogens, and underlying thyroid dysfunction. Doerge emphasized the need for further research into the safety of soy isoflavones.

Many other foods contain thyroid-disrupting compounds, such as millet (containing epigenin and luteolin) and the cabbage family (containing goitrin). In parts of Africa where goiter is endemic, such as Sudan and the Republic of Guinea, it probably results from the combination of underlying iodine deficiency and large amounts of millet in the diet.

Radiation: Out, In, High, Low?

The thyroid can be affected by ionizing radiation through the skin by gamma radiation, including x-rays; by fission products, such as cesium; or by ingestion or inhalation of iodine-131 (I-131), an isotope present in nuclear fission products. I-131 emits mostly beta radiation, which penetrates surfaces more shallowly than gamma radiation. It has a half-life of only about eight days, but in fallout form it can be inhaled directly or taken up by plants eaten by cows and goats, in whose milk it is then expressed. The thyroid cannot distinguish I-131 from the nonradioactive form.

Ionizing radiation is at present the only known cause of human thyroid cancer. Thyroid tumors, or nodules, rarely result in detectable disruption of thyroid function. About 1% of these tumors are malignant and are treated with surgery, radiation, or both.

Most radiation research has focused on exposures from nuclear bomb tests, wartime bomb drops, and nuclear power plant accidents. Bomb drops and tests occurred from 1945 until aboveground testing was phased out in 1963. Possibly the most famous nuclear events were the Hiroshima and Nagasaki bombings in 1945. Other significant exposures occurred as the result of weapons production and testing in the Marshall Islands from 1946 to 1958, in the American West north and east of the Nevada bomb tests—principally in Utah and Idaho—from 1951 to 1963, and near the Hanford Nuclear Site in eastern Washington state from 1944 to 1957 (lesser releases continued at Hanford until 1972). The 1986 explosion and fire at the Chernobyl nuclear power plant exposed some 5 million people in Belarus, Ukraine, and Russia to radiation.

Of the fallout victims studied, the Japanese victims received high doses of mixed external radiation in a very short time, the Marshall Islanders and Utah residents received primarily I-131 exposure periodically over about 12 years, and those downwind from Hanford probably received relatively lower doses, primarily of I-131, from multiple releases over a slightly longer period. The Chernobyl accident produced an acute, rapid exposure, mostly to I-131, but also to a mixture of other fission products. Thus, in none of these events was there a clear-cut relationship among radiation type, duration of exposure, and internal versus external exposure.

High doses of external gamma radiation can damage thyroid gland tissue and lead to hypothyroidism as well as benign or malignant nodules, but the effects of low doses, especially of beta radiation such as I-131, are less certain. There was some increase in the incidence of both benign and malignant nodules among weapons-exposed populations, and Chernobyl victims, primarily children, suffered a striking spike in thyroid cancer incidence. According to the United Nations Scientific Committee on the Effects of Atomic Radiation's 2000 report, *Sources and Effects of Ionizing Radiation*, 1,791 children under 18 at the time of the accident were diagnosed with thyroid cancer between 1990 and 1998 in Belarus, Russia, and Ukraine, representing a four-fold increase in incidence. In Belarus, the incidence in children under 15 at diagnosis jumped from 0.2 per 100,000 to 5.6 per 100,000 in 1995, then tapered to 3.9 per 100,000 by 1998. Because some Chernobyl victims were iodine-deficient, their risk of cancer may have been magnified.

Although Chernobyl provided strong evidence that high I-131 exposure increases cancer risk, it did not answer the question of whether low chronic doses do so, but research on those downwind from Hanford seems to indicate low risk from low chronic doses. Yet, "nothing's crystal-clear regarding radiation effects," says Scott Davis, chairman of the Department of Epidemiology at the University of Washington School of Public Health and Community Medicine in Seattle.

Davis directed the *Hanford Thyroid Disease Study* (HTDS), which was conducted in response to a 1988 congressional mandate to the U.S. Centers for Disease Control and Prevention (CDC). The study asked whether exposure to I-131 from Hanford resulted in increased incidence of thyroid disease among 3,441 subjects identified as having lived in the highest-exposure areas during the relevant period. The study found that the risk of thyroid disease did not vary with radiation dose and that those downwind from Hanford were at no higher risk of thyroid disease than the general population. The preliminary HTDS results were released by the CDC in its 1999 *Hanford Thyroid Disease Study Draft Final Report* to a chorus of criticism from those downwind of Hanford, antinuclear activists, and some scientists. The final CDC report was issued in 2002, but the HTDS results have not yet been published in a peer-reviewed journal; papers based on HTDS data are currently under review by several journals, according to Davis.

The 2000 National Academy of *Sciences Review of the Hanford Thyroid Disease Study Draft Final Report* supported the study's methodology, but noted the report's reliance on highly uncertain dose amounts. In addition, Keith Baverstock, a prominent Chernobyl researcher with the WHO European Center for Environment and Health in Bonn, Germany, noted in a comment posted at the HTDS website (http://www.cdc.gov/nceh/radiation/hanford/htdsweb/index.htm) that the results could indicate an excess of thyroid cancer cases, and that "there are certainly more cases detected than would be expected on the basis of the national rates for invasive thyroid cancer." Follow-up research on the Hanford and Chernobyl victims is ongoing.

Next Steps

At this point in the understanding of environmental effects on the thyroid, there are far more questions than answers, but whether the toxicant under consideration is chemical or radioactive, most of the questions have to do with the effects of low-level exposures rather than acute ones. A further critical issue is whether combinations of toxicants have synergistic effects or sometimes even cancel each other out. Because the effects of low-level exposure may be subtle, Schettler thinks the precautionary principle should be implemented long before unambiguous results accumulate from laborious laboratory and epidemiologic studies.

As researchers implement the EPA mandate to study endocrine disruption, they must tackle some difficult procedural issues. For example, the rat thyroid system has been well characterized, but because rats and humans may metabolize certain toxicants differently (and thus, for example, rats may receive non-comparable doses of hydrophobic toxicants such as PCBs via breast milk), it is not certain how confidently researchers can extrapolate rat results to humans.

Kevin Crofton, a behavioral neurotoxicologist at the EPA National Health and Environmental Effects Research Laboratory in Research Triangle Park, North Carolina, points to other problems: "One of the big issues is potential difference in susceptibility of the developing rat brain versus the developing human brain," he says. "For example, epidemiologic studies have shown that a twenty-five percent decrease in maternal T4 during the first trimester results in decreased IQ in children, [but] there are no rat models that demonstrate this level of sensitivity to T4 decreases. . . . Alternatively, the measures of neurological development in the rat may be crude compared to IQ testing in children."

Many features of brain development are strongly conserved in vertebrates, however. Howdeshell is working to develop a model of the African clawed frog, *Xenopus laevis*, to shed light on gene regulation by thyroid hormone in human processes including brain development. *Xenopus* provides a good model for thyroid hormone effects because the metamorphosis from tadpole to frog is heavily mediated by thyroid hormone. "While *Xenopus* studies cannot be directly extrapolated to human development," says Howdeshell, "the thyroid hormone system is conserved across all vertebrates, including rats and humans, and *Xenopus* undergo thyroid hormone-directed brain maturation similar to the brain development of more complex vertebrates."

The lack of certainty regarding circulating hormone levels as a measure of toxicant effects is also vexing, and researchers are busy devising better assays and end points. Crofton has identified one such end point that he thinks may be a reliable indicator. In research currently under review, he has correlated postnatal T4 concentrations with hearing loss in rats. These data demonstrate that, at a minimum, a 50% decrease of thyroid hormone in developing rats is needed to adversely impact hearing function.

A further issue is that endocrine disruption research involves to some extent a culture clash between toxicologists and endocrinologists; the methods and typical questions of interest peculiar to each must be harmonized with the other. For example, toxicologists tend to focus on dose-response determinations, whereas endocrinologists historically haven't considered dose response with respect to hormones at all, says Zoeller.

The thyroid system is so complex that understanding its normal function is difficult enough, but deciphering environmental disruptions to it is staggeringly convoluted. Yet, the more research reveals, the more pressing the questions become. The thyroid affects nearly every bodily system, and its role in fetal development makes protection of healthy thyroid function imperative. The increasing body of research indicating subtle and possibly additive or synergistic effects of environmental contaminants only adds salience to the issue.

Chapter 14

Radiation Emergencies Can Damage the Thyroid Gland

Chapter Contents

107

Section 14.1

Frequently Asked Questions about a Radiation Emergency

"Frequently Asked Questions (FAQs) about a Radiation Emergency,"
Centers for Disease Control and Prevention (CDC), June 2003.

What is radiation?

- Radiation is a form of energy that is present all around us.

- Different types of radiation exist, some of which have more energy than others.

- Amounts of radiation released into the environment are measured in units called curies. However, the dose of radiation that a person receives is measured in units called rem.

How can exposure occur?

- People are exposed to small amounts of radiation every day, both from naturally occurring sources (such as elements in the soil or cosmic rays from the sun), and man-made sources. Man-made sources include some electronic equipment (such as microwave ovens and television sets), medical sources (such as x-rays, certain diagnostic tests, and treatments), and from nuclear weapons testing.

- The amount of radiation from natural or man-made sources to which people are exposed is usually small; a radiation emergency (such as a nuclear power plant accident or a terrorist event) could expose people to small or large doses of radiation, depending on the situation.

- Scientists estimate that the average person in the United States receives a dose of about one-third of a rem per year. About 80% of human exposure comes from natural sources and the remaining 20% comes from man-made radiation sources— mainly medical x-rays.

- Internal exposure refers to radioactive material that is taken into the body through breathing, eating, or drinking.

- External exposure refers to an exposure to a radioactive source outside of our bodies.

- Contamination refers to particles of radioactive material that are deposited anywhere that they are not supposed to be, such as on an object or on a person's skin.

What happens when people are exposed to radiation?

- Radiation can affect the body in a number of ways, and the adverse health effects of exposure may not be apparent for many years.

- These adverse health effects can range from mild effects, such as skin reddening, to serious effects such as cancer and death, depending on the amount of radiation absorbed by the body (the dose), the type of radiation, the route of exposure, and the length of time a person was exposed.

- Exposure to very large doses of radiation may cause death within a few days or months.

- Exposure to lower doses of radiation may lead to an increased risk of developing cancer or other adverse health effects later in life.

What types of terrorist events might involve radiation?

- Possible terrorist events could involve introducing radioactive material into the food or water supply, using explosives (like dynamite) to scatter radioactive materials (called a dirty bomb), bombing or destroying a nuclear facility, or exploding a small nuclear device.

- Although introducing radioactive material into the food or water supply most likely would cause great concern or fear, it probably would not cause much contamination or increase the danger of adverse health effects.

- Although a dirty bomb could cause serious injuries from the explosion, it most likely would not have enough radioactive material in a form that would cause serious radiation sickness among large numbers of people. However, people who were exposed to radiation scattered by the bomb could have a greater risk of developing cancer later in life, depending on their dose.

- A meltdown or explosion at a nuclear facility could cause a large amount of radioactive material to be released. People at the facility would probably be contaminated with radioactive material and possibly be injured if there was an explosion. Those people who received a large dose might develop acute radiation syndrome. People in the surrounding area could be exposed or contaminated.

- Clearly, an exploded nuclear device could result in a lot of property damage. People would be killed or injured from the blast and might be contaminated by radioactive material. Many people could have symptoms of acute radiation syndrome. After a nuclear explosion, radioactive fallout would extend over a large region far from the point of impact, potentially increasing people's risk of developing cancer over time.

What preparations can I make for a radiation emergency?

- Your community should have a plan in place in case of a radiation emergency. Check with community leaders to learn more about the plan and possible evacuation routes.

- Check with your child's school, the nursing home of a family member, and your employer to see what their plans are for dealing with a radiation emergency.

- Develop your own family emergency plan so that every family member knows what to do.

- At home, put together an emergency kit that would be appropriate for any emergency. The kit should include the following items:
  - A flashlight with extra batteries
  - A portable radio with extra batteries
  - Bottled water
  - Canned and packaged food
  - A hand-operated can opener
  - A first-aid kit and essential prescription medications
  - Personal items such as paper towels, garbage bags, and toilet paper

How can I protect myself during a radiation emergency?

- After a release of radioactive materials, local authorities will monitor the levels of radiation and determine what protective actions to take.

- The most appropriate action will depend on the situation. Tune to the local emergency response network or news station for information and instructions during any emergency.

- If a radiation emergency involves the release of large amounts of radioactive materials, you may be advised to shelter in place, which means to stay in your home or office; or you may be advised to move to another location.

- If you are advised to shelter in place, you should do the following:
  - Close and lock all doors and windows.
  - Turn off fans, air conditioners, and forced-air heating units that bring in fresh air from the outside. Only use units to recirculate air that is already in the building.
  - Close fireplace dampers.
  - If possible, bring pets inside.
  - Move to an inner room or basement.
  - Keep your radio tuned to the emergency response network or local news to find out what else you need to do.

- If you are advised to evacuate, follow the directions that your local officials provide. Leave the area as quickly and orderly as possible. In addition:
  - Take a flashlight, portable radio, batteries, first-aid kit, supply of sealed food and water, hand-operated can opener, essential medicines, and cash and credit cards.
  - Take pets only if you are using your own vehicle and going to a place you know will accept animals. Emergency vehicles and shelters usually will not accept animals.

Should I take potassium iodide during a radiation emergency?

- Potassium iodide (KI) should only be taken in a radiation emergency that involves the release of radioactive iodine, such as an accident at a nuclear power plant or the explosion of a nuclear bomb. A dirty bomb most likely will not contain radioactive iodine.

- A person who is internally exposure to radioactive iodine may experience thyroid disease later in life. The thyroid gland will absorb radioactive iodine and may develop cancer or abnormal growths later on.

- KI will saturate the thyroid gland with iodine, decreasing the amount of harmful radioactive iodine that can be absorbed. KI only protects the thyroid gland and does not provide protection from any other radiation exposure.

- Some people are allergic to iodine and should not take KI. Check with your doctor about any concerns you have about potassium iodide.

Websites for Additional Information

Radiation Information
http://www.epa.gov/radiation
http://www.orau.gov/reacts/define.htm

Health Effects from Radiation Exposure
http://www.bt.cdc.gov/radiation/healthfacts.asp

Terrorist Events and Radiation
http://www.bt.cdc.gov/radiation/terrorismqa.asp

Emergency Response
http://www.fema.gov
http://www.redcross.org
http://www.epa.gov/swercepp

Potassium Iodide (KI)
http://www.bt.cdc.gov/radiation/ki.asp
http://www.fda.gov/cder/drugprepare/KI_Q&A.htm
http://www.fda.gov/cder/guidance/4825fnl.htm

Section 14.2

Frequently Asked Questions on Potassium Iodide (KI)

"Frequently Asked Questions on Potassium Iodide (KI)," Center for Drug Evaluation and Research, U.S. Food and Drug Administration (FDA), March 18, 2003.

In November 2001, the Food and Drug Administration (FDA) issued a final "Guidance on Potassium Iodide as a Thyroid Blocking Agent in Radiation Emergencies." The objective of the document is to provide guidance to other Federal agencies, including the Environmental Protection Agency (EPA) and the Nuclear Regulatory Commission (NRC), and to state and local governments regarding the safe and effective use of potassium iodide (KI) as an adjunct to other public health protective measures in the event that radioactive iodine is released into the environment. The adoption and implementation of the recommendations are at the discretion of the state and local governments responsible for developing regional emergency-response plans related to radiation emergencies. The recommendations in the guidance address KI dosage and the projected radiation exposure at which the drug should be used. This guidance updates FDA's 1982 recommendations.

What does potassium iodide (KI) do?

The effectiveness of KI as a specific blocker of thyroid radioiodine uptake is well established. When administered in the recommended dose, KI is effective in reducing the risk of thyroid cancer in individuals or populations at risk for inhalation or ingestion of radioiodine. KI floods the thyroid with non-radioactive iodine and prevents the uptake of the radioactive molecules, which are subsequently excreted in the urine.

Can potassium iodide (KI) be used to protect against radiation from bombs other than radioactive iodine?

Potassium iodide (KI) works only to prevent thyroid uptake of radioactive iodine. It is not a general radioprotective agent.

113

Who really needs to take potassium iodide (KI) after a nuclear radiation release?

The FDA guidance prioritizes groups based on age, which primarily determines risk for radioiodine-induced thyroid cancer. Those at highest risk are infants and children, as well as pregnant and nursing females, and the recommendation is to treat them at the lowest threshold (with respect to predicted radioactive dose to the thyroid). Anyone over age 18 and up to age 40 should be treated at a slightly higher threshold. Finally, anyone over 40 should be treated with KI only if the predicted exposure is high enough to destroy the thyroid and induce lifelong hypothyroidism (thyroid deficiency).

What potassium iodide (KI) products are currently available?

As of March 2003, the FDA has approved three KI products (Thyro-Block, Iosat, and ThyroSafe). You can find out more about these KI products and any other KI products the agency may approve in the future in "Approved Drug Products with Therapeutic Equivalence Evaluations" (the Orange Book) at http://www.fda.gov/cder/ob/default.htm. Please be aware that only the KI products approved by FDA may be legally marketed in the United States.

How are these products available?

MedPointe, Inc., is distributing Thyro-Block strictly to state, local, and federal agencies, nuclear power plants, and hospitals. In addition to distributing to state, local, and federal agencies, Anbex, Inc. has made its product available to the general public via the Internet.

What dosages of potassium iodide (KI) should be taken for specific exposure levels?

Exposures greater than 5 centigrays (cGy):

- Birth through 2 mos.–16 milligrams (mg).
- 1 mo. through 3 yrs.–32 mg.
- 3 yrs. through 18 yrs.–65 mg. (Adolescents over 150 pounds should take adult dose.)

Exposures greater than 10 cGy:

- 18 yrs. through 40 yrs.–130 mg

Exposures greater than 500 cGy:

- Adults over 40 yrs.–130 mg.

How long should potassium iodide (KI) be taken?

Since KI protects for approximately 24 hours, it should be dosed daily until the risk no longer exists. Priority with regard to evacuation and sheltering should be given to pregnant females and neonates because of the potential for KI to suppress thyroid function in the fetus and neonate. Unless other protective measures are not available, we do not recommend repeat dosing in pregnant females and neonates.

Who should not take potassium iodide (KI) or have restricted use?

Persons with known iodine sensitivity should avoid KI, as should individuals with dermatitis herpetiformis and hypocomplementemic vasculitis, extremely rare conditions associated with an increased risk of iodine hypersensitivity. Individuals with multinodular goiter, Graves disease, and autoimmune thyroiditis should be treated with caution—especially if dosing extends beyond a few days.

What are the possible risks and side effects of taking potassium iodide (KI)?

Thyroid side effects of KI at recommended doses rarely occur in iodine-sufficient populations such as the U.S. As a rule, the risk of thyroid side effects is related to dose and to the presence of underlying thyroid disease (e.g., goiter, thyroiditis, Graves). FDA recommends adherence to the *Guidance* for intervention threshold and dose, though it is recognized that the exigencies of any particular emergency situation may mandate deviations from those recommendations. With that in mind, it should be understood that as a general rule, the risks of KI are far outweighed by the benefits with regard to prevention of thyroid cancer in susceptible individuals.

Should I check with my doctor first?

Potassium iodide (KI) is available over-the-counter (OTC). However, if you have any health concerns or questions, you should check with your doctor.

Should I go out and buy potassium iodide (KI) to keep on hand?

KI works best if used within 3–4 hours of exposure. Although FDA has not made specific recommendations for individual purchase or use of KI, the Nuclear Regulatory Commission has contracted to purchase KI for states with nuclear reactors and states that have population within the 10-mile emergency planning zone, (e.g., Delaware or West Virginia).

How do I know that potassium iodide (KI) will be available in case of an emergency?

FDA will continue to work with interested pharmaceutical manufacturers to assure that high quality, safe, and effective KI products are available for purchase by consumers, by state and local authorities, and by federal government agencies electing to do so.

Section 14.3

Home Preparation Procedure for Emergency Administration of KI Tablets

"Home Preparation Procedure for Emergency Administration of Potassium Iodide Tablets to Infants and Small Children," Center for Drug Evaluation and Research, U.S. Food and Drug Administration (FDA), October 2002.

In the event of accidental release of radioactive iodine into the atmosphere, potassium iodide (KI) is recommended for use as an aid to other emergency measures, such as evacuation and food control measures. When used correctly, potassium iodide can prevent or reduce the amount of radioactive iodine taken up by the thyroid gland. The government stockpiles potassium iodide for emergency uses, such as in the event of an unexpected release of radioactive iodide.

Potassium iodide (KI) is stockpiled as tablets because tablets are easier to store; however, infants and small children cannot swallow tablets. In an emergency such as an unexpected release of radioactive iodine, the potassium iodide tablets may need to be given to infants and children by their parents or caregivers. Since potassium iodide dissolved in water may be too salty to drink, the Food and Drug Administration (FDA) has provided parents or caregivers with instructions on how to mix the potassium iodide tablets with a food or a drink to disguise the taste so infants and small children will take the medicine in an emergency. To see what worked best to disguise the taste of potassium iodide, FDA asked adults to taste the following six mixtures of potassium iodide and drinks.

- Water
- Low fat white milk
- Low fat chocolate milk
- Orange juice
- Flat soda (For example, cola)
- Raspberry syrup

The mixture of potassium iodide with raspberry syrup disguises the taste of potassium iodide best. The mixtures of potassium iodide with low fat chocolate milk, orange juice, and flat soda (for example, cola) generally have an acceptable taste. Low fat white milk and water did not hide the salty taste of potassium iodide.

Ingredients and Supplies Needed to Prepare Potassium Iodide (KI) Tablets

- Potassium iodide (KI) 130 mg tablet
- Metal teaspoon
- Small bowl
- One of the drinks from the list or infant formula.

Preparation for 130 MG Potassium Iodide Tablet

1. Grind the potassium iodide tablet into powder.

   - Put one 130 mg potassium iodide tablet into a small bowl and grind it into a fine powder using the back of the metal teaspoon against the inside of the bowl. The powder should not have any large pieces.

117

2. Mix potassium iodide powder into a drink.

    - Add four teaspoonful of water to the potassium iodide powder in the small bowl. Use a spoon to mix them together until the potassium iodide powder is dissolved in the water.

3. Mix drink of choice with potassium iodide powder and water solution

    - Add four teaspoonful of drink to the potassium iodide powder and water mixture described in Step 2.

The amount of potassium iodide in the drink is 16.25 mg per teaspoon. The number of teaspoonful of the drink to give your child depends on your child's age. Table 14.2. of this section tells you how much to give your child.

The potassium iodide in any of the six drinks listed and infant formulas will keep for up to seven days in the refrigerator. FDA recommends that the potassium iodide drink mixtures be prepared weekly; unused portions should be discarded.

Table 14.1. Threshold thyroid radioactivity exposures and the recommended dose of potassium iodide (KI) for different groups.[1]

If you are:	And your predicted thyroid exposure is	Then you should take:	Number of 130 mg tablets
An adult over the age of 40	Equal to or greater than 500 centigray (cGy)	a 130 mg dose of potassium Iodide (KI)	1
An adult between the ages of 18 and 40	Equal to or greater than 10 cGy	a 130 mg dose of potassium Iodide (KI)	1
A pregnant or lactating woman	Equal to or greater than 5 cGy	a 130 mg dose of potassium Iodide (KI)	1

[1] FDA, *Guidance: Potassium Iodide as a Thyroid Blocking Agent in Radiation Emergencies*, December 2001.

Administration

FDA recommends doses for potassium iodide based on age, predicted thyroid exposure to radioiodine, and whether a woman is pregnant or nursing (see Table 14.1). Adults over 18 years of age and pregnant or lactating women should take the potassium iodide 130 mg tablet. Infants, children, and adolescents through 18 years of age should take potassium iodide in a drink prepared according to the procedure previously described. Table 14.2 shows how many teaspoonsful of potassium iodide mixture to give to an adolescent, child, or infant. The dose of potassium iodide should be taken once a day until a risk of significant exposure to radioiodine no longer exists.

Table 14.2. Recommended doses of KI for adolescents, children, and infants with predicted thyroid radioactivity exposures equal to or greater than 5 cGy,[1] using 130 mg tablet preparations.

If your child is:	Give your child this amount of potassium iodide (KI) *	Which is
An adolescent between 12 and 18 years old**	4 teaspoonsful (not tablespoonsful)	65 mg of potassium iodide (KI)
Between 4 and 12 years old	4 teaspoonsful (not tablespoonsful)	65 mg of potassium iodide (KI)
Over 1 month through 3 years	2 teaspoonsful (not tablespoonsful)	32.5 mg of potassium iodide (KI)
An infant from birth through 1 month	1 teaspoonful (not a tablespoonful)	16.25 mg of potassium iodide (KI)

* This is the amount to give your child for one dose. You should give your child one dose each day.

** Adolescents approaching adult size [equal to or greater than 154 pounds (70 kg)] should receive the full adult dose (130 mg tablet or 8 teaspoonsful of KI mixture).

[1] FDA, *Guidance: Potassium Iodide as a Thyroid Blocking Agent in Radiation Emergencies*, December 2001.

Preparation for 65 MG Potassium Iodide Tablet

If you have potassium iodide 65 mg tablets, then prepare the mixture as follows:

1. Grind the potassium iodide 65 mg tablet into powder.

   - Put one 65 mg potassium iodide tablet into a small bowl and grind it into a fine powder using the back of the metal teaspoon against the inside of the bowl. The powder should not have any large pieces.

2. Mix potassium iodide powder into a drink.

   - Add four teaspoonsful of water to the potassium iodide powder in the small bowl. Use a spoon to mix them together until the potassium iodide powder is dissolved in the water.

3. Mix drink of choice with potassium iodide powder and water solution.

   - Add four teaspoonsful of drink to the potassium iodide powder and water mixture described in Step 2.

Table 14.3. Recommended doses of KI for children and infants with predicted thyroid radioactivity exposures equal to or greater than 5 cGy,[1] using 65 mg tablet preparations.

If your child is:	Give your child this amount of potassium iodide (KI) *	Which is
Between 4 and 12 years old	8 teaspoonsful (not tablespoonsful)	65 mg of potassium iodide (KI)
Over 1 month through 3 years	4 teaspoonsful (not tablespoonsful)	32.5 mg of potassium iodide (KI)
An infant from birth through 1 month	2 teaspoonsful (not tablespoonsful)	16.25 mg of potassium iodide (KI)

* This is the amount to give your child for one dose. You should give your child one dose each day.

[1] FDA, *Guidance: Potassium Iodide as a Thyroid Blocking Agent in Radiation Emergencies*, December 2001.

The amount of potassium iodide in the drink is 8.125 mg per teaspoon. The number of teaspoonsful of the drink to give your child depends on your child's age. Table 14.3 shows how many teaspoonsful of potassium iodide mixture to give to an adolescent, child, or infant.

Please pay attention to the number of teaspoonsful recommended when using a potassium iodide 65 mg tablet as it is different from the number of teaspoonsful given when using a potassium iodide 130 mg tablet.

Information on Obtaining Approved Potassium Iodide Pills

If you wish to obtain potassium iodide pills approved by the FDA, you may do so by contacting:

Anbex, Inc. for Iosat Tablets
35246 U.S. Highway 19 N.
PMB 284
Palm Harbor, FL 34684-1931
Phone: 212-580-2810
Website: http://www.anbex.com
E-mail: info@anbex.com

MedPointe Inc. for Thyro-Block
265 Davidson Ave., Suite 300
Somerset, NJ 08873-2200
Phone: 732-564-2200
Website: http://www.medpointeinc.com

If you have any questions about the availability of potassium iodide tablets in your area, please contact your state officials.

Chapter 15

Potential Effects of Chemicals on the Endocrine System

In recent years, increasing scientific and public attention has been focused on the potential effects of synthetic chemicals on the hormone system. In March 1996, Theo Colborn, Dianne Dumanoski, and John Peterson Myers published a book entitled *Our Stolen Future* that addressed this issue. According to the book, hormone disrupting chemicals are widespread and can cause adverse effects even at low levels, resulting in potentially serious risks to the environment and public health.

This chapter summarizes EPA's understanding of this issue and the action it is taking, as well as discussing some of the book's recommendations.

What is the endocrine system, and what are endocrine disruptors?

The endocrine system consists of a set of glands and the hormones they produce that help guide the development, growth, reproduction, and behavior of animals including human beings. Some of the endocrine glands include the pituitary, thyroid, and adrenal glands, the female ovaries and male testes. Hormones are chemicals, produced by endocrine glands, which travel through the bloodstream and cause responses in other parts of the body. Examples of hormones include adrenaline, which helps stimulate physical activity, and estrogen, which is essential for female reproductive function. Hormones can

"Potential of Chemicals to Affect the Endocrine System," U.S. Environmental Protection Agency (EPA), May 19, 2003.

produce both positive and negative effects. For example, some types of breast cancer are exacerbated by estrogen, but studies also indicate that estrogen has a protective effect in combating heart disease and osteoporosis-related fractures.

Chemicals that interfere with the normal functioning of this complex system are known as endocrine disruptors. Disruption of the endocrine system can occur in various ways. For example, some chemicals may mimic a natural hormone, fooling the body into over-responding to the hormone. Other chemicals may block the effects of a hormone in parts of the body normally sensitive to it. Still others may directly stimulate or inhibit the endocrine system, leading, to overproduction or underproduction of hormones. Certain drugs are used to intentionally cause some of these effects, such as birth control pills.

What is EPA's position on this issue, and what is EPA doing to address endocrine disruptors?

EPA is concerned about the growing body of evidence that some man-made chemicals may be interfering with normal endocrine system functioning in humans and other animals. Considerable scientific uncertainty remains, however, as to which chemicals may be involved, patterns of exposure, mechanisms of action in humans and wildlife, and the best means for testing to predict or screen for these effects. EPA is investing significant resources to resolve these uncertainties.

In addition to conducting research, EPA has taken and is taking a number of steps to reduce chemical risks. The Agency has already banned the use in the United States of a number of the more environmentally persistent chemicals that have raised concerns about possible hormonal effects (PCBs, and such organochlorine pesticides as DDT, chlordane, aldrin/dieldrin, endrin, kepone, toxaphene, and 2,4,5-T) and is working with the international community to limit production and use of these chemicals worldwide. The Agency is also revising its testing guidelines for reevaluating the effects of pesticides and toxic substances on reproduction and the developing fetus, which will enable EPA scientists to more readily identify chemicals with hormone-disrupting effects.

EPA continues to encourage actions to reduce unnecessary chemical exposure and use, and more generally, to promote pollution prevention. For example, EPA is working with pesticide user groups to reduce pesticide use and risk, and encouraging the design and use of safer industrial chemicals and pesticides. EPA is also implementing the Worker Protection Standard which requires appropriate protective equipment and other measures to reduce exposure to pesticides in agriculture. Through expansion of the Toxics Release Inventory, the Agency is providing the public with more information and fostering constructive dialogue between citizens and industry on reducing and preventing chemical releases into the environment. Other informational efforts include the development of practical guides for consumers who wish to reduce their exposure to pesticides in their homes, schools, and other settings.

Specifically, what research effort is EPA undertaking to learn more about endocrine disruptors?

EPA has developed its own research strategy and is working with other agencies to develop a comprehensive research strategy for the Federal Government. This effort is being expanded in the hope that an international strategy can be established, coordinated with both the public and private sectors.

The goals of EPA's overall research strategy are to (1) establish priorities for the allocation of the Agency's research funds; (2) serve as a basis for coordination and communication among other principally involved Federal agencies; and (3) provide a basic research framework for regulatory programs within EPA.

With respect to specific projects, research on various aspects of hormone disruptors has been ongoing at EPA's laboratories and in collaboration with non-EPA scientists. Some of the work has looked at the reproductive effects of certain pesticides, evaluated human sperm count and fertility relationships, and studied reproductive problems among alligators and fish populations in Lake Apopka, Florida. EPA will continue to support relevant research through its grants program.

EPA is also collaborating in two major studies being conducted by the National Cancer Institute and National Institute of Environmental Health Sciences: the *Long Island Breast Cancer Study*, which is evaluating various environmental and occupational factors in breast cancer, and the *Agricultural Health Study*, which will assess pesticide exposure and health risks, including potential reproductive effects and effects on child growth and development.

Does EPA require testing of chemicals for endocrine effects?

EPA routinely screens new industrial chemicals prior to their introduction into commerce and seeks to control any, including suspected hormonal disruptors, which may pose an unreasonable risk to human health and the environment. New pesticides are routinely tested in animals for effects on reproduction, fertility, and the developing fetus before they are approved for use. Older pesticides are tested as part of EPA's ongoing re-registration program, a comprehensive reevaluation of all pesticides first approved before 1984. The growth and development of offspring are also evaluated, including an assessment of birth defects or other abnormalities. Although these tests are not specifically designed to identify endocrine disruption, they can detect certain reproductive and developmental effects which may result from endocrine disruption.

EPA's Office of Prevention, Pesticides, and Toxic Substances has proposed revised testing guidelines for evaluating the developmental and reproductive effects of pesticides and industrial chemicals. Although current tests can detect some hormonal effects of chemicals, the proposed revisions would increase the sensitivity of the tests, thereby increasing the Agency's capacity to screen for potential effects of chemicals on mating, fertility, pregnancy, delivery, and care of young by laboratory animals. The revised tests will also look at effects on reproductive organ structure and functioning in parents and offspring. Examples include an examination of female hormonal cycling and male sperm count, shape, and activity.

Does EPA agree with the recommendations in Our Stolen Future?

EPA agrees with many of the concerns raised in *Our Stolen Future* and has already taken steps to address a number of its recommendations. For example, EPA agrees that pesticides should only be used when necessary and is working with other agencies and groups to reduce pesticide use and risk. These efforts include promoting integrated pest management programs and safer pest control alternatives. EPA is also working to implement recommendations from the National Academy of Sciences and others to provide greater assurance that our safety standards protect vulnerable populations, especially infants and young children, and improving the ability to screen for potential endocrine effects. New legislation is being implemented that strengthens efforts in this regard and develops an expanded research agenda. Finally, as the book points out, many of the chemicals of greatest concern have already been banned in the U.S. but may continue to be used in other countries. EPA has taken a leadership role in international efforts to eliminate such persistent organic pollutants.

The book also contains many practical suggestions and recommendations for people seeking to reduce their exposure to chemical risks. As with all suggestions affecting consumer choice, the final decisions will appropriately be made by individuals. Thus, the Agency does not necessarily believe that all of the book's suggestions will be equally practical or appropriate for every person.

Does EPA regulate endocrine disruptors in drinking water? Does EPA require any testing for the presence of endocrine disruptors in public water systems and reporting of the results?

EPA regulates certain chemicals that are suspected of being endocrine disruptors in drinking water. The drinking water regulations contain testing, reporting, and public notification requirements for regulated contaminants. Regulation of potential endocrine disruptors under the Safe Drinking Water Act (SDWA) generally has been based on adverse health effects such as cancer and other chronic adverse effects. Most regulatory levels are protective for the individual chemicals but uncertainty remains in specific cases and for the cumulative effect of multiple exposures.

Maximum contaminant levels (MCLs) have been established under the SDWA for pesticides (e.g., chlordane, dichloro-diphenyl-trichloroethane (DDT), endrin, toxaphene, lindane, atrazine, simazine), non-pesticide organics (e.g., polychlorinated biphenyls (PCBs), dioxin, polycyclic aromatic hydrocarbons (PAH)) and inorganic chemicals (e.g., mercury, lead) that are suspected endocrine disruptors.

Does EPA recommend that people drinking from private wells test their water for the presence of endocrine disruptors, and if so, how should they do that?

The Safe Drinking Water Act (SDWA) does not regulate private wells. However, EPA recommends that if a private well owner suspects that there is a potential for contamination, the water should be tested for those contaminants of potential concern. For example, a shallow well in an agricultural area with heavy pesticide use should be tested for the presence of those pesticides of concern. Private well owners can request assistance from the appropriate State authority to have their water tested for the presence of those potential endocrine disruptors that are currently regulated in drinking water. There are laboratories throughout the United States certified to conduct testing for regulated drinking water contaminants. States can provide information on laboratories that are certified. Certified laboratories should be used to ensure that the testing results are reliable.

Is bottled water in plastic containers safe to drink?

The Food and Drug Administration (FDA) regulates bottled water, not EPA. FDA investigates the potential toxicity of leaching chemicals and establishes safe levels for contaminants in bottled water. There is currently no indication that contaminants from leaching or from the water source are a problem in bottled water. Therefore, EPA believes that bottled water is generally safe to drink.

Does EPA recommend the use of water purification devices if people are worried about contamination?

EPA believes that a public water supply or a private well that meets the Federal drinking water standards provides drinking water which is safe for human consumption. Individuals should make a judgement as to whether they are willing to invest resources on a water purification device for additional peace of mind.

Am I at risk of being exposed to PCBs and DDT/dichloro-diphenyldichloro-ethylene (DDE) by eating fish?

The fish we eat can come from many different environments. Some fish are harvested by ocean fishing vessels; others are freshwater fish caught in lakes, rivers, and streams, or raised in ponds on aquaculture establishments. Most fish sold in the grocery store and in restaurants come from the ocean and are much less likely to have detectable levels of PCBs and DDT/DDE than freshwater fish.

The U.S. Food and Drug Administration (FDA) monitors the safety of fish sold at retail establishments and those shipped in interstate commerce. When PCBs and DDT/DDE are detected in commercially sold species, they usually occur at low levels that should not be of concern to the consumer.

Freshwater fish caught by sport fishermen or by those who subsist on freshwater fish in areas where PCBs have historically been found in the environment sometimes contain levels exceeding federal limits established to protect the public. The greatest potential of exposure to these chemicals in fish comes from recreational fishing in areas where PCBs and DDT/DDE are found at elevated levels. People who catch and eat freshwater fish should ensure that the waters they are fishing in are safe from environmental hazards by checking with their state authorities. Local advisories are sometimes implemented if state authorities feel that it is unsafe to consume high quantities of fish from a certain source.

Usually these advisories contain recommendations to reduce the risk of chemical exposure from fish caught in contaminated waters. These recommendations include proper cleaning procedures, such as removing the skin and fatty tissues where chemicals may concentrate.

Should people avoid animal fats in their diet?

EPA and other public health experts agree that people can best protect their health by eating a varied and balanced diet, eating more fruits and vegetables, and reducing excess fat and calories. This advice has been consistently reaffirmed in scientific studies and reports, such as in the report from the National Academy of Sciences (NAS) on *Carcinogens and Anti-Carcinogens in Food*. Controlling fat and calories, while increasing fruit and vegetable consumption, appears to have many advantages independent of potential hormonal effects, for example in reducing risk of heart disease and cancer.

Most health and nutrition experts advise trimming excess fat from meat and poultry as a general practice. Since some chemical residues concentrate in fatty tissues, people who wish to minimize their exposure to these residues should follow this advice.

Should people be concerned about pesticides in food?

As pointed out by the NAS and others, pesticide residues in food are generally present at low levels unlikely to present significant risks. Individuals who wish to minimize pesticide residues can take steps to reduce traces of residues in the food they consume. EPA advises rinsing fruits and vegetables thoroughly with water, scrubbing them with a brush, and peeling when appropriate. Cooking and baking will reduce residues of some pesticides even further.

Many people prefer organically grown food for a number of reasons. EPA does not think that consumers need to switch to organic food based on dietary risk concerns, but choice of organic food is a personal matter for consumers to decide for themselves.

Should people stop using plastic containers and plastic wrap when storing or heating up food?

The Food and Drug Administration (FDA) regulates food packaging materials. Plastics for food packaging undergo tests to determine the extent of migration and the potential toxicity of leaching chemicals. These data are reviewed by FDA prior to marketing, and specific regulations are developed listing the chemicals that are permitted for use in contact with food. FDA has found currently approved food packaging plastics to be safe, primarily because they migrate to food in only trivial amounts.

FDA is continuing to investigate the migration levels of certain food packaging materials into food and will take additional regulatory action should the data indicate potential health risks.

Because food package components are tested under conditions reflecting each container's intended use, it is important to use plastic food containers only as intended. Food should be heated only in containers that are clearly intended for use at elevated temperatures. Packaged food with labeling instructions for heating in the package or storage containers sold for use in microwave ovens are two examples of such containers.

Will frequent hand washing reduce exposure to endocrine disruptors?

As a matter of good hygiene and proper pesticide use, EPA advises individuals to wash their hands after applying any pesticide and before handling food. This practice will help minimize unnecessary exposure and prevent contamination of foods with chemical or microbial agents. It is also important to follow other precautions on product labels carefully, for example, to wear gloves when directed to do so on the label, and to store pesticides and other household chemicals out of the reach of children.

Should consumers avoid using pesticides?

Pesticides are designed to be biologically active and should never be used unless necessary. Pesticides have risks as well as benefits, and it is important to use them properly. When they are used according to label directions, EPA believes pesticides are generally safe.

Should golfers be concerned about pesticides used on golf courses?

The Agency is working with the golf industry as well as many other pesticide user groups to reduce the risks from the use of pesticides through the Pesticide Environmental Stewardship Program (PESP). PESP is a broad effort by EPA, USDA, and FDA to work with pesticide users and others to reduce pesticide use and risk in both agricultural and nonagricultural settings by developing use/risk reduction strategies that include reliance on biological pesticides and increasing adoption of integrated pest management (IPM) programs.

The Golf Course Superintendents Association of America and the Professional Lawn Care Association are both partners in PESP through the New York Audubon Society's Cooperative Sanctuary Program. The Sanctuary Program encourages property owners, both corporate and private, to improve wildlife habitat on their property and to adopt IPM programs to control problems that may occur. Through this partnership, EPA aims to reduce the risk and use of pesticides. in the turf grass industry, specifically in golf course planning and siting, design, construction, maintenance and facility operations.

Golfers who seek to reduce their exposure to pesticides may wish to ask if the golf course follows IPM practices and what pesticides are used. Some golf courses may have a list of pesticides they use and when they are applied. Golfers may want to schedule their play to avoid recent pesticide applications.

What is integrated pest management (IPM)?

IPM is an effective and environmentally sensitive approach to pest management that relies on a combination of common sense practices. IPM weighs costs, benefits, and impacts on health and the environment, thus identifying the most suitable way to control pests. Options include prevention, monitoring, mechanical trapping devices, natural predators, biological pesticides, and, if appropriate, chemical pesticides. The goal is to get the best long-term results with the least disruption of the environment.

Should parents try to keep infants and children from playing with or chewing on plastic objects?

Our Stolen Future raises important questions about the relationship of chemicals used in plastics and possible effects on the endocrine system, but the book acknowledges that much more research is necessary. At present, EPA does not believe the scientific evidence supports this recommendation, which would also be very difficult to achieve in practical terms.

Does EPA agree with the recommendations to a) greatly reduce the number of chemicals on the market; b) reduce the number of chemicals in a product; and c) disallow products if we do not understand how they degrade in the environment?

EPA does not necessarily equate fewer chemicals in commerce with greater safety for public health and the environment. One can not

131

arbitrarily restrict the numbers of chemicals on the market or in products. Chemicals in products have a function in the performance of the product or else they wouldn't be there. Fundamentally, EPA's role is to encourage the use of safer chemicals and processes in the operations of the industrial sector. Clearly our success depends on industry incorporating the principles of pollution prevention into its basic technological and developmental decisions. The majority of existing chemicals do not pose significant risk to human health or the environment in their current uses and many new chemicals appear to be safer than the ones that they displace.

EPA's new chemicals program under TSCA [Toxic Substances Control Act] plays a major role in screening chemicals before they reach the marketplace to ensure that use of commercial chemicals will not pose unreasonable risks to human health or the environment. For chemicals already in commerce, we are increasingly recognizing the advantages of looking at clusters of chemicals, rather than single chemicals, in evaluating alternative products and processes, and we are working cooperatively with a variety of industries to encourage them to turn to products and processes that are safer and more effective. We believe that our new chemical review process, which scrutinizes every new chemical entering the market, is sophisticated enough to prevent substantial harm from known types of hazards. We need to better understand what types of chemicals disrupt endocrine function, but we believe we have an adequate legal and regulatory framework to deal with these risks.

Does EPA think it is realistic for society to use dramatically lower amounts of pesticides?

We believe substantial progress has been made in the U.S. to reduce reliance on chemical pesticides, but agree that more can be done, especially as safer pest management tools are developed and approved, for use. EPA is accelerating the registration of biological pesticides and chemical pesticides that are safer than products currently in use. In 1993 EPA, the Food and Drug Administration, and the U.S. Department of Agriculture entered into a joint effort to expand the use of integrated pest management to 75% of the crop acres in agriculture, the sector of our society which uses the most pesticides. Key to the success of this effort is the assurance that farmers will be able to meet their pest control needs economically and efficiently. When this effort is complete, the Agency expects there will be not only less pesticide use, but safer and smarter use as well.

In addition, EPA is working to reduce nonagricultural pesticide use and risk through the PESP program and efforts to provide homeowners and others with practical information on lawn care and effective pest control strategies in the home and other nonagricultural settings.

Additional Information

National Service Center for Environmental Publications (NSCEP),
P.O. Box 42419
Cincinnati, OH 45242-2419
Toll-Free: 800-490-9198
Phone: 513-489-8190
Fax: 513-489-8695
Website: http://www.epa.gov/ncepihom

National Pesticides Information Center (NPIC)
Oregon State University
333 Weniger Hall
Corvallis, OR 97331-6502
Toll-Free: 800-858-7378 (7 days/week, except holidays, 6:30 a.m. to 4:30 p.m. Pacific Time)
Website: http://npic.orst.edu
E-mail: npic@ace.orst.edu

Chapter 16

Iodine: Beneficial and Harmful Effects

Chapter Contents

Section 16.1

Health Questions about Iodine

"ToxFAQs™: Iodine," Agency for Toxic Substances and Disease Registry (ATSDR), updated May 25, 2004.

This section answers the most frequently asked health questions about iodine. This information is important because this substance may harm you. The effects of exposure to any hazardous substance depend on the dose, the duration, how you are exposed, personal traits and habits, and whether other chemicals are present.

Iodine is a naturally occurring element that is required for good health. Exposure to high levels of stable or radioactive iodine can cause damage to the thyroid.

What is iodine?

Iodine is a naturally occurring element found in sea water and in certain rocks and sediments. There are nonradioactive and radioactive forms of iodine.

Iodine is used as a disinfectant for cleaning surfaces and storage containers and is used in skin soaps and bandages, and for purifying water. Iodine is also added to some table salt to ensure that all people in the United States have enough iodine in their diet.

Radioactive iodine also occurs naturally. It is used in medical tests and to treat certain diseases. Most radioactive forms of iodine change very quickly (seconds to days) to stable elements that are not radioactive. However, I-129 (read as iodine 129) changes very slowly (over millions of years).

What happens to iodine when it enters the environment?

The primary source of nonradioactive iodine is the ocean. It enters the air from sea spray or as iodine gas. Once in the air, iodine can combine with water or with particles in air and can enter the soil and surface water, or land on vegetation when these particles fall to the ground or when it rains. Iodine can remain in soil for a long time. It can also be taken up by some plants that grow in the soil, but plants are considered a poor source of dietary iodine.

Radioactive iodine forms naturally from chemical reactions high in the atmosphere. Small amounts of radioactive iodine can enter the air from nuclear power plants. Larger amounts of radioactive iodine have been released to the air from accidents at nuclear power plants and from explosions of nuclear bombs.

How might I be exposed to iodine?

The general population is exposed to low levels of iodine in air, some food, and some beverages. Food (iodized salt, bread, and milk) is the largest sources of exposure to iodine. The general population is rarely exposed to radioactive iodine, unless they undergo certain medical tests or are given it for the treatment of thyroid disease. People who work at facilities using radioactive iodine may be exposed to higher than normal levels.

How can iodine affect my health?

Iodine has both beneficial and harmful effects on human health. Iodine is needed by your thyroid gland to produce thyroid hormones. However, exposure to unnecessarily high levels of nonradioactive and radioactive iodine can damage the thyroid. Damage to the thyroid gland can result in effects in other parts of your body, such as your skin, lung, and reproductive organs.

How likely is iodine to cause cancer?

Some human studies have found an increased risk of thyroid cancer in certain populations, particularly populations with iodine deficient diets receiving iodine supplements. Other human studies have not found an association between exposure to high levels of iodine and cancer risk. Neither the EPA nor the International Agency for Research on Cancer (IARC) has reviewed the carcinogenicity of iodine.

Exposure to high levels of radioactive iodine may also increase the risk of thyroid cancer. However, the evidence is inconclusive.

How can iodine affect children?

Iodine is essential for the growth and development of children. However, children are more sensitive to the harmful effects of excessively high levels of stable and radioactive iodine than adults because their thyroid glands are still growing and they need a healthy thyroid gland for normal growth. If babies and children receive too much iodine, they can develop an enlarged thyroid gland (called a goiter), which does not produce enough thyroid hormone for normal growth. Too much iodine from the mother can cause a baby's thyroid gland to be so large that it makes breathing difficult or impossible.

Radioactive iodine in food can be more harmful to babies and children than to adults. Because a child's thyroid gland is smaller than that of an adult, a child's thyroid gland will receive a higher radiation dose than the adult exposed to the same amount of iodine.

How can families reduce the risk of exposure to iodine?

The general population is exposed to iodine in some food and beverages. We do not want to prevent exposure to iodine, but we do want to try to prevent exposure to too much iodine. Foods are not normally expected to have enough iodine to harm your health. Unless you are exposed to radioactive waste or emissions, you generally do not have to worry about excessive exposure.

Is there a medical test to show whether I've been exposed to iodine?

There are reliable tests that can measure iodine in the blood, urine, and saliva. These tests are not available at your doctor's office, but your doctor can send the samples to a laboratory that can perform the tests. However, these tests cannot predict whether you will experience any health effects.

Radiation detectors can measure radioactive iodine inside your body using the radiation coming from the thyroid gland in your neck. Your body quickly eliminates iodine and radioactive iodine, so tests should be done shortly after exposure.

Has the federal government made recommendations to protect human health?

The National Research Council has established a recommended dietary allowance (RDA) for iodine of 150 micrograms per day (150 μg/day), with additional allowances of 25 μg/day during pregnancy and 50 μg/day during nursing. These dietary intake levels are sufficient to satisfy the metabolic needs of the body.

The Nuclear Regulatory Commission (NRC), the National Council of Radiation Protection and Measurement (NRCP), and the International

Commission of Radiological Protection (ICRP) have established recommended limits for worker exposures to radioactive iodine and for releases of radioactive iodine to the environment.

References

Agency for Toxic Substances and Disease Registry (ATSDR). 2001. *Toxicological Profile for iodine. Draft for Public Comment.* Atlanta, GA: U.S. Department of Health and Human Services, Public Health Service.

Additional Information

Agency for Toxic Substances and Disease Registry (ATSDR)
Division of Toxicology Information Center
1600 Clifton Road N.E., Mailstop F-32
Atlanta, GA 30333
Toll-Free: 888-422-8737
Phone: 404-498-0110
Fax: 404-498-0093
Website: http://www.atsdr.cdc.gov
E-mail: ATSDRIC@cdc.gov

Section 16.2

Use of Iodine for Water Disinfection

Excerpted from "Use of Iodine for Water Disinfection: Iodine Toxicity and Maximum Recommended Dose," by Howard Backer and Joe Hollowell, *Environmental Health Perspectives* Volume 108, Number 8, August 2000, National Institute of Environmental Health Sciences (NIEHS).

Introduction

Iodine is an essential nutrient for optimal thyroid function in adults and for fetal, infant, and child development. Dietary supplementation, generally via iodized salt but occasionally via iodinated water, has decreased goiter and hypothyroidism due to iodine deficiency in most of the world. Data from supplementation programs and elsewhere indicate that adults need to ingest at least 150–200 micrograms (µg) iodine per day.[1-3] Hollowell et al. [4] reported that the average American intake of iodine is near optimal. Nonetheless, ingestion of iodine in excess of the recommended daily intake level is common because of iodine in dietary sources such as dairy, eggs, meat, bread, and seaweed, or that in pharmacologic sources such as the cardiac antiarrhythmic drug amiodarone. Excess iodine may also disrupt normal thyroid function, but the maximum safe level for long-term ingestion remains undetermined. Experts suggest that 1–2 mg/day is safe for most people, yet empiric evidence suggests that much higher amounts are usually tolerated without problems.[1, 5]

The use of iodine to improve the microbiologic quality of drinking water in areas without safe public sources of potable water also contributes iodine levels in excess of the recommended maximum daily intake. Field water treatment is a necessity for millions of travelers, campers, military troops, and people living and working in underdeveloped areas, in addition to entire populations in disaster and medical relief situations.[6] Published data was reviewed on the effects of consuming more than the daily recommended dose of iodine in an attempt to identify the maximum safe dose and duration of ingestion when iodine is used for water disinfection.

Iodine for Water Treatment

Iodine is a halogen, like chlorine, that exerts a biocidal effect through its chemical property as a strong oxidant. The active disinfectant species are elemental iodine and hypoiodous acid.[7, 8] Iodide has no disinfectant activity; however, iodine is rapidly converted to iodide in the stomach and absorbed into the blood. Water disinfection with halogens is a first-order chemical reaction: the primary variables are aqueous concentration of halogen and the time it is in contact with the microorganism.[9, 10] In addition, different classes of microorganisms vary in their susceptibility to halogens. Bacteria are very sensitive, viruses are intermediate, and protozoan cysts are more resistant. Doses of iodine below 1 (milligram per liter) mg/L are effective for bacteria within minutes; however, at this concentration, it would take many hours to kill Giardia cysts. Although low doses can be used in controlled situations, recommended levels of iodine for point-of-use water disinfection in unmonitored field situations are higher to allow for unanticipated reactions with organic contaminants (halogen demand) and to allow a relatively short contact time.[6]

Iodine has several advantages over chlorine for field use—including greater chemical stability of the product and less reactivity with organic nitrogenous contaminants of residual concentrations in water—leaving higher free residual concentration in water and more acceptable taste in equipotent doses.[11, 12] Iodine is available in a variety of forms, including solutions (tincture of iodine, povidone, Lugol's, and saturated aqueous solution with iodine crystals), tablets, and iodine resins.

Iodine resins offer additional advantages for field use because the resins are an extremely stable form of iodine that can be incorporated into a wide range of filters and act as a demand disinfectant with limited dissolution in water.[13] Little iodine is released into aqueous solution, however; as water passes through and microorganisms contact the resin, iodine is aided by electrostatic forces and binds to microorganisms. The residual iodine concentration with iodine resins is much less than concentrations from the recommended doses of tablet or liquid forms of iodine. Iodine resin filters usually incorporate two additional stages: microfiltration to remove Cryptosporidium oocysts that are resistant to halogen disinfection, and granular activated charcoal to further reduce the concentration of iodine in effluent water.

Iodine has been used to ensure the safety of potable water since the 1940s, when the military developed a tablet formulation for use by troops in the field.[10] Widespread use followed in the civilian population.

There are no accurate figures for the number of civilian or military personnel who use iodine for water disinfection. A survey of manufacturers reveals that in 1998 approximately 60,000 iodine resin devices were sold for individual or small-group civilian use. In addition, the leading manufacturer sold more than 300,000 bottles of iodine tablets. This does not include iodine sold in other forms, such as tincture of iodine, povidone, or iodine crystals in aqueous solution.

Because of the ill-defined risk of iodine affecting thyroid function and because other means of water treatment are often available, the World Health Organization (WHO) and the U.S. Environmental Protection Agency recommend that iodine be used for short-term or emergency use only for water treatment.[16-18] However, many people use iodine for much longer periods because of the convenience and effectiveness of the products. Despite the extensive use of iodine for both pharmacologic preparations and water disinfection over the past 50 years, there are remarkably few reports of resulting clinical thyroid disorders.[19] Recently, goiters discovered among a group of Peace Corps volunteers in Africa were linked epidemiologically to the use of iodine resin filters for water disinfection.[20]

Thyroid Effects of Excess Iodine Ingestion

Physiologic effects. The physiologic regulation of the thyroid gland by iodine is complex, involving feedback mechanisms at several biochemical and physiologic steps that depend on the amount of iodine and the rate of administration. In most instances, these autoregulatory mechanisms effectively handle excess iodine intake.

In humans, iodide intake of greater than 2 mg/day results in a proportionate decrease in the organification of thyroidal iodide, but there is no evidence that the overall amount of organic iodination is decreased.[24] There are adequate data to demonstrate that thyroid I-131 uptake or thyroid clearance of iodide decreases with increases in serum iodide levels. Studies to limit radioactive iodine uptake in the event of a nuclear accident or fallout have demonstrated rapid suppression of uptake after the administration of iodide.[25, 26] Single doses greater than 10 mg suppress the uptake of radioactive iodine to 1.5% within 24 hours, and daily doses of 15 mg will maintain uptake below 2%.[25]

The limitations of in vivo measurement make it difficult to demonstrate the same biochemical mechanism of the Wolff-Chaikoff (W-C) effect and escape from it in humans.[27] Regardless of the mechanism, an escape from the inhibitory effects of prolonged excess levels of iodine is also seen in humans. For this reason, most people can tolerate high doses of iodine without developing thyroid abnormalities.

Clinical Effects

Hyperthyroidism. Iodine-induced hyperthyroidism can be caused by underlying thyroid disease or by the consumption of iodine by people with prior iodine deficiency.[5, 28, 29] During the worldwide campaign to eliminate endemic goiter and associated cretinism, Stanbury et al.[30] reported that some people would develop hyperthyroidism after receiving only small amounts of iodine supplements. The average incidence of hyperthyroidism was 1.7%, but ranged as high as 7% in Sweden. Any increase in iodine intake will cause some increase in the incidence of hyperthyroidism in a previously iodine-deficient population.[31, 32] Most cases result from underlying multinodular thyroid disease when autonomous nodules that are not suppressed by increased iodine uptake produce excessive thyroid hormone.[31, 32] Most of these cases resolve spontaneously and the incidence of hyperthyroidism drops to pre-supplementation levels within a few years. The elderly are at more risk because they have a higher incidence of multinodular goiter. In areas without endemic goiter, hyperthyroidism as a result of iodine is much less common. Hyperthyroidism may also be induced in people with Graves disease, especially after antithyroid therapy, and in approximately 2% of patients taking amiodarone[33] or other pharmacologic sources of iodine. There is also concern that iodine may induce autoimmune thyroid disease and both papillary and follicular thyroid cancer.[1, 29]

Reports of hyperthyroidism from the ingestion of iodine used for water disinfection are rare. Liel and Alkan[34] reported on two travelers who became hyperthyroid, presumably because of using iodine tablets for water disinfection. Both were from iodine-sufficient areas and tested positive for antithyroid peroxidase antibodies and negative for antithyroglobulin antibodies. The mother and sister of one of the travelers had Hashimoto thyroiditis.[34] The course of the thyroid dysfunction for both travelers was relatively mild and self-limited.

A female Swiss traveler developed mild and reversible hyperthyroidism after using iodine for water purification. The traveler had a previous hemithyroidectomy for a nontoxic nodule, had evidence of autoimmune disease, and tested positive for antithyroid peroxidase antibodies. The traveler's transient hyperthyroidism was followed briefly by subclinical hypothyroidism but reverted to euthyroid status a few months later, when her iodine intake was reduced.[35]

Iodine-induced hypothyroidism and/or goiter. Hypothyroidism from excessive iodine intake is much more common than hyperthyroidism. Hypothyroidism is attributed to the prolonged suppression of thyroid hormone production as the result of excess iodine levels, but the mechanism through which iodide goiter is produced is not well understood.[36, 37] Apparently, patients with iodide goiter require less iodide to inhibit the organic binding of iodine and do not escape the inhibitory effects of iodides as do those who do not develop goiter.[38, 39] The problem may result from the thyroid gland's inability to limit the uptake of iodine when large amounts are available, after which the accumulated iodine inhibits the synthesis of hormone.[36] Histologic studies suggest that many people who develop iodide goiter have underlying thyroid disease.[40] Iodine-induced hypothyroidism or goiter is more common in several groups, but may occur with or without underlying thyroid disease. The following people are at increased risk for iodine-induced hypothyroidism:[5, 28, 37, 41]

- those with underlying thyroid problems, including current or prior thyroiditis, previous treatment for Graves disease, previous subtotal thyroidectomy for benign nodules, and previous treatment with interferon

- fetuses, preterm neonates, and newborn infants who are at risk because of the placental transfer of iodide from mothers treated with iodides

- those with endemic goiter due to very high dietary iodine intake—mainly described in coastal areas of Japan

- those with other conditions, including:
  - elderly people without clinical thyroid disease who may have subclinical hypothyroidism (i.e., elevated TSH but normal free T4 levels) (subclinical hypothyroidism is very common, affecting 5–10% of adults over the age of 50)
  - patients with certain non-thyroid diseases such as chronic dialysis and cystic fibrosis, especially those taking sulfasoxazole
  - patients taking medications containing iodine, formerly iodide expectorants, but, more recently, amiodarone
  - patients taking lithium
  - people with a family history of goiter or thyroiditis (suggested by a few case reports)

Excess iodine ingestion may be causally related to autoimmune thyroid disease.[1, 5] However; a recent study of Japanese subjects who excreted an average of 1.5 mg/day iodine in their urine demonstrated no correlation between antithyroglobulin antibodies or hypothyroidism and levels of urinary iodine.[42]

Recommendations for Iodine Use in Water Treatment

We are not advocating raising the daily minimum requirements of iodine, nor are we promoting the use of iodine for routine community water treatment in small remote communities or in developing countries, where there would be a higher incidence of adverse effects. Despite alternative methods of disinfection alternatives, iodine remains popular for individual and small-group field water treatment in situations where surface water is ingested or water quality from a distribution system is questionable. This discussion should be useful for the development of policy and procedures for agencies that place personnel in remote locations and for stimulation of policy debate at agencies that regulate products containing iodine.

When iodine is considered the best means of water treatment, the following is recommended:

- Do not use an iodine-based water treatment method for people with increased susceptibility to iodine-induced thyroid disorders:
  - pregnant women (fetus susceptible to goiter)
  - people with known hypersensitivity to iodine
  - people with a history of thyroid disease, even if controlled on medication
  - people with a strong family history of thyroid disease
  - people from countries or localities with chronic iodine deficiency

- Examine the thyroid and do thyroid function tests on anyone planning to use iodine for prolonged periods (longer than 3 months) to ensure that they are initially euthyroid. It is not clear whether the presence of antithyroid antibodies is a contraindication to iodine use.

- Limit the use of water disinfection methods that produce moderately high levels of iodine (5–32 mg/L), such as iodine tablets, to 3 months.

145

- Euthyroid people can safely use iodine treatments that produce a low residual (1 mg/L) level, even for long periods of time. Current products containing iodine resin devices with a charcoal scavenger to remove residual iodine can meet this standard when used properly. Likewise, a two-step process of water treatment with iodine tablets or iodine solutions, then filtration by a device containing charcoal, can ensure safe levels of iodine and effective water treatment.

- Standards are needed to ensure the efficacy and safety of iodine-containing water purification products intended for prolonged use:
  - The products must contain an effective iodine scavenger (usually granular activated charcoal) sufficient to decrease the residual to a level safe for long-term use (years).
  - The iodine scavenger must be effective throughout the life span of the device or there must be a reliable method to indicate when the iodine scavenger no longer has adsorptive capacity so that it can be replaced.
  - The product must perform adequately without the need for high levels of residual iodine.

In summary, the use of iodine for water disinfection requires a risk-benefit decision similar to other medical interventions that are used to prevent illness in high-risk populations. The paucity of accurate water quality data for most parts of the world, and known issues of water quality where it is measured, mandate additional measures to ensure potable water in many situations. [44] The risk for enteric infection[45] and the availability of other means of producing potable water should be weighed against the risk for and severity of thyroid disorder from iodine. Enteric disease rates from water with microbiologic contamination may be high and repeat infections can be anticipated because only limited immunity develops.[46] Iodine is an effective, simple, and cost-efficient means of water disinfection. For temporary residents, relief workers, and travelers in areas where municipal water treatment is not reliable, the benefit of use exceeds the risk.

Although there is fair evidence that the current recommended upper limits of daily iodine ingestion are safe, there are limited data to suggest that this upper limit is the maximum safe level. Coupled with periodic monitoring of thyroid function, techniques that generate low levels (1–2 mg/L) of iodine in water can be safely used for years.

References and Notes

1. Dunn J. What's happening to our iodine [Editorial]. *J Clin Endocrinol Metab* 83:3398-3400 (1998).

2. Review of Findings from *Seven-Country Study in Africa on Levels of Salt Iodization in Relation to Iodine Deficiency Disorders, Including Iodine-Induced Hyperthyroidism.* WHO/AFRO/NUT/97.2. Geneva: Joint World Health Organization/United Nations Children's Fund (UNICEF)/International Council for Control of Iodine Deficiency Disorders, 1996.

3. International Council for Control of Iodine Deficiency Disorders. Iodized Water to Eliminate Iodine Deficiency. *IDD Newsletter*, Volume 13 Number 3, August 1997. Available: http://www.people.virginia.edu/~jtd/iccidd/ idddocs/idd897.htm [cited 24 May 2000].

4. Hollowell J, Staehling N, Hannon H, Flanders D, Gunter E, Marberly G, Braverman L, Pino S, Miller D, Garbe P, et al. Iodine nutrition in the United States. Trends and public health implications: iodine excretion data from National Health and Nutrition Examination Surveys I and III (1971-1974 and 1988-1994*). J Clin Endocrinol Metab* 83:3401-3408 (1998).

5. Braverman L. Iodine and the thyroid: 33 years of study. *Thyroid* 4:351-355 (1994).

6. Backer H. Field water disinfection. In: *Wilderness Medicine: Management of Wilderness and Environmental Emergencies* (Auerbach P, ed). St. Louis, MO: Mosby, 1995;1061-1110.

7. Gottardi W. Iodine and iodine compounds. In: *Disinfection, Sterilization, and Preservation* (Block S, ed). Philadelphia: Lea & Febiger, 1991;152-167.

8. White G. *Handbook of Chlorination*. New York: Van Nostrand Reinhold, 1992.

9. Black A, Kinman R, Thomas W, Freund G, Bird E. Use of iodine for disinfection. *J Am Water Works Assoc* 57:1401-1421 (1965).

10. Chang S, Morris J. Elemental iodine as a disinfectant for drinking water. *Ind Eng Chem* 45:1009-1012 (1953).

11. National Academy of Science Safe Drinking Water Committee. The disinfection of drinking water. In: *Drinking Water and*

Health, Vol 2. Washington, DC: National Academy Press, 1980;5-139.

12. O'Connor J, Kapoor S. Small quantity field disinfection. *J Am Water Works Assoc* 62:80-84 (1970).

13. Marchin G, Fina L. Contact and demand-release disinfectants. *Crit Rev Environ Control* 19:227-290 (1989).

14. Powers E. *Inactivation of Giardia Cysts by Iodine with Special Reference to Globaline: A Review.* Tech Rpt Natick/TR-91/022. Natick, MA: U.S. Army Natick Research, Development and Engineering Center, 1991.

15. Marchin G, Fina L. Contact and demand-release disinfectants. *Crit Rev Environ Control* 19:277-290 (1989).

16. Zoeteman B. *The Suitability of Iodine and Iodine Compounds as Disinfectants for Small Water Supplies.* Tech Paper No 2. The Hague: World Health Organization International Reference Center for Community Water Supply, 1972.

17. Water and Sanitation for Health Project. Water Supply and Sanitation in Rural Development: Proceedings of a Conference for Private and Voluntary Organizations. *WASH Tech Rpt No 14.* Washington, DC: Water and Sanitation for Health, 1981.

18. Cotruvo J, Jones G. *Policy on Iodine Disinfection.* Washington, DC: U.S. Environmental Protection Agency, 1982.

19. Morgans M, Trotter W. Two cases of myxoedema attributed to iodide administration. *Lancet* ii: 1355-1357 (1953).

20. Kettel-Khan L, Li R, Gootnick D, Peace Corps Thyroid Investigation Group. Thyroid abnormalities related to iodine excess from water purification units [Research Letter]. *Lancet* 352: 1519 (1998).

21. Nagataki S, Ingbar S. Relation between qualitative and quantitative alterations in thyroid hormone synthesis induced by varying doses of iodide. *Endocrinology* 74:731 (1964).

22. Wolff J, Chaikoff I. Plasma inorganic iodide as a homeostatic regulator of thyroid function. *J Biol Chem* 174:555-564 (1948).

23. Wolff J, Chaikoff I, Goldberg R, Meier J. The temporary nature of the inhibitory action of excess iodine on organic iodine synthesis in the normal thyroid. *Endocrinology* 45:504-513 (1949).

24. Nagataki S, Shizume K, Nakao K. Thyroid function in chronic excess iodide ingestion: comparison of thyroidal absolute iodine uptake and degradation of thyroxine in euthyroid Japanese subjects. *J Clin Endocrinol Metab* 27:638-647 (1967).

25. Sternthal E, Lipworth L, Stanley B, Abreau C, Fang S, Braverman L. Suppression of thyroid radioiodine uptake by various doses of stable iodide. *N Engl J Med* 303:1083-1088 (1980).

26. Saxena K, Chapman E, Pryles C. Minimal dosage of iodide required to suppress uptake of iodine-131 by normal thyroid. *Science* 138:430-431 (1962).

27. Nagataki S, Yokoyami N. Other factors regulating thyroid function. Autoregulation effects of iodide. In: Werner and Ingbar's *The Thyroid* (Braverman L, Utiger R, eds). Philadelphia: Lippincott-Raven, 1996;241-247.

28. Roti E, Vagenakis A. Effect of excess iodide: clinical aspects. In: Werner and Ingbar's *The Thyroid* (Braverman L, Utiger R, eds). Philadelphia: Lippincott-Raven, 1996;316-327.

29. Koutras D. Control of efficiency and results, and adverse effects of excess iodine administration on thyroid function. *Ann Endocrinol* 57:463-469 (1996).

30. Stanbury J, Ermans A, Bourdoux P, Todd C, Oken E, Tonglet R, Vidor G, Braverman LE, Medeiros-Neto G. Iodine-induced hyperthyroidism: occurrence and epidemiology. *Thyroid* 8:83-100 (1998).

31. Corvilain B, Sande J, Dumont J, Bourdoux P, Ermans A. Autonomy in endemic goiter. *Thyroid* 8:107-113 (1998).

32. Boyages S, Bloot A, Maberly G, Eastman C, Mu L, Qidong A, Derun L, VanderGaag R, Drexhage H. Thyroid autoimmunity in endemic goitre caused by excessive iodine intake. *Clin Endocrinol* 31:453-465 (1989).

33. Kishore J, Licata A. Effects of amiodarone on thyroid function. *Ann Intern Med* 126:63-73 (1997).

34. Liel Y, Alkan M. Travelers' thyrotoxicosis: transitory thyrotoxicosis induced by iodinated preparations for water purification. *Arch Intern Med* 156:807-810 (1996).

35. Mueller B, Diem P, Burgi U. Travelers' thyrotoxicosis revisited [Letter]. *Arch Int Med* 158:1723 (1998).

36. Harrison M, Alexander W, Harden R. Thyroid function and iodine metabolism in iodine-induced hypothyroidism. *Lancet* i:238-241 (1963).

37. Wolff J. Iodide goiter and the pharmacologic effects of excess iodide. *Am J Med* 47:101-124 (1969).

38. Paris J, McConahey W, Owen C, Woolner L, Bahn R. Iodide Goiter. *J Endocrinol* 20:57-67 (1960).

39. Tajiri J, Higashi K, Mority M, Umeda T, Sato T. Studies of hypothyroidism in patients with high iodide intake. *J Clin Endocrinol Metab* 63:412-417 (1986).

40. Mizukami Y, Michigishi T, Nonomura A, Hashimoto T, Tonami N, Matsubara F, Takazakura E. Iodine-induced hypothyroidism: a clinical and histological study of 28 patients. *J Clin Endocrinol Metab* 76:466-471 (1993).

41. Braverman L, Roti E. Effects of iodine on thyroid function. *Acta Med Austriaca* 23:4-9 (1996).

42. Nagata K, Takasu N, Akamine H, Ohshiro C, Komiya I, Murakami K, Suzawa A, Nomura T. Urinary iodine and thyroid antibodies in Okinawa, Yamagata, Hyogo, and Nagano, Japan: the differences in iodine intake do not affect thyroid antibody positivity. *Endocr J* 45:797-803 (1998).

43. Konno N, Makita H, Yuri K, Iizuka N, Kawasaki K. Association between dietary iodine intake and prevalence of subclinical hypothyroidism in the coastal regions of Japan. *J Clin Endocrinol Metab* 78:393-397 (1993).

44. Cooper R, Olivieri A, Danielson R, Badger P, Spear R, Selvin S. *Infectious Agent Risk Assessment Water Quality Project.* UCB/SEEHRL Rpt No 84-4 and 84-5. Berkeley, CA: University of California, 1984.

45. Hurst C, Clark R, Regli S. Estimating the risk of acquiring infectious disease from ingestion of water. In: *Modeling Disease Transmission and its Prevention by Disinfection* (Hurst C, ed). Melbourne, Australia: Cambridge University Press, 1996;99-139.

46. Ericsson C, DuPont H. Travelers' diarrhea: approaches to prevention and treatment. *Clin Infect Dis* 16:616-624 (1993).

Part Three

Thyroid Tests

Chapter 17

Neck Check Home Test

The thyroid gland is a small, butterfly-shaped gland located in the base of the neck just below the Adam's apple. Although relatively small, the thyroid gland influences the function of many of the body's most important organs including the heart, brain, liver, kidneys, and skin. Ensuring that the thyroid gland is healthy and functioning properly is important to the body's overall well-being.

Thyroid disease affects an estimated 13 million Americans of all ages, yet more than half remain undiagnosed. Undiagnosed thyroid disease can lead to elevated cholesterol levels and subsequent heart disease, infertility, and osteoporosis. Research also shows that there is a strong genetic link between thyroid disease and other autoimmune diseases including certain types of diabetes, anemia, and arthritis. That's why the American Association of Clinical Endocrinologists (AACE) has launched a new public education initiative called *The Neck's Generation*. The campaign aims to educate Americans about the genetic links associated with thyroid disease, and encourage them to investigate their family health history to uncover any at-risk conditions.

Because many of thyroid disease's symptoms are vague, AACE is working to increase awareness of the flagship signs such as fatigue, depression, forgetfulness, changes in growth or cognitive function, or changes in hair, skin, and nails. As a first step in identifying an underlying thyroid problem, AACE recommends that patients experiencing these symptoms conduct a simple thyroid self-exam.

"How to Take the Thyroid 'Neck Check'," © 2002 American Association of Clinical Endocrinologists. Reprinted with permission.

Take the Neck Check™ to help determine whether or not you have an enlarged thyroid gland, which may require further examination by an endocrinologist and testing with the highly sensitive TSH test.

How to Take the Thyroid "Neck Check"

Five Easy Steps That Could Save Your Life

All you will need is:

- a glass of water
- a handheld mirror

1. Hold the mirror in your hand, focusing on the area of your neck just below the Adam's apple and immediately above the collarbone. Your thyroid gland is located in this area of your neck.

2. While focusing on this area in the mirror, tip your head back.

3. Take a drink of water and swallow.

4. As you swallow, look at your neck. Check for any bulges or protrusions in this area when you swallow. Reminder: don't confuse the Adam's apple with the thyroid gland. The thyroid gland is located further down on your neck, closer to the collarbone. You may want to repeat this process several times.

5. If you do see any bulges or protrusions in this area, see your physician. You may have an enlarged thyroid gland or a thyroid nodule, and should be checked to determine whether cancer is present or if treatment for thyroid disease is needed.

Additional Information

American Association of Clinical Endocrinologists (AACE)
1000 Riverside Ave., Suite 205
Jacksonville, FL 32204
Phone: 904-353-7878
Fax: 904-353-8185
Website: http://www.aace.com
E-mail: info@aace.com

Chapter 18

Thyroid Function Blood Tests

Chapter Contents

Section 18.1

Triiodothyronine (T3)

"T3: The Test Sample, The Test," © 2004 American Association for Clinical Chemistry. Reprinted with permission. For additional information on clinical lab testing, visit the Lab Tests Online website at www.labtests online.org.

The Test Sample

What is being tested?

The test measures the amount of triiodothyronine, or T3 in your blood. T3 is one of two major hormones produced by the thyroid gland (the other hormone is called thyroxine, or T4). T3 makes up less than 10% of what we call thyroid hormone, while T4 makes up the rest. T3, however, is about four times as strong as T4, and is thought to cause most, if not all, the effects of thyroid hormones.

Many of your body's cells can turn T4 into T3; T4 may be mainly a reservoir used to make T3 available. Thyroid hormones help regulate the body's metabolism (how the body functions).

About 99.7% of the T3 in blood is attached to a protein, and the rest is unattached. The blood test can measure either the total (both bound and unattached) or free (unattached) T3 hormone in the blood.

How is the sample collected for testing?

A blood sample is obtained from a needle placed in a vein in your arm.

T3: The Test

Formally known as: triiodothyronine

How is it used?

A T3 test determines whether the thyroid is performing properly, and is used mainly to help diagnose hyperthyroidism, since T3 can become abnormal earlier than T4 and return to normal later than T4.

T3 is not usually helpful if your doctor thinks you have hypothyroidism.

When is it ordered?

A total or free T3 test may be ordered if you get an abnormal T4 test result.

What does the test result mean?

A high total or free T3 result may indicate an overactive thyroid gland (hyperthyroidism).

Low total or free T3 results may indicate an underactive thyroid gland (hypothyroidism).

Please Note: Numerically reported test results are interpreted according to the test's reference range, which may vary by the patient's age, sex, as well as the instrumentation or kit used to perform the test. A specific result within the reference (normal) range—for any test—does not ensure health just as a result outside the reference range may not indicate disease. To learn the reference range for your test, consult your doctor or laboratorian. Lab Tests Online recommends you consult your physician to discuss your test results as a part of a complete medical examination.

Is there anything else I should know?

Many medications—including estrogen, certain types of birth control pills, and large doses of aspirin—can interfere with total T3 test results, so tell your doctor about any drugs you are taking. In general, free T3 levels are not affected by these medications.

When you are sick, your body decreases production of T3 from T4. Most people who are sick enough to be in the hospital will have a low T3 or free T3 level. For this reason, doctors do not usually use T3 as a routine thyroid test for patients in hospitals.

Section 18.2

Thyroxine (T4)

T4 Test Sample

Formally known as: thyroxine

What is being tested?

This test identifies thyroxine, or T4, in your blood. T4 is one of two major hormones produced by the thyroid gland (the other is called triiodothyronine, or T3).

T4 makes up nearly all of what we call thyroid hormone, while T3 makes up less than 10%. Thyroid hormones help regulate the body's metabolism (that is, how the body functions).

Most T4 in blood is attached to a protein; less than 1% is unattached. The blood test can measure either the total (both bound and unattached) or free (unattached) T4 hormone in your blood. Scientists believe that free hormone is responsible for all the effects of thyroid hormone.

How is the sample collected for testing?

A blood sample is obtained from a needle placed in a vein in your arm.

T4: The Test

How is it used?

A T4 test tells whether the thyroid is performing properly. Newborns are commonly screened for T4 levels as well as TSH concentrations to check for hypothyroidism, which can cause mental retardation.

In adults, the T4 test generally aids in the diagnosis of hypothyroidism or hyperthyroidism. The test may also be used to help evaluate a patient with an enlarged thyroid gland, called a goiter. It may also aid in the diagnosis and monitoring of female infertility problems.

When is it ordered?

Thyroid hormone screening is commonly performed in newborns. In adults, a total T4 or free T4 test usually is ordered in response to an abnormal TSH test result.

What does the test result mean?

High free or total T4 results may indicate an overactive thyroid gland (hyperthyroidism).

Low free or total T4 results may indicate an underactive thyroid gland (hypothyroidism).

Please Note: Numerically reported test results are interpreted according to the test's reference range, which may vary by the patient's age, sex, as well as the instrumentation or kit used to perform the test. A specific result within the reference (normal) range—for any test—does not ensure health just as a result outside the reference range may not indicate disease. To learn the reference range for your test, consult your doctor or laboratorian. Lab Tests Online recommends you consult your physician to discuss your test results as a part of a complete medical examination.

Is there anything else I should know?

Many medications—including estrogen, certain types of birth control pills, and large doses of aspirin—can interfere with total T4 test results, so tell your doctor about any drugs you are taking. In general, free T4 levels are not affected by these medications. In addition, total T4 levels may be affected by contrast material used for certain x-ray imaging tests.

Section 18.3

Thyroid-Stimulating Hormone (TSH)

"TSH: Test Sample, The Test," © 2004 American Association for Clinical Chemistry. Reprinted with permission. For additional information on clinical lab testing, visit the Lab Tests Online website at www.labtestsonline.org

Test Sample

What is being tested?

The test measures the amount of thyroid-stimulating hormone (TSH) in your blood, which is an indicator of thyroid disease. TSH is made by the pituitary gland located in your brain. TSH is the pituitary gland's messenger—it tells the thyroid gland to start making thyroid hormone.

How is the sample collected for testing?

A blood sample obtained from a needle placed in a vein in your arm.

TSH: The Test

Formally known as: thyroid-stimulating hormone, thyrotropin

How is it used?

TSH testing is used to:

- diagnose a thyroid disorder in a person with symptoms
- screen newborns for an underactive thyroid
- monitor thyroid replacement therapy in people with hypothyroidism
- diagnose and monitor female infertility problems

- screen adults for thyroid disorders as recommended by some organizations, such as the American Thyroid Association

When is it ordered?

Your doctor orders this test if you show symptoms of a thyroid disorder. For example, symptoms of hyperthyroidism include heat intolerance, weight loss, rapid heartbeat, nervousness, insomnia, and breathlessness.

Common symptoms of hypothyroidism include fatigue, weakness, weight gain, slow heart rate, and cold intolerance.

The blood test may be ordered with other thyroid hormone tests and after a physical examination of your thyroid. TSH screening is routinely performed in newborns. The American Thyroid Association recommends that adults older than age 35 be screened for thyroid disease every five years although other organizations, such as the U.S. Preventive Services Task Force, challenge this recommendation. Several organizations recommend instead screening women over 50, asymptomatic adults over 60, or those at high risk for thyroid disorders, such as pregnant and postpartum women.

What does the test result mean?

A high TSH result often means an underactive thyroid gland caused by failure of the gland (hypothyroidism). Rarely, a high TSH result can indicate a problem with the pituitary gland, such as a tumor producing unregulated levels of TSH, in what is known as secondary hyperthyroidism. A high TSH value can also occur in people with underactive thyroid glands who have been receiving too little thyroid hormone medication.

A low TSH result can indicate an overactive thyroid gland (hyperthyroidism). A low TSH result can also indicate damage to the pituitary gland that prevents it from producing TSH. A low TSH result can also occur in people with an underactive thyroid gland who are receiving too much thyroid hormone medication.

Please note: Numerically reported test results are interpreted according to the test's reference range, which may vary by the patient's age, sex, as well as the instrumentation or kit used to perform the test. A specific result within the reference (normal) range—for any test—does not ensure health just as a result outside the reference range may not indicate disease. To learn the reference range for your test, consult your doctor or laboratorian. Lab Tests Online recommends you consult your physician to discuss your test results as a part of a complete medical examination.

Is there anything else I should know?

Many medications—including aspirin and thyroid-hormone replacement therapy—may interfere with thyroid gland function test results, so tell your doctor about any drugs you are taking. When your doctor adjusts your dose of thyroid hormone, it is important to wait at least one to two months before you check your TSH again, so that your new dose can have its full effect. Extreme stress and acute illness may also affect TSH test results, and results may be low during the first trimester of pregnancy.

Section 18.4

Calcium Test

The Test

Related tests: Phosphorus, Vitamin D, parathyroid hormone (PTH), magnesium, albumin, and comprehensive metabolic panel

How is it used?

Blood calcium is tested to screen for, diagnose, and monitor a range of conditions relating to the bones, heart, nerves, kidneys, and teeth. Blood calcium levels do not directly tell how much calcium is in the bones, but rather, how much total calcium or ionized calcium is circulating in the blood.

Doctors can get a better picture of your health by comparing your calcium result with the results of other tests. Calcium levels in the blood are regulated and stabilized by a feedback loop that includes:

calcium, PTH, vitamin D, phosphorus, and magnesium. Your doctor is looking at the balance among all of these elements. Conditions and diseases that disrupt this feedback loop can cause inappropriate elevations or decreases in calcium and lead to symptoms of hyper- or hypocalcemia. For example, when parathyroid hormone (PTH) from the parathyroid gland is released, PTH level rises, calcium also rises, and phosphorus drops. In some kidney problems, a high phosphorus level in blood can depress calcium levels. Depending on the levels you have, these two tests can help your doctor discover whether you have a parathyroid problem or another condition.

Directly measuring free or ionized calcium is important during major surgery (particularly if blood or blood products are transfused), in critically ill patients, and when protein levels are very abnormal. Large fluctuations in free calcium can cause the heart to slow down or to beat too rapidly, can cause muscles to go into spasm (tetany), and can cause confusion or even coma.

When is it ordered?

Calcium is often used as a screening test as part of a general medical examination. It is typically included in the comprehensive metabolic panel.

Calcium can be used as a diagnostic test if you go to your doctor with symptoms that suggest:

- kidney stones
- bone disease
- neurologic (nerve-related) disorders

Your doctor also may order a calcium test if:

- you have kidney disease, because low calcium is especially common in those with kidney failure;
- you have symptoms of too much calcium, such as fatigue, weakness, loss of appetite, nausea, vomiting, constipation, abdominal pain, urinary frequency, and increased thirst;
- you have symptoms of low calcium, such as cramps in your abdomen, muscle cramps, or tingling fingers; or
- you have other diseases that can be associated with abnormal blood calcium, such as thyroid disease, intestinal disease, cancer, or poor nutrition.

Your doctor may order an ionized calcium test if you have numbness around the mouth and in the hands and feet, and muscle spasms in the same areas, which are symptoms of low levels of ionized calcium. If calcium levels fall slowly, however, many people have no symptoms at all.

You may need calcium monitoring as part of your regular laboratory tests if you have certain kinds of cancer (particularly breast, lung, head and neck, kidney, and multiple myeloma), kidney disease, or kidney transplant. You may also need to be monitored for calcium level if it is clear that you have abnormal calcium levels, or if you are receiving calcium or vitamin D supplements.

What does the test result mean?

A normal calcium result with other normal lab results means that you have no problems with calcium metabolism (use by the body).

Because about half of the calcium in your blood is bound by albumin (a protein), these two tests are usually ordered together. Calcium values must be interpreted in combination with albumin to determine if the calcium concentration of serum is appropriate. As albumin levels rise, calcium rises as well, and vice versa.

A high calcium level is called hypercalcemia. You have too much calcium in your blood and will need treatment for the underlying condition. This usually is caused by:

- **Hyperparathyroidism (increase in parathyroid gland function):** This condition is usually caused by a benign (not cancerous) tumor on the parathyroid gland. This form of hypercalcemia is usually mild and can be present for many years before being noticed.

- **Cancer:** Cancer can cause hypercalcemia when it spreads to the bones, which releases calcium into the blood, or when cancer causes a hormone similar to PTH to increase calcium levels.

Other causes of hypercalcemia include:

- hyperthyroidism
- sarcoidosis
- tuberculosis
- bone breaks combined with bed rest or not moving for a long period of time

- excess vitamin D intake
- kidney transplant
- high protein levels (for example, if a tourniquet is used for too long while blood is collected)—in this case, free or ionized calcium remains normal

High levels of ionized calcium occur with all the above, except high protein levels.

Low calcium levels, called hypocalcemia, mean that you do not have enough calcium in your blood or that you don't have enough protein in your blood. The most common cause of low total calcium is low protein levels, especially low albumin. When low protein is the problem, the ionized calcium level remains normal.

Low calcium, known as hypocalcemia, is caused by many conditions:

- low protein levels
- underactive parathyroid gland (hypoparathyroidism)
- decreased dietary intake of calcium
- decreased levels of vitamin D
- magnesium deficiency
- too much phosphorus
- acute inflammation of the pancreas
- chronic renal failure
- calcium ions becoming bound to protein (alkalosis)
- bone disease
- malnutrition
- alcoholism

Causes of low ionized calcium levels include all the above, except low protein levels.

Please note: Numerically reported test results are interpreted according to the test's reference range, which may vary by the patient's age, sex, as well as the instrumentation or kit used to perform the test. A specific result within the reference (normal) range—for any test—does not ensure health just as a result outside the reference range may not indicate disease. To learn the reference range for your test, consult your doctor or laboratorian. Lab Tests Online recommends you consult your physician to discuss your test results as a part of a complete medical examination.

Is there anything else I should know?

Two hormones control blood calcium within a small range of values. Parathyroid hormone (PTH) is produced by a group of small glands in the neck (near the thyroid gland), stimulated by a decrease in ionized calcium. PTH causes the release of calcium from bone and decreases calcium losses from the kidneys, so that calcium levels rise. PTH also stimulates activation of vitamin D by the kidneys.

Vitamin D, in turn, increases calcium absorption in the intestine, but decreases calcium lost from the kidneys in urine. Overall, as vitamin D levels rise, calcium levels rise and PTH falls. In healthy people, these two hormones keep blood calcium at normal levels, even though maintaining that balance in the blood may cause calcium to be released from bones.

Newborns, especially premature and low birthweight infants, often are monitored during the first few days of life for neonatal hypocalcemia. This can occur because of an immature parathyroid gland and doesn't always cause symptoms. The condition may resolve itself or may require treatment with supplemental calcium, given orally or intravenously.

Blood and urine calcium measurements cannot tell how much calcium is in the bones. A test similar to an x-ray, called a bone density or Dexa Scan, is needed for this purpose.

Taking thiazide diuretic drugs (drugs that encourage urination) is the most common drug-induced reason for a high calcium level.

Should I be concerned if my doctor only orders a regular calcium and not free or ionized calcium?

No. The total calcium is sufficient for most screening purposes. Free or ionized calcium is particularly important during surgery as well in severely ill patients, when changes in total calcium do not reliably tell how abnormal the free calcium level is.

What foods are high in calcium?

Dairy products are the main source of calcium, but lesser amounts are found in eggs, green leafy vegetables, broccoli, legumes, nuts, and whole grains. Many fruit juices are now fortified with calcium.

If I consume foods fortified with calcium, would it change my laboratory results?

In general, consuming fortified foods will not affect your calcium test results.

Can I perform this test at home?

No. While there are handheld instruments available, these are intended for use in a hospital or medical office setting and must be operated by trained personnel.

Section 18.5

Calcium-Pentagastrin Test

"Calcium-Pentagastrin Test," Warren Grant Magnuson Clinical Center, National Institutes of Health (NIH), 1999. Reviewed in November 2004 by David A. Cooke, M.D., Diplomate, American Board of Internal Medicine.

You are scheduled for a calcium-pentagastrin test. It helps your doctor assess how your glands are working. Specifically, the test shows the activity of special cells in your thyroid. Throughout the test, blood samples will be taken to measure how your body responds to calcium and pentagastrin.

Preparation

- Do not eat or drink after midnight on the day of the test.
- An I.V. (intravenous line) will be placed in a vein in each arm. Calcium and pentagastrin will be given through one line; blood samples will be taken through the other.

Procedure

- You will be asked to rest in a reclining chair.

- Calcium will be given through the I.V. You may feel muscle weakness, numbness, tingling, or changes in your heartbeat.

- One minute after you have been given calcium, you will be given pentagastrin. You may feel like you have heartburn, an unusual taste in your mouth, tiredness, flushing, warmth, and nausea.

- Blood samples will be taken after calcium and pentagastrin have been given.

- The test lasts 20 minutes.

After the Procedure

- The I.V. lines will be removed, and you may eat breakfast. You may continue your usual activities.

- The side effects from calcium and pentagastrin will go away when the test is over. There are usually no long-term effects from these substances.

If you have questions about the procedure, please ask. Your nurse and doctor are ready to assist you.

Section 18.6

Antithyroid Microsomal Antibody

"Antithyroid Microsomal Antibody," © 2003 A.D.A.M., Inc.
Reprinted with permission.

Alternative names: Thyroid antimicrosomal antibody; Antimicrosomal antibody; Microsomal antibody

Definition: This is a test to measure antithyroid microsomal antibodies in the blood. Microsomes are small cell particles.

How the Test Is Performed

Blood is drawn from a vein, usually on the inside of the elbow or the back of the hand. The puncture site is cleaned with antiseptic, and an elastic band is placed around the upper arm to apply pressure and restrict blood flow through the vein. This causes veins below the band to fill with blood.

A needle is inserted into the vein, and the blood is collected in an air-tight vial or a syringe. During the procedure, the band is removed to restore circulation. Once the blood has been collected, the needle is removed, and the puncture site is covered to stop any bleeding.

For an infant or young child: The area is cleansed with antiseptic and punctured with a sharp needle or a lancet. The blood may be collected in a pipette (small glass tube), on a slide, onto a test strip, or into a small container. Cotton or a bandage may be applied to the puncture site if there is any continued bleeding.

How to Prepare for the Test

Fasting may be required for 6 to 8 hours before the test (usually overnight). Medications that affect the test will be monitored or discontinued during the test.

How the Test Will Feel

When the needle is inserted to draw blood, some people feel moderate pain, while others feel only a prick or stinging sensation. Afterward, there may be some throbbing.

Why the Test Is Performed

This test is performed to confirm the cause of thyroid problems or other autoimmune disorders. The body produces microsomal antibodies in response to microsomes escaping from damaged thyroid cells. Such autoantibodies are usually present in Hashimoto thyroiditis. However, they can also be increased in other autoimmune disorders.

Normal Values

A negative test is normal.

What Abnormal Results Mean

A positive test may indicate:

- autoimmune hemolytic anemia
- granulomatous thyroiditis
- Hashimoto thyroiditis
- nontoxic nodular goiter
- rheumatoid arthritis
- Sjögren's syndrome
- systemic lupus erythematosus
- thyroid carcinoma

Additional conditions under which the test may be performed:

- autoimmune hepatitis

What the Risks Are

- excessive bleeding
- fainting or feeling light-headed
- hematoma (blood accumulating under the skin)
- infection (a slight risk any time the skin is broken)
- multiple punctures to locate veins

Special Considerations

Veins and arteries vary in size from one patient to another and from one side of the body to the other. Obtaining a blood sample from some people may be more difficult than from others.

Section 18.7

Parathyroid Hormone (PTH)

"PTH: The Test Sample, The Test," © 2004 American Association for Clinical Chemistry. Reprinted with permission. For additional information on clinical lab testing, visit the Lab Tests Online website at www.labtestsonline.org

The Test Sample

Also known as: Intact PTH, Parathormone

Formally known as: Parathyroid Hormone

Related tests: Calcium, Phosphorus, Magnesium, Vitamin D

The Test Sample

What is being tested?

Parathyroid hormone (PTH) helps the body maintain stable levels of calcium in the blood. It is part of a feedback loop that includes calcium, PTH, vitamin D, and to some extent phosphorus and magnesium. Conditions and diseases that disrupt this feedback loop can cause inappropriate elevations or decreases in calcium and PTH levels and lead to symptoms of hypercalcemia or hypocalcemia.

PTH is produced by four parathyroid glands that are located in the neck beside the thyroid. Normally, these glands secrete PTH into the bloodstream in response to low blood calcium levels. Parathyroid hormone then works in three ways to help raise blood calcium levels back to normal. It takes calcium from the body's bone, stimulates the activation of vitamin D in the kidney (which in turn increases the absorption of calcium from the intestines), and suppresses the excretion of calcium in the urine (while encouraging excretion of phosphorus). As calcium levels begin to increase in the blood, PTH normally decreases.

How is the sample collected for testing?

A blood sample is obtained by inserting a needle into a vein in the arm.

The Test

How is it used?

PTH is ordered to diagnose the cause of a low or high calcium level. PTH is used to differentiate between a parathyroid and non-parathyroid problem and to diagnose a parathyroid tumor.

PTH is also used to diagnose hyperparathyroidism. Hyperparathyroidism is separated into primary, secondary, and tertiary hyperthyroidism. Primary hyperparathyroidism is most frequently due to a parathyroid tumor (usually benign, but very rarely cancerous) that secretes PTH without feedback control. This puts PTH constantly in the "on" position, where it can cause hypercalcemia, and can lead to kidney stones, calcium deposits in organs, and decalcification of bone. With primary hyperparathyroidism, patients will generally have high calcium and high PTH levels.

Secondary and tertiary hyperparathyroidism are usually due to kidney failure. In patients with kidney disease and/or failure, phosphorus may not be excreted efficiently, disrupting its balance with calcium. As phosphorus levels build up, PTH is secreted. Depending on the severity of the condition and the state of the kidneys the imbalance may be mild (secondary—causing high PTH levels and low or normal calcium levels), or severe (tertiary—causing high PTH and high calcium).

Along with other tests, PTH can be used to diagnose hypoparathyroidism and be used to monitor patients who have conditions or diseases that cause chronic calcium imbalances, and monitor those who have had surgery or other treatment for parathyroid tumors.

Calcium should be monitored at the same time as PTH: It is not just their levels in the blood that is important, but the balance between the two and the response of the parathyroid to changing levels of calcium. Usually doctors are concerned about either severe imbalances in calcium metabolism (that may require medical intervention), or in persistent imbalances (that indicate an underlying problem).

When is it ordered?

PTH is not part of a general screen, but is often ordered when a screen for calcium is abnormal. PTH may be ordered when you have hypercalcemia, which may cause symptoms such as: fatigue, nausea, abdominal pain, and thirst. PTH may also be ordered when you have hypocalcemia, which may cause symptoms such as: abdominal pain, muscle cramps, and tingling fingers. One uncommon cause of hypocalcemia is hypoparathyroidism. Your doctor may order a PTH, along with calcium (and other tests) as a monitoring tool when you have had treatment for diseases or conditions that affect calcium regulation, such as the removal of a parathyroid tumor, or when you have chronic conditions such as kidney disease.

What does the test result mean?

A PTH level needs to be evaluated relative to a calcium level; the doctor will look to see if they are in balance as they should be. If both PTH and calcium levels are normal, then it is likely that the body's calcium regulation system is functioning properly.

Low levels of PTH may be due to conditions causing hypercalcemia, or to an abnormality in PTH production causing hypoparathyroidism. Excess PTH secretion may be due to hyperparathyroidism, which is most frequently caused by a benign parathyroid tumor.

Calcium and PTH Relationship

- If calcium levels are low and PTH levels high, then PTH is responding as it should. Depending on the degree of hypocalcemia, your doctor may investigate the low calcium further by looking at your vitamin D, phosphorus, and magnesium levels.

- If calcium levels are low and PTH levels are normal or low, then PTH is not responding and you probably have hypoparathyroidism.

- If calcium levels are high and PTH levels are high, then your parathyroid gland is producing inappropriate amounts of PTH and your doctor may order x-rays or other imaging studies to check for the cause and severity of hyperparathyroidism.

- If calcium levels are high and PTH levels are low, then your calcium regulation system is functioning, but your doctor will do further investigation to check for non-parathyroid related reasons for your elevated calcium.

173

Table 18.1. Calcium–PTH Relationship

Calcium	PTH	Interpretation
Normal	Normal	Calcium regulation system functioning okay.
Low	High	PTH is responding correctly; may run other tests to check hypocalcemia.
Low	Normal/Low	PTH not responding correctly; probably have hypoparathyroidism.
High	High	Parathyroid gland producing too much PTH, may do imaging studies to check for hyper-parathyroidism.
High	Low	PTH is responding correctly; may run other tests to check for non-parathyroid-related reasons for elevated calcium.

Please note: Numerically reported test results are interpreted according to the test's reference range, which may vary by the patient's age, sex, as well as the instrumentation or kit used to perform the test. A specific result within the reference (normal) range—for any test—does not ensure health just as a result outside the reference range may not indicate disease. To learn the reference range for your test, consult your doctor or laboratorian. Lab Tests Online recommends you consult your physician to discuss your test results as a part of a complete medical examination.

Is there anything else I should know?

- Intact PTH is broken down into several molecular fragments including: an N-terminal, a C-terminal, and a midregion. While each of these fragments can give the doctor information about calcium regulation, intact PTH is measured most frequently as it is the major biologically active form.

- PTH levels will vary during the day, peaking about 2 a.m. Specimens are usually drawn about 8 a.m.

- Drugs that may increase PTH levels include: phosphates, anticonvulsants, steroids, isoniazid, lithium, and rifampin.

- Drugs that may decrease PTH include cimetidine and propranolol.

Section 18.8

Thyroglobulin (Tg)

The Test

Formally known as: Thyroglobulin (Tg)

Related tests: Thyroglobulin antibody, Tumor markers

The Test

How is it used?

The main use of the thyroglobulin test is as a tumor marker to determine the effectiveness of thyroid cancer treatment and to monitor for recurrence. Since thyroglobulin normally is made only in the thyroid, it should drop to very low or undetectable levels in patients who have had their thyroid completely removed as part of thyroid cancer treatment. There are several types of thyroid cancer; only the most common types (papillary and follicular thyroid cancer) that arise from the follicle cells can make thyroglobulin. Thyroglobulin testing also is used at times to help determine the cause of hyperthyroidism.

Based on the results of a thyroglobulin test, your doctor may follow-up with a radioactive iodine scan (iodine is needed to make thyroid hormones) and/or radioactive iodine treatments to identify and/or destroy any remaining normal thyroid tissue or thyroid cancer. Your thyroglobulin levels will be checked again in a few weeks or months to verify that the therapy has worked.

When is it ordered?

A thyroglobulin test may be ordered after the surgical removal of your thyroid gland for cancer so your doctor can check for any normal and/or cancerous thyroid tissue that may have been left behind.

It is often ordered on a regular basis, even if negative after surgery, to make sure that the tumor has not come back or spread.

A thyroglobulin test also may be ordered if your doctor suspects that you have symptoms of Graves disease or thyroiditis, such as hyperthyroidism and/or an enlarged thyroid gland.

What does the test result mean?

Thyroglobulin levels should be undetectable or very low after a thyroidectomy (surgical removal of the thyroid) and/or after subsequent radioactive iodine treatments. If levels are still detectable, there may be normal or cancerous thyroid tissue remaining in your body.

If the level is low a few weeks or months after surgery and then begins to rise over time, the cancer is probably recurring.

Please note: Numerically reported test results are interpreted according to the test's reference range, which may vary by the patient's age, sex, as well as the instrumentation or kit used to perform the test. A specific result within the reference (normal) range—for any test—does not ensure health just as a result outside the reference range may not indicate disease. To learn the reference range for your test, consult your doctor or laboratorian. Lab Tests Online recommends you consult your physician to discuss your test results as a part of a complete medical examination.

Is there anything else I should know?

Elevated levels of thyroglobulin do not in themselves imply a poor prognosis. In monitoring for cancer recurrence, change over time is more important than one particular thyroglobulin test result.

It is important to have serial thyroglobulin tests performed at the same laboratory because test methods may produce different results in different laboratories.

Fifteen to twenty percent of thyroid cancer patients have antibodies to thyroglobulin called thyroglobulin antibodies or thyroglobulin autoantibodies. These antibodies can interfere with thyroglobulin testing, leading to falsely low or high results depending on the method used. For this reason, many laboratories will measure anti-thyroglobulin antibodies at the same time as thyroglobulin.

Chapter 19

Thyroid Ultrasound

Once a thyroid nodule has been detected (or suspected), there are a few things that the physician wants to know before any recommendations can be made regarding what actions to take. Remember, the vast majority of thyroid nodules are benign and nothing to worry about, so the focus is on determining which ones have any reasonable chance of being cancerous. It is those few worrisome nodules which will need to be operated upon with that portion of the thyroid removed.

One of the first tests which is routinely performed is the fine needle aspiration (FNA) biopsy. The FNA will usually (but not always) tell if a nodule is benign or malignant. Often this is the only test which is needed.

Another test which is routinely performed is the ultrasound. This simple test uses sound waves to image the thyroid. The sound waves are emitted from a small hand-held transducer which is passed over the thyroid. A lubricant jelly is placed on the skin so that the sound waves transmit easier through the skin and into the thyroid and surrounding structures. This test is quick, accurate, cheap, painless, and completely safe. It usually takes only about 10 minutes and the results can be known almost immediately. Not all nodules need this test, but it is almost routine.

During an ultrasound of the thyroid gland, the probe is placed on the skin and sound waves are directed deep into the neck and thyroid. As sound waves hit structures they bounce back like an echo. The probe

"Thyroid Nodule Ultrasound: What is it, what does it tell me?" by James Norman, M.D., Norman Endocrine Surgery Clinic, Tampa, Florida. © 2003 Endocrine Surgery Clinic. Reprinted with permission.

detects these reflections to make pictures. An ultrasound of the thyroid can show a nodule or be programmed to detect blood flow. If it is a simple cyst filled with serous fluid, then it will not show blood flow.

There are certain characteristics of thyroid nodules seen on ultrasound which are more worrisome than others. Keep in mind, however, that ultrasound alone cannot make the diagnosis of cancer. This test will usually help tell that the nodule has a low chance of being cancer (has characteristics of a benign nodule), or that it has some characteristics of a cancerous nodule and therefore a biopsy is indicated.

Ultrasound Characteristics Which Suggest a Benign Nodule

- Nice sharp edges are seen all around the nodule
- Nodule filled with fluid and not live tissue (a cyst)
- Lots of nodules throughout the thyroid (almost always a benign multi-nodular goiter)
- No blood flowing through it (not live tissue, likely a cyst)

If a nodule does have a few worrisome characteristics, a fine needle aspirate biopsy may be performed. In this test, a very small needle is passed into the nodule and some cells are aspirated out and then placed on a glass slide for a pathologist to stain and determine if they are malignant or not. This test is very simple, takes less than 30 seconds, is virtually pain free, and can be very accurate. If it is read as cancer, this test is almost always right. Sometimes, however, there are not enough cells removed, or some but not all cells look abnormal. In this case, the pathologist will not be able to tell cancer from a benign nodule. This situation usually dictates that the test be repeated or that the patient undergoes surgical removal of this part of the thyroid. Remember, the vast majority of nodules are benign, and even if it is cancer, most thyroid cancers are extremely curable.

Additional Information

Norman Endocrine Surgery Clinic
505 South Boulevard
Tampa, FL 33606
Phone: 813-991-6922
Fax: 813-991-6918
Website: http://www.endocrineweb.com

Chapter 20

Thyroid Fine Needle Aspiration Biopsy

You are scheduled for a thyroid fine needle aspiration biopsy (FNAB). During this procedure, your doctor takes cells from your thyroid gland to diagnose your thyroid problem. This procedure is usually done in a treatment room by your doctor(s), with the help of a nurse. A technician with a microscope is also present in the room. Sometimes, this procedure is done by a radiologist.

Before the procedure, the doctor will explain everything to you, including the risks and benefits. When you have a good understanding of what will be done, you will be asked to sign a consent form giving permission to do the procedure. Please feel free to ask any questions you may have.

Preparation

There is no special preparation. You may eat or drink whatever you like right up to the time of the procedure. But for your comfort, please empty your bladder before the procedure.

In some cases, your doctor may ask you to have a blood test done within 7 days before your biopsy. The purpose of this is to check your bleeding times to make sure that your blood clots normally.

If you are taking medications that contain aspirin (such as Anacin, Bayer, Bufferin, Ecotrin, Excedrin, or cough/cold remedies) or nonsteroidal antiinflammatory medications (such as Advil, Aleve, Celebrex,

"Thyroid Fine Needle Aspiration Biopsy (FNAB)," Warren Grant Magnuson Clinical Center, National Institutes of Health (NIH), November 2001.

ibuprofen, Mobic, Motrin, or Naproxen), please inform your doctor before the biopsy. If you don't know whether your medication contains these ingredients, please ask your doctor, nurse, or pharmacist.

Procedure

- You will be helped to lie on your back on the treatment room table. A towel or small blanket will be placed under your shoulders so that your head and neck will be tilted back. This position gives the doctor the best access to your neck.

- Your doctor will look closely at your neck, and will also feel your neck with his or her fingers and hands. Then the skin on your neck will be cleansed with a liquid containing iodine and alcohol.

- A thin needle attached to a syringe will be inserted through the skin of your neck and into your thyroid gland. The size of the needle is the same as the one used for blood draws from your forearm.

- As the needle is inserted into your neck, you may feel pushing, pressure, or slight pain. (Most patients say that this feels like having a blood draw from the forearm.) While the needle is in your neck, you will not be allowed to swallow, talk, laugh, cough, sneeze, or move your neck or upper body.

- Your doctor will aspirate (pull back) thyroid cells into the syringe. The syringe will then be passed to a technician who will prepare the cells to be seen under a microscope. For your biopsy to be useful, enough thyroid cells must be taken. It usually takes between four and eight needle passes to obtain enough thyroid cells. The procedure takes about 1 hour.

After the Procedure

After the biopsy, an ice pack may be placed over the site to decrease any swelling or bleeding. A small bandage will be put on your neck. You will stay in the treatment room for about an hour so that your nurse can observe you for any complications.

When you are released from the treatment room, you may resume your normal activities. If you have neck discomfort, you may take an over-the-counter pain reliever containing acetaminophen (such as Tylenol), if this does not conflict with other medical conditions or treatments. Do not take medications containing aspirin or nonsteroidal anti-inflammatory for 5 days after the biopsy.

To prevent infection, keep the biopsy site clean and dry by wearing the bandage for 8 hours. After this time, you may remove the bandage and shower or bathe as usual.

Complications

Complications from this procedure are rare, but check the biopsy site regularly. If any of the following occurs, contact your doctor immediately. If the symptoms are severe, go immediately to your nearest emergency department:

- difficulty swallowing
- bleeding
- increased redness
- increased swelling
- persistent or increasing pain
- discharge (pus) from the site
- persistent cough

Please be aware that it is not possible for the doctor or technician to give you a firm diagnosis at the time of the biopsy. In most cases, final biopsy results are ready in 1 to 2 weeks. Your doctor will contact you to discuss the test results and recommend treatments.

If you have any questions about the procedure, ask your doctor or nurse. They are always ready to assist you.

Chapter 21

Thyroid Scan Uptake Study

You are scheduled for a thyroid scan/thyroid uptake study. These studies help your doctor learn if there is a change from normal in your thyroid gland. They are safe, effective, and painless ways to get picture information of your thyroid gland.

The scans use a compound containing a small amount of radioactive material. The scans are done for diagnostic purposes, and will take place in the nuclear medicine department.

Preparation

Do not eat or drink 2 hours before or 1 hour after you receive the dose of the compound.

Procedure

You may have only a thyroid scan, or a thyroid scan with thyroid uptakes.

Thyroid Scan

You will be given a small amount of radioactive iodine to take by mouth 4 hours before the scan. After this time, the scan will be started. You will lie down on an examination table. A pillow will be placed

"Thyroid Scan/Thyroid Uptake Study," Warren Grant Magnuson Clinical Center, National Institutes of Health (NIH), March 2000.

under your shoulders to extend your neck so that the thyroid can be easily scanned. Pictures will be taken with a very sensitive machine called a gamma camera that receives and records the radiation in your thyroid gland.

Thyroid Scan and Thyroid Uptake

You will be given a small amount of radioactive iodine by mouth. You will be asked to return either 4 hours and 24 hours later, or only 24 hours later. You will be asked to sit in a chair while a small probe is placed in front of your neck. This probe detects any change from normal in your thyroid gland.

- The scan, without uptake, lasts about one hour.
- The scan, with uptake, lasts about one and a half hours.

After the Procedure

There are no adverse effects. Your body rids itself of the compound as it does the food you eat. If you have questions about the procedure, please ask. Your nurse and doctor are ready to assist you at all times.

Special Instructions

- You should not have had any I.V. contrast for at least 4 weeks before this study.
- Do not eat any seaweed (as in sushi) for 4 weeks before the scan. (I.V. contrast and seaweed contain a lot of iodine, which will interfere with the test.)
- If you take thyroid medications, these should usually be stopped before this test. Ask your doctor if and when you should stop taking these medications.
- Because it uses radioactivity, this study is not performed in pregnant women. If you are pregnant or think you might be pregnant, please inform your doctor immediately so that a decision can be made about this study.
- Also, please inform your doctor immediately if you are breastfeeding. Some studies can be performed in breastfeeding women if they are willing to stop breastfeeding for a while.

Chapter 22

Parathyroid Scans

Parathyroid Scan for Information about Parathyroid Glands

You are scheduled for a parathyroid scan. This scan will help your doctor locate any abnormal parathyroid glands. The scan is a safe, effective, and painless way to get information about your parathyroid glands.

The scan uses two compounds containing a small amount of radioactive material, and is done for diagnostic purposes. This scan will be done in the nuclear medicine department.

Preparation

There is no special preparation. You may eat and drink whatever you like before the scan.

Procedure

- You will be asked to lie down on an examination table.
- A pillow may be placed under your shoulders with your neck extended.

"Parathyroid Scan," Warren Grant Magnuson Clinical Center, National Institutes of Health, March 2000. And "Sestamibi Scan for Parathyroid Disease," by James Norman, M.D., Norman Endocrine Surgery Clinic, Tampa, Florida. © 2004 Norman Endocrine Surgery Clinic. Reprinted with permission.

- You will be given two injections by vein: technetium pertechnetate and technetium sestamibi.

- After each injection, pictures will be taken with a very sensitive camera, called a gamma camera. This device receives and records the radiation in your thyroid and parathyroid glands. Please lie very still so that clear pictures can be taken.

- The scan lasts about 3 hours.

After the Procedure

- Drink plenty of liquids to flush the radioactive tracer from your body. The fluids also help keep your kidneys healthy.

- If you have questions about the procedure, please ask. Your nurse and doctor are ready to assist you at all times.

Special Instructions

- Because it uses radioactivity, this scan is not performed in pregnant women. If you are pregnant or think you might be pregnant, please inform your doctor immediately so that a decision can be made about this scan.

- Also, please inform your doctor immediately if you are breastfeeding. Some scans can be performed in breastfeeding women if they are willing to stop breastfeeding for a while.

Sestamibi Scanning for Parathyroid Tumors

The sestamibi scan locates problem parathyroid glands and parathyroid tumors. The sestamibi scan will show which parathyroid gland is bad.

Sestamibi scanning is the preferred way to localize diseased parathyroid glands prior to an operation. This scan was invented in the early 1990s and now is widely available at essentially every hospital in the United States. Sestamibi is a small protein which is labeled with the radio-pharmaceutical technetium-99. This very mild and safe radioactive agent is injected into the veins of a patient with parathyroid disease (hyperparathyroidism) and is absorbed by the overactive parathyroid gland. Since normal parathyroid glands are inactive when there is high calcium in the bloodstream, they do not take up the radioactive particles. When an x-ray machine is placed over the patient's neck an accurate picture will show the overactive gland.

When a parathyroid gland is making too much parathyroid hormone it will become radioactive during the scan, making a bright yellow spot on the patient's sestamibi scan. Since the normal parathyroids are not producing any hormone, they do not absorb radioactivity and therefore do not show up on this scan. Only the overactive parathyroid gland shows up—a very accurate test.

A parathyroid tumor that is making too much parathyroid hormone will show up as a "hot" spot in the neck on the sestamibi scan. When performing a minimally invasive radioguided parathyroid (MIRP) surgery, or mini parathyroid operation, the little radioactive probe that the surgeon uses in the operating room will find this radioactive tumor allowing the operation to be performed under local anesthesia, typically in less than 30 minutes.

Remember, a sestamibi scan is a very safe procedure. There is no cross-reactivity for other types of x-ray dye, so parathyroid patients with allergies to x-ray dye can have a sestamibi scan. Also note that the sestamibi drug used to show the over-active parathyroid gland is the exact same drug that is used to perform cardiac stress tests—it

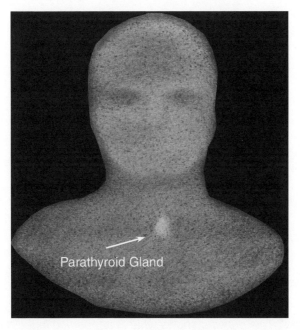

Figure 22.1. *Sestamibi scanning will reveal an overactive parathyroid gland.*

is very safe. The type of radioactivity used is the mildest radioactive agent used in all of medicine. You are in no danger and your family can stay with you—it is not dangerous to them (or your doctor).

Parathyroid Surgery and Mini Parathyroid Surgery Uses Sestamibi Scanning

The sestamibi scan will display the hyperactive parathyroid gland which is causing hyperparathyroidism in about 90 percent (90% sensitivity) of all patients. When it does show a single hot gland, it is correct about 98% of the time. When combined with the probe in the operating room (the MIRP mini parathyroid operation), the cure rate can be over 99%. It takes approximately two hours to perform the

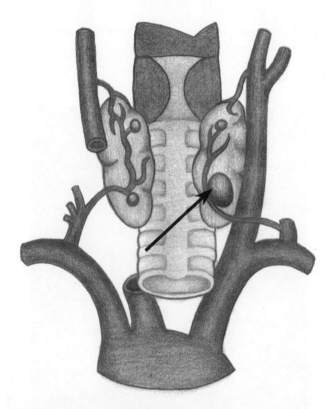

Figure 22.2. *This drawing shows what is happening in the patient undergoing the Sestamibi scan depicted in Figure 22.1. One of the parathyroid glands is enlarged.*

sestamibi scan. Pictures of the neck and chest are usually taken immediately after the injection and again in 1.75 to 2.0 hours.

The biggest problem with sestamibi scanning is the variability in scans from hospital to hospital. Because most hospitals and radiology departments see only a few parathyroid patients per year, they do not get many opportunities to perform this test.

There is a very high correlation between hospitals that do a lot of sestamibi scanning (more than 100 per year) and their accuracy. Like other aspects of treating parathyroid disease, the experience of the doctors involved makes a difference.

Additional Information

Norman Endocrine Surgery Clinic
505 South Boulevard
Tampa, FL 33606
Phone: 813-991-6922
Fax: 813-991-6918
Website: http://www.endocrineweb.com

Chapter 23

Diagnostic Positron Emission Tomography (PET) Scan

You are scheduled for a diagnostic PET (positron emission tomography) scan. A PET scan uses small amounts of radioactivity to take detailed pictures of different areas inside the body. Diagnostic PET scans use one type of radioactive compound: fluorinated deoxyglucose (F18-FDG). They can help your health care team do one of the following:

- diagnose and treat cancer

- locate parts of the brain causing epileptic seizures

- check the brain for recurrent cancer or damage from radiation therapy

What does PET mean?

The letters P E stand for positron emission. This is the scientific term for the type of radioactivity attached to the compound you will be given. T stands for tomography. Tomography means that the radioactivity can be detected at many angles as you move through the scanner. By using many angles, the scanner can make detailed pictures of sections of your body.

"Positron Emission Tomography (PET) Scan–Diagnostic," Warren Grant Magnuson Clinical Center, National Institutes of Health, October 2003.

How does PET differ from other scans, like CT?

Computerized tomography (CT) shows the shape and structure of your body's organs and tissues; PET shows how they work. Because of this, PET scans can often find changes in the body's tissues before changes can be seen in their structure.

Will the scan hurt?

The scan, itself, is painless. But you may feel sore after lying still for the time needed to complete the scan. You may also feel discomfort as a soft tube or small needle is placed into your vein (usually in the arm). The compound will be given to you through this tube or needle.

What if I cannot stay still for the scan?

If you are concerned about lying still for a long time, or if you have claustrophobia, you may need a sedative before the scan. The sedative may be given to you as a tablet. If you need sedation, make sure someone can drive you home.

How should I prepare for the scan?

- Be on time for your scan. The dose of compound you get is made precisely for the time of your injection.
- Do not eat for 4 to 6 hours before your appointment. However, you are encouraged to drink water and take your prescribed medications. Please note: You may drink water only. No gum, mints, or sugarless foods may be eaten.
  - For diagnostic brain scans: Do not eat for 4 hours before your appointment.
  - For diagnostic whole body scans: Do not eat for at least 6 hours before your appointment.
- If you have diabetes, follow your daily routine by eating small, normal meals. Take your insulin or oral medications as usual. Your blood sugar should be between 100 and 200 mg/dL before the scan. You may be asked to have your blood drawn in phlebotomy to measure your blood sugar level.
- If you are a woman of childbearing age, you will be asked to give a urine or blood sample to test for pregnancy. You will also

be asked to sign a card in the nuclear medicine department stating that you are not pregnant or breastfeeding a child.

What will happen?

- A soft, flexible tube (intravenous, or I.V.) or needle will be placed into one of your veins. You will receive the compound through this tube.

- After the compound is given, you will be asked to rest in a reclining chair in a quiet, darkened room. If you are having a brain scan, you will rest for 30 minutes; if you are having a body scan, you will rest for 50 minutes. This time allows your body to absorb the compound.

- To prevent the compound from going to your tongue and vocal cords, you may be asked not to speak. Take a book or CD player to help pass the time.

- When it is time for your scan, you will be asked to lie on your back on a table. This table slides into the PET scanner, a donut-shaped machine that looks like a CT scanner. Because scanning is almost noiseless, the room will stay quiet.

- For part of the scan, you may be asked to keep your arms raised above your head. This may be uncomfortable for some people, especially those with arthritis. Please be assured that every effort will be made to keep you comfortable. Pillows or cushions may be used to help you stay positioned.

- You will be asked to lie as still as possible so that the scanner can take clear pictures. Depending on which part of your body is being scanned, the test will last from 30 to 90 minutes.

What happens after the scan is complete?

- If you were not sedated, you may resume your usual routine. If you were sedated, do not drive yourself home—have someone else drive you. Even if you plan to take a taxi or other public transportation, please arrange for someone to go with you.

- Continue to drink plenty of fluids for the next 4 hours. You may drink any kind of liquid after the scan—you are not limited to water.

Part Four

Underactive Thyroid Gland Disorders

Chapter 24

Hypothyroidism

Chapter Contents

Section 24.1

Underactive Thyroid: Overview

Note: The recommendations given here are those of the American Thyroid Association (ATA). This advice cannot apply to every patient, and your doctor may make different suggestions. If you have any questions or concerns, check with your doctor.

What Is the Thyroid?

The thyroid gland is a butterfly-shaped endocrine gland that is normally located in the lower front of the neck. The thyroid's job is to make thyroid hormone. The main thyroid hormone is thyroxine, also called T4 because it contains four iodine molecules. Thyroid hormone is carried through the blood to every tissue in the body. Thyroid hormone is essential to help each cell in each tissue and organ to work right. For example, thyroid hormone helps the body use energy, stay warm, and keep the brain, heart, muscles, and other organs working as they should.

What Is Hypothyroidism?

Hypothyroidism is an underactive thyroid gland (hypo means under or below normal). Hypothyroidism means that the thyroid gland cannot make enough thyroid hormone to keep the body running normally. People are hypothyroid if they have too little thyroid hormone in their blood. Common causes are autoimmune disease, surgical removal of the thyroid, and radiation treatment. Low thyroid hormone levels cause the body's functions to slow down, leading to general symptoms like dry skin, fatigue, loss of energy, and memory problems. Hypothyroidism is diagnosed by a simple blood test for thyroid-stimulating hormone (TSH). Hypothyroidism is treated by replacing the missing thyroid hormone with synthetic thyroxine pills, which the person must take every day for life. With daily treatment, most patients recover completely.

Symptoms

When thyroid hormone levels are too low, the body's cells cannot get enough thyroid hormone and the body's processes start slowing down. For example, the body makes less heat and less energy, and organs like the brain and bowels move more slowly. As the body slows, you may notice that you feel colder, you tire more easily, your skin is getting drier, you are becoming forgetful and depressed, and you have started getting constipated.

You may also have body changes that you cannot feel. For example, you may not know that cholesterol is building up in your blood and plaque is hardening your arteries, increasing your risk for heart attack. So hypothyroidism doesn't just cause symptoms. It can make other conditions worse. Some people develop hypothyroidism quickly over a few months.

Some people develop it slowly over many years. In general, the lower thyroid hormone levels become and the longer they stay low, the more severe the symptoms will be. Subclinical (mild) hypothyroidism may cause mild symptoms or none at all. Severe hypothyroidism usually causes severe symptoms. But no one can predict exactly which symptoms a person will develop or how severe they will be. Some people are very sick by the time they learn their diagnosis; others whose blood tests show severe hypothyroidism have few if any symptoms.

Because the symptoms are so variable, the only way to know for sure whether you have hypothyroidism is with blood tests.

Common Features of Hypothyroidism

- Less energy
- More fatigue, trouble awakening in the morning, need for more sleep, and tendency to fall asleep during the day
- Feeling cold when other people feel warm
- Less sweating
- Drier, itchier skin
- Yellow or orange skin, caused by a build-up of the pigment carotene from fruits and vegetables

- Drier, coarser, more brittle hair
- More hair loss (the amount differs in different people; patients do not go bald, but their hair can look thin)
- Loss of appetite
- Mild weight gain (5–20 pounds) and difficulty losing weight (hypothyroidism doesn't cause obesity)
- New or worsening problems with memory, slower thinking
- New snoring
- More frequent and severe muscle cramps and joint aches
- New feeling of pins and needles in the hands and feet (paresthesia)
- New constipation
- New puffiness around the face (especially the eyes), hands, ankles, and feet because of fluid build-up
- Carpal tunnel syndrome
- Heavier and/or more frequent menstrual periods, worse cramps, worse premenstrual symptoms
- Feeling irritable
- New depression—sadness or not caring about anything
- New hoarse voice
- New hearing loss
- Goiter (swelling in the front of the neck, caused by enlargement of the thyroid; goiter is most likely to be part of Hashimoto thyroiditis)
- Shrinking thyroid (most likely in atrophic thyroiditis)
- Slowing of heart rate, reducing the blood flow and oxygen delivered to body tissues
- Slightly higher blood pressure, caused by stiffening of arteries
- Higher cholesterol levels

Causes

There can be many reasons why the cells in the thyroid gland can not make enough thyroid hormone. Here are the major causes, from the most to least common:

Autoimmune Disease

The immune system normally protects the body against bacterial and viral invaders. In autoimmune diseases (auto means self), the immune system mistakenly attacks a normal part of the body. In autoimmune hypothyroidism, the immune system accidentally attacks cells in the thyroid gland, interfering with their ability to make thyroid hormone. When enough thyroid cells have been destroyed, too few are left to meet the body's need for thyroid hormone. Autoimmune thyroid disease is more common in women than men. It can start at any age, but becomes more common as people get older. In women, it often begins during pregnancy, after delivery, or around menopause. The cause is probably a combination of an inherited tendency and an as yet unknown trigger. No one knows whether stress plays a role. Autoimmune thyroiditis can begin suddenly, but in most patients it develops slowly over years. The most common forms are Hashimoto thyroiditis and atrophic thyroiditis.

Surgical Removal of Part or All of the Thyroid Gland

Some people with thyroid nodules, thyroid cancer, or Graves disease need to have part or all of their thyroid removed. If the whole thyroid is removed, people will definitely become hypothyroid. If only part of the thyroid is removed, the remaining part may:

- Work well enough to keep thyroid hormone blood levels normal throughout the person's life.
- Never make enough thyroid hormone to keep blood levels normal.
- At first make enough thyroid hormone, but later become unable to meet the body's need for hormone.

Radiation Treatment

Some people with Graves disease, nodular goiter, or thyroid cancer are given radioactive iodine (I-131) to destroy their thyroid gland purposely. Patients with Hodgkin's disease, lymphoma, or cancers of the head or neck are treated with radiation. All these patients can lose part or all of their thyroid function.

Congenital Hypothyroidism (Hypothyroidism at Birth)

A few babies are born without a thyroid or with a partly formed thyroid. A few babies have part or all of their thyroid in the wrong place (ectopic thyroid). In some babies, the thyroid cells or their enzymes do not work right. Babies with any of these problems may be hypothyroid from birth. In some, the thyroid may make enough hormone for a while and then may no longer be able to keep up with the need, so the person becomes hypothyroid as an older child or even as an adult.

Thyroiditis

Thyroiditis is an inflammation of the thyroid gland, usually caused by an autoimmune attack (in postpartum thyroiditis or silent thyroiditis) or by a viral infection. Thyroiditis can make the thyroid release its whole supply of stored thyroid hormone into the blood at once, causing brief hyperthyroidism (an overactive thyroid); once all of the stored hormone has been released, the thyroid becomes underactive. Almost all patients with viral thyroiditis recover their thyroid function, but about one-fourth of patients with autoimmune thyroiditis have permanent hypothyroidism.

Medicines

Medicines like amiodarone, lithium, interferon alpha, and interleukin-2 can interfere with the thyroid gland's ability to make thyroid hormone. These drugs are most likely to trigger hypothyroidism in patients who have a genetic tendency to autoimmune thyroid disease. It is also possible that treatment with thalidomide for multiple myeloma can cause hypothyroidism.

Too Little or Too Much Iodine

The thyroid gland must have iodine to make thyroid hormone. Iodine comes into the body in foods, mainly dairy products, chicken, beef, pork, fish, and iodized salt. The iodine then travels through the blood to the thyroid. Keeping thyroid hormone production in balance requires the right amount of iodine. People who live in undeveloped parts of the world may not get enough iodine in their diet. Worldwide, iodine deficiency is the most common cause of hypothyroidism, although it is a rare cause in the U.S. Taking in too much iodine can also cause or worsen hypothyroidism. The major source of too much iodine is dietary supplements containing kelp, a kind of seaweed. Most such supplements are sold with the false promise of helping people lose weight. Other sources of too much iodine are x-ray dyes, medicines like amiodarone, and some older expectorants (medicines that help clear the lungs and throat).

Damage to the Pituitary Gland

The pituitary tells the thyroid how much hormone to make. If the pituitary is damaged by a tumor, radiation, or surgery, it may no longer be able to give the thyroid the right instructions, and the thyroid may stop making enough hormone.

Rare Disorders That Infiltrate the Thyroid

In a few people, diseases deposit abnormal substances in the thyroid. For example, amyloidosis can deposit amyloid protein, sarcoidosis can deposit granulomas, and hemochromatosis can deposit iron. These deposits can prevent the thyroid from working right.

What Does Not Cause Hypothyroidism?

- Soy does not cause hypothyroidism, but it does interfere with the body's ability to absorb thyroid replacement therapy.

- The amounts of broccoli, cabbage, and brussel sprouts that people eat in a normal diet do not cause hypothyroidism.

- There is no evidence that some people's thyroid gland makes enough hormone, but it does not get to the body's cells.

Who Is at Risk?

Hypothyroidism is one of the most common thyroid disorders. It affects people all over the world, of every age, sex, race, and level of wealth and education. About 2–3% of Americans have pronounced hypothyroidism, and as many as 10–15% have subclinical (mild) hypothyroidism. More than half of people who have hypothyroidism don't know it.

The most common cause of hypothyroidism is autoimmune disease. Risk factors for autoimmune hypothyroidism are:

- Family history: Having a relative with autoimmune thyroid disease.

- Older age: Hypothyroidism can start at any age, but the risk keeps growing as people get older.

- Being female: Hypothyroidism is more common in women than men. It is much more common in young women than young men, but as men get older, they start to catch up.

- Being white or Asian: Hypothyroidism is common in whites and Asians. African-Americans are at lower risk.

- Having another autoimmune disorder, such as type 1 diabetes, rheumatoid arthritis, multiple sclerosis, celiac disease, Addison's disease, pernicious anemia, vitiligo, or even prematurely gray hair.
- Having Down syndrome or Turner's syndrome.
- Having bipolar disease (manic-depression).

The rate of hypothyroidism goes up:

- During pregnancy
- After delivery
- Around menopause

Can Hypothyroidism Be Prevented?

In countries where the diet does not contain enough iodine, taking iodine supplements can prevent hypothyroidism. In developed countries like the U.S., where most people's diet contains enough iodine, there is no known way to keep from getting hypothyroidism.

The best way to prevent hypothyroidism from becoming severe is to diagnose it early by testing newborn babies, pregnant women, and people who have symptoms or risk factors. The biggest risk factor is having relatives with thyroid disease.

Diagnosis

The correct diagnosis of hypothyroidism depends on:

- the patient's symptoms, medical history, risk factors, and family history
- the physical exam
- blood tests for TSH and the free T4 or free T4 index

Symptoms

Hypothyroidism has no characteristic symptoms. There are no symptoms that everyone with hypothyroidism always has, but that no one with another disease ever has. This makes hypothyroidism hard to diagnose just by its symptoms. Most hypothyroid symptoms are common complaints that many people with a normal thyroid can have. These symptoms may not signal any serious underlying disease, or they might be clues to a number of serious conditions related, or unrelated to the thyroid.

If people have hypothyroidism but do not know it, they may go to many doctors trying to find out what is wrong with them. They may go to the dermatologist saying that their skin is dry, or to the gynecologist worrying about why their periods have gotten heavier, or to a psychiatrist saying they are depressed. It can work the other way, too: People might have some of the symptoms of hypothyroidism and think that is what is wrong with them, but it turns out that the symptoms are being caused by some other condition. For example, tiredness might really be caused by anemia. Hypothyroidism can also be hard to diagnose because in most people it develops slowly. One way to help figure out whether your complaints are symptoms of hypothyroidism is to think about whether you have always had a symptom (hypothyroidism is less likely), or whether the symptom is a change from the way you used to feel (hypothyroidism is more likely).

Medical and Family History

You should tell your doctor

- about changes in your health
- if you have ever had thyroid surgery
- if you have ever had radiation to your neck to treat cancer
- if you are taking any of the medicines that can cause hypothyroidism: amiodarone, lithium, interferon alpha, interleukin-2, and maybe thalidomide
- whether anyone in your family has thyroid disease; this makes it more likely that you do, too

Physical Exam

The doctor will check your thyroid gland and look for changes like dry skin, swelling, slower reflexes, and a slower heart rate.

Blood Tests

TSH Test

TSH (thyroid-stimulating hormone) is the most important and sensitive test for hypothyroidism. TSH is a simple blood test that measures how much T4 the thyroid gland is being asked to make. An abnormally high TSH means hypothyroidism: The thyroid gland is being asked to make more T4 because there is not enough T4 in the blood.

Your thyroid needs to be told how much thyroid hormone to make. The instructions come from the pituitary gland below your brain. The system works as a feedback loop: Special cells in your pituitary gland determine the normal T4 range for your body—your set point. As blood flows through your pituitary, these cells measure the T4 levels and can tell whether or not they are at your set point.

The pituitary cells communicate with your thyroid gland by sending their own hormone, TSH (thyroid-stimulating hormone), into the blood. When your T4 levels are at your set point, the pituitary sends out enough TSH to tell the thyroid gland to keep making the same amount of T4. If your T4 levels get low, the pituitary sends out more TSH to tell the thyroid to make more T4. The lower your T4 levels go, the higher your TSH goes, as your pituitary asks your thyroid to work harder and make more T4. The opposite is also true: If your T4 levels get too high, the pituitary sends out less TSH, telling your thyroid to make less T4.

Table 24.1. Normal and Abnormal TSH Levels (Milliunit per Liter–mU/L)

Thyroid Condition	TSH Level (m/U/L)
hyperthyroidism or suppressed TSH	0.0–0.4
normal range	0.4–4.0
at risk: repeat TSH test at least once a year	2.5–4.0
subclinical (mild)hypothyroidism	4.0–10.0
hypothyroidism	10.0 and above

In most labs, the normal range for TSH is 0.4 mU/L to 4.0 mU/L (Table 24.1). If your TSH is above 4.0 mU/L on both a first test and a repeat test, you probably have hypothyroidism.

Most people whose thyroid works normally have a TSH between 0.4 and 2.5 mU/L. If your TSH is above 2.5 mU/L, your doctor should test your blood for anti-thyroid peroxidase (anti-TPO) antibodies. If you have these antibodies, your immune system may be attacking your thyroid and you may be at risk for developing hypothyroidism. You should have the TSH test repeated at least once a year. There is no need to repeat a positive anti-TPO test.

Remember: As the T4 falls, the TSH rises (as the thyroid hormone supply falls, the demand increases). As the T4 rises, the TSH falls (as the supply rises, the demand falls).

There is one exception to the rule that everyone with hypothyroidism has a high TSH. If the pituitary stops working right, it may not be able to send out normal amounts of TSH. The thyroid may be healthy, but if it does not get enough TSH, it won't make enough T4. This disorder is called secondary hypothyroidism. Fortunately, it is quite rare.

T4 Tests

Most of the T4 in the blood is attached to a protein called thyroxine-binding globulin. This bound T4 cannot get into body cells. Only about 1–2% of T4 in the blood is unattached (free) and can get into cells. The free T4 and the free T4 index are both simple blood tests that measure how much unattached T4 is in the blood and available to get into cells.

Ways That Hypothyroidism Cannot Be Diagnosed

- **Low body temperature** is not a reliable measure of hypothyroidism. Some hypothyroid patients—but also many healthy people—regularly have a temperature well below 98.6 degrees Fahrenheit (F).

- **Reflexes** may be slowed in hypothyroidism, but in many other conditions, too.

- **Saliva tests** for thyroid disease are not accurate.

- **Swelling in the base of the neck:** An underactive thyroid may look like a normal thyroid, or it may be larger or smaller. Even if your thyroid looks normal, you can have thyroid disease.

Treatment

Thyroxine (T4) Replacement

Hypothyroidism cannot be cured. No one has discovered a way to make the thyroid gland start to work normally again. But with daily treatment, taken every day for life, hypothyroidism can be completely controlled in almost every patient. It is treated by replacing the amount of hormone that your own thyroid can no longer make, to bring your T4 and TSH back to normal levels. So even if your thyroid gland cannot work right, T4 replacement can restore your body's thyroid hormone levels and your body's function. Synthetic thyroxine pills (also called L-thyroxine or levothyroxine) contain hormone exactly like the T4 that the thyroid gland itself makes.

One reason that thyroxine treatment works so well is that, like the T4 that your own thyroid gland makes, each dose of synthetic thyroxine keeps working in your blood for a very long time—about a week. This lets your blood T4 levels stay steady so a constant supply of T4 is available to your body cells. (Thyroxine takes about 4 weeks to clear completely from the body.) All hypothyroid patients except those with severe hypothyroidism (myxedema) can be treated as outpatients, not needing to go into the hospital.

Who Should Treat You?

Many hypothyroid patients can be treated effectively by their primary care doctor. You might need to see an endocrinologist or thyroidologist for a second opinion or for regular care if:

- You have congenital hypothyroidism or another unusual cause for your hypothyroidism.

- You have autoimmune polyglandular syndrome—autoimmune hypothyroidism combined with one or more other autoimmune conditions, most often type 1 diabetes, Addison's disease, or premature ovarian failure.

- You have another condition, like epilepsy, heart disease, or bowel disease that affects the treatment of your hypothyroidism.

- You have trouble settling into the right dose of thyroxine.

- You have many questions and concerns that your regular doctor cannot answer or cannot take the time to answer.

How Your Thyroxine Dose Is Decided

When you are first diagnosed with hypothyroidism, your doctor will choose your starting dose of thyroxine based on your:

- **Weight:** The heavier you are, the higher the dose may be.

208

- **Age:** Older people should start on a low dose and raise it slowly, to give their body time to adjust. Because older people's bodies clear drugs more slowly, they generally stay on lower doses.

- **Cause of your hypothyroidism:** If your thyroid has been removed, all of your T4 must be replaced. If your hypothyroidism is caused by autoimmune disease, your thyroid is still probably making some hormone, so you can take a lower dose. If you have had thyroid cancer, you need a higher-than-usual dose to keep your TSH near zero (suppressive treatment) and prevent the cancer from growing back.

- **Other conditions that you have:** If you have celiac disease or Crohn disease, you may have trouble absorbing thyroxine and you many need a higher dose. If you have heart disease, you should start with a very low dose and raise it slowly.

- **Other medicines that you are taking:** If you take birth control pills, hormone replacement therapy, Zoloft®, Tegretol®, Dilantin®, or phenobarbital, you may need a higher dose. If you take testosterone, or possibly niacin, you may need a lower dose.

Your starter dose will probably have to be changed later—not necessarily because your hypothyroidism has worsened, but because that first dose was just your doctor's educated guess. Your doctor may purposely start you on a low dose to prevent you from getting symptoms of too much thyroxine, like anxiety, restlessness, nervousness, and a racing heart. The doctor may then raise your dose gradually.

Because thyroxine is a slow-acting hormone, it may take several weeks before your body adjusts to the pills and you start to feel their effects. After about 6 to 10 weeks, your body will have adjusted enough that your doctor can test your TSH again to see whether it has gone down. If your TSH is still high and you still have symptoms, your doctor may raise your thyroxine dose and then give you 6 weeks or more to adjust to it before testing your TSH again.

This pattern may repeat several times before you settle into the right dose. Every patient responds differently to thyroxine replacement, and you may need a higher or lower dose than someone else who started out with the same TSH as you. You will reach a stable dose, and you may stay on that dose for many, many years.

You must take your assigned dose every day. (It might be the same dose every day, or you might be told to take different doses on different days.) That is the only way that your doctor can measure accurately how your TSH is responding to treatment—and it is the only way that you will get and stay better. Some patients who have hypothyroidism without any symptoms say that they do not want to have to take pills because they feel fine. They still need to be treated because their body functions are slowing down even if they cannot feel it.

Many hypothyroid people are taking too high or too low a dose of thyroxine. Getting the right dose for you is just a matter of taking your pills as prescribed and getting regular blood tests. A small change in your thyroxine dose can make a big change in how you feel and function. If you're on the right dose, all your symptoms caused by hypothyroidism should disappear.

How to Take Your Pills

What is most important is that you start treatment right away and remember to take your pill every day. Thyroxine is not like an antibiotic that you take for a few days until you feel better. Thyroxine replaces the hormone that your thyroid can no longer make. The only way to control your hypothyroidism is to take your pill every day for the rest of your life. If you stop taking your pills for any reason, your hypothyroidism will return.

You should take your pill at about the same time every day. First thing in the morning or last thing at night works well for many people. You may remember to take your pill more easily if you combine it with a routine like brushing your teeth.

When you are supposed to take a pill every day, it is easy to forget whether you have taken today's pill. To keep track more easily, you can store your pills in a container that has a little box marked for each day of the week. Whatever container you use, keep it tightly closed so your pills stay dry. Store your pills in the room where you will best remember to take them. As with all medicines, keep thyroxine out of the reach of children.

You can take your pill with any liquid except soy milk. Cow's milk is probably fine. Grapefruit juice is fine. Do not try to swallow your pill without liquid; it can dissolve in your mouth or throat, and then not enough medicine will be absorbed into your blood.

It does not matter whether you take your pill on an empty stomach or with food, as long as you always do the same thing. If you always take your pill with food, you will probably need a higher dose than if you always take it on an empty stomach. Foods and medicines can interfere with the body's ability to absorb thyroxine. In particular, wait 4 hours after taking thyroxine before you:

- Eat foods that contain soy, including soy formula for babies.

- Take calcium supplements (regular amounts of cow's milk are probably okay), iron supplements, or antacids that contain either calcium or aluminum hydroxide.

- Take medicines like cholestyramine (Questran®), colestipol (Colestid®), or sucralfate (Carafate®).

Thyroxine does not interfere with the body's ability to absorb other drugs.

Giving Thyroxine to Babies

You can crush the pill between two spoons, mix it with a little water or breast milk, and immediately squirt it inside the baby's cheek with a medicine dropper. Then you should nurse or bottle-feed the baby. (Do not crush the pill in a milk bottle. It does not dissolve; it just sits in the bottle, losing its strength and clogging up the nipple. Thyroxine weakens quickly when it is put in liquid.)

Giving Thyroxine to Children Who Cannot Swallow Pills

You can give the pill the same way that you would to a baby. Or you can put the pill in a small paper cup, with just enough water to dissolve the pill. Have the child drink the solution. Then put a little more water in the cup to catch any more bits of the pill, and have the child drink that.

Why You Should Always Take the Same Brand of Thyroxine

The available brands of thyroxine are Synthroid®, Levothroid®, Levoxyl®, and Unithroid®. The U.S. Food and Drug Administration (FDA) regulates all four brands. All are safe and effective. Each brand contains the same active ingredient—thyroxine (T4)—but each is made a little differently. Because these small differences affect the way that the body absorbs the drug, the FDA has not ruled that these products are interchangeable (you cannot just substitute one for another). If you change from one brand to another, even at the same dose, your body may absorb and respond to it differently. This means that if you switch to a new drug, you need a TSH test 6 to 12 weeks later and your new dose may need to be adjusted.

The American Thyroid Association recommends that once you get used to one brand of thyroxine, you stick with that brand. The Association also recommends that you be given a brand name drug rather than a generic, because every time you fill your generic prescription, you may be given a different product. Every time you pick up your pills, you should make sure that the pharmacist has given you the same brand.

Thyroxine comes in many different strengths, each with its own pill color. When you get your pills, make sure you've been given the right strength.

Many patients have to take two thyroxine pills—sometimes of two different strengths—to get the right dose. For example, thyroxine pills are not made in a strength of 163 micrograms (mcg). If your dose needs to be 163 mcg, your doctor might give you prescriptions for 75-mcg pills and for 88-mcg pills. Some pharmacies charge the two strengths as two separate prescriptions. If you check around, you may find a pharmacy that charges the two strengths as a single prescription.

If You Miss a Pill

If you miss just one pill, it is not too serious because thyroxine stays in your blood for such a long time. If this afternoon you remember that you did not take this morning's pill, take it now. If today you re-member that you didn't take yesterday's pill, you can take two pills in one day. But you might feel better if you do not take both doses at once. If possible, take one of the pills in the morning and the other one in the evening. You can probably also safely skip one pill.

If you vomit up a pill because you have the flu, do not take an ex-tra pill. Wait and take your next regular dose tomorrow. If you vomit up a pill because you are pregnant, you might want to try taking your pills at bedtime, when you are less likely to feel sick.

If you miss one thyroxine pill every week, it is much more serious. It is as though you are taking a lower dose of thyroxine. (For example, say that you are supposed to take 100 mcg a day, which adds up to 700 mcg a week. If you miss one pill every week, you are taking only 600 mcg a week or 86 mcg a day. If you miss two pills every week, you are taking only 500 mcg a week or 71 mcg a day. If your doctor prescribed 100 mcg a day, your body needs all that thyroxine.)

If you miss lots of pills, do not try to make them all up. Just start over with daily pills and figure out how you will best remember to take them.

Keep track of how often you miss your pills, so you can tell your doctor next time your TSH is tested.

If You Get Pregnant

Keep taking your regular thyroxine dose. Thyroxine is completely safe when you are pregnant. In fact, you need it more than ever because you must provide T4 for both yourself and your developing fetus.

You should see your doctor as soon as you find out you are pregnant—or, even better, before you decide to become pregnant. You should work closely with your doctor throughout your pregnancy to ensure the best possible health for yourself and your baby. Your doctor should test your TSH several times while you are pregnant, and may raise your thyroxine dose by as much as 30 to 50% because your body needs more T4 to handle the physical demands of pregnancy. After your baby is born, your body returns to needing the same amount of T4 as before you got pregnant, so your thyroxine dose should be lowered.

Many experts recommend that all women be tested for thyroid disease if they are thinking of becoming pregnant or as soon as they learn that they are pregnant. If you are diagnosed with hypothyroidism during your pregnancy, you must begin thyroxine treatment right away and continue treatment and testing at least every 6 to 8 weeks until you deliver. Then your TSH levels will determine whether you need to continue treatment.

Should patients with subclinical (mild) hypothyroidism be treated?

Subclinical (also called mild) hypothyroidism is now defined as a T4 in the normal range, but with a slightly high TSH of 4.0 to 10.0 mU/L, usually causing few or no symptoms. Experts do not agree on whether to treat people with subclinical hypothyroidism. Some doctors treat all of these people. Some treat only those who have symptoms. Some treat those with anti-TPO antibodies or a high cholesterol. Some do not treat at all, but keep testing patients to see whether their TSH rises higher.

There is no harm in treating patients with subclinical hypothyroidism, as long as they are given the correct thyroxine dose. Research is still needed on whether patients do better if they are treated and whether they are harmed if they are not treated. It is possible that even subclinical hypothyroidism can increase people's risk for heart problems.

People with a TSH in the high-normal range of 2.6 and 4.0 mU/L should also keep being tested to see whether their levels rise to the level of hypothyroidism.

How helpful are treatments combining T4 with T3?

A normal thyroid gland makes two thyroid hormones, T4 and T3—but 14 times as much T4 as T3. When tissue cells remove T4 from the bloodstream, they change some of it into T3. In fact, more than 80% of the T3 in your blood is made from T4 that has been changed by the liver and other tissues outside the thyroid. Underactive thyroids still make both T4 and T3—just not enough. Because the failing thyroid still makes some T3, and because body tissues turn some T4 into T3, most hypothyroid patients need to be treated only with T4. In most such patients, having the right amount of T4 allows the body to make the right amount of T3. All the U.S. thyroxine brands contain only T4.

Some researchers and patients have wondered whether a combination of T4 and T3 might be better. Early studies have shown that some patients felt better on the combination, but the improvement did not last.

One problem is that the only FDA-approved brand of T3 works in the body for just a few hours—unlike T4, which works for a week. This means that patients taking T3 need several doses a day. Another problem is that taking T3 pills interferes with the body's normal ability to adjust T3 levels, so the T3 levels that the pills give to patients cannot match the body's normal patterns. This makes some patients actually feel worse on combined therapy.

A T4-T3 combination might be of some help to people who have had their whole thyroid removed and cannot make any T4 or T3 of their own. If patients want to try a T4-T3 combination, the American Thyroid Association recommends that their doctor give them at most 5 mcg of T3 twice a day, and, in turn, reduce their T4 dose. Taking too much T3 can seriously harm the heart.

Thyroxine from Animals

Thyroid hormone taken from pigs has been used for about 100 years to treat hypothyroidism. Dried, powdered bovine (cow) thyroid is now also available. People can buy it over the Internet—legally if it is sold as a food supplement, but illegally if it's sold as a medicine. Before synthetic forms of thyroxine became available, animal thyroid saved many lives. Now patients are safer taking synthetic thyroxine. Some patients argue that pills made from animal thyroids are more natural, but these pills pose several dangers:

- Pills made from animal thyroid are not purified. They contain some proteins that never normally appear in the human bloodstream. Thyroxine made in a lab is exactly the same hormone that a human thyroid gland makes, but in a pure form.

- The balance of T4 to T3 in animals is not the same as in humans, so the hormones in animal thyroid pills are not necessarily natural for the human body.

- The amounts of both T4 and T3 can vary in every batch of animal thyroid, making it harder to keep blood levels right.

In sum, synthetic thyroxine is much safer than animal thyroid.

Thyroxine and Weight Loss

Hypothyroidism can cause a mild weight gain of 5 to 20 pounds, but does not cause obesity. People who have gained a lot of weight should find the real cause. Hypothyroid patients who are started on the right thyroxine dose will not suddenly lose weight, but they should find it easier to lose if they try. Patients who take too high a thyroxine dose in the hope of losing weight in a hurry can weaken their muscles and bones and can get serious heart trouble—all of which makes it harder for them to exercise. Worse yet, the high dose can make them hungrier. So instead of losing weight, they may gain.

People with a normal TSH should never take thyroxine pills to help them lose weight. Taking a low thyroxine dose will not speed up their metabolism. Taking a high dose can weaken their muscles and bones, and cause serious heart trouble.

Ineffective Treatments

Most hypothyroidism is permanent. Chinese herbs, selenium, iodine-tyrosine supplements, kelp (a kind of seaweed), and other herbal remedies at the health food store may promise to jump-start the thyroid, but they do not work. Once the thyroid stops doing its job, taking extra iodine or other substances will not help it work better. In fact, taking too much iodine can worsen both hypothyroidism and hyperthyroidism. Worse yet, taking false remedies can prevent patients from getting the thyroxine treatment that they really need.

Side Effects and Complications of Treatment

The only dangers of thyroxine are caused by taking too little or too much. If you take too little, your hypothyroidism will continue. If you take too much, you will develop the symptoms of hyperthyroidism—

an overactive thyroid gland. The most common symptoms of too much thyroid hormone are fatigue and an inability to sleep, greater appetite, nervousness, shakiness, feeling hot when other people are cold, and trouble exercising because of weak muscles, shortness of breath, and a racing, skipping heart. Hyperthyroidism can also cause changes that you cannot feel, like bone loss (osteoporosis) and irregular heart beat. Patients who have hyperthyroid symptoms should have their TSH tested. If it is below normal, their thyroxine dose needs to be lowered. People who have had thyroid cancer need to take higher-than-usual (suppressive) thyroxine doses, which increase their risk for osteoporosis. They should take in plenty of calcium through food and supplements, even though supplements cannot correct the bone loss caused by too much thyroxine. These people should also be checked regularly for thinning of their bones. Thyroxine pills do not harm the thyroid gland.

Follow-Up

Repeat Blood Tests

You will need to have your TSH checked about every 6 to 10 weeks after a thyroxine dose change. You may need tests more often if you are pregnant or you are taking a medicine that interferes with your body's ability to use thyroxine. The goal of treatment is to get and keep your TSH in the normal range. The American Thyroid Association recommends that your doctor try to keep your TSH within a narrow range of 0.5 to 2.0 mU/L. Within this range, your body gets the best possible amount of thyroxine and you are likely to feel the best. Babies must get all their daily treatments and have their TSH levels checked as they grow, to prevent mental retardation and stunted growth (cretinism).

Normal Variation in TSH Levels

Do not worry if you get a result of 0.8 on one TSH test, and 1.1 on your next test—both of them while you are taking the same thyroxine dose. It does not mean that your hypothyroidism is getting worse. Differences in test results are expected:

- It is normal for your TSH levels to vary because the pituitary sends out TSH in pulses rather than a steady stream, and because TSH levels normally go up at night and come down during the day.

- Labs cannot measure every test exactly the same way. If a lab runs two tests on one blood sample, they may get two slightly different results.

There is some evidence that T4 levels also normally vary a little bit through the day.

Reasons for Needing Extra TSH Tests

Once you have settled into a regular thyroxine dose, you can return for TSH tests only about once a year. You need to return sooner if:

- Your symptoms return or get worse. If your TSH turns out to be high, hypothyroidism is probably causing your symptoms. But if your TSH is normal, it means that your thyroxine dose has your body working right and something else is causing your symptoms.

- You want to change your thyroxine dose or brand, or change to taking your pills with or without food.

- You gain or lose a lot of weight. If you did not weigh much to begin with, you should be tested after a gain or loss of as little as 10 pounds.

- You start or stop taking a drug that can interfere with absorbing thyroxine, or you change your dose of such a drug. For example, if you start taking estrogen in a birth control pill or in hormone replacement therapy, you may need to raise your dose. If you stop taking the drug, you may need to lower your dose.

- You are not taking your thyroxine pill every day. Tell your doctor honestly how many pills you have missed. If you have missed pills, but you say that you have been taking all of them, and if your TSH test is then high, your doctor may mistakenly think that your hypothyroidism is getting worse and may raise your thyroxine dose.

- You want to try stopping thyroxine treatment. If ever you think you are doing well enough not to need thyroxine treatment any longer, try it only under your doctor's close supervision. Rather than stopping your pills completely, you might ask your doctor to try lowering your dose. If your TSH goes up, you will know that you need to continue treatment. You should never stop thyroxine treatment on your own. If you do, your hypothyroid symptoms will return. You must take your thyroxine every day, most likely for the rest of your life.

If Hypothyroidism Is Not Treated or If Treatment Is Stopped

Babies and Children

Thyroid hormone is essential for the brain to develop normally. Early in a healthy pregnancy, a mother supplies her fetus with thyroid hormone. During the second trimester, the fetus's thyroid gland starts to make its own hormone. Once babies are born, they must depend completely on their own thyroid gland.

Too little thyroid hormone can keep the brain from developing normally. If the mother is hypothyroid, she cannot give her fetus enough thyroid hormone. When a mother with untreated or under-treated hypothyroidism bears a child who has a normal thyroid, the baby's IQ may be a few points lower than it would have been otherwise, but the child is not at higher-than-normal risk for birth defects. If a fetus is hypothyroid, it cannot maintain normal thyroid hormone levels before or after birth.

Hypothyroidism that begins before birth or up to age 3 and goes untreated puts babies at risk for mental retardation. Untreated severe hypothyroidism retards both brain development and physical growth (cretinism).

In the United States and some other developed countries, all babies are tested for hypothyroidism a few days after birth so that they can be diagnosed and begin treatment right away.

Hypothyroidism Caused by Iodine Deficiency

The body needs iodine to make thyroid hormone. In underdeveloped parts of the world where people cannot get enough iodine from their food, their body cannot make enough thyroid hormone and they may be hypothyroid. This puts babies at double risk. Hypothyroid mothers cannot give their fetuses enough thyroid hormone before they are born, and once the babies are born, their own thyroid cannot make enough hormone. Hypothyroidism prevents the brain and body from developing normally. Worldwide, iodine deficiency is the major cause of hypothyroidism and preventable mental retardation.

Patients of All Ages

No one can predict whether hypothyroidism will worsen. Subclinical (mild) hypothyroidism may never get worse, or it may progress over months or years to become moderately or very severe (myxedema). If people with autoimmune hypothyroidism also have high levels of anti-TPO antibodies, their hypothyroidism is more likely to progress, although there is no way to predict how quickly. Anti-TPO antibodies attack the enzyme within the thyroid gland that helps thyroid cells make hormone. No one knows whether treating hypothyroidism prevents it from worsening.

Severe Hypothyroidism (Myxedema)

The worse untreated hypothyroidism becomes, the less the body is able to cope with stressors like cold weather, infections, or even minor surgery. Severe hypothyroidism is called myxedema. Usually it takes years for hypothyroidism to reach the point of myxedema, but patients who do not have a thyroid (because of surgery or radioactive iodine treatment) can progress to myxedema in months. In patients with myxedema, the body slows to the point that it starts to shut down. At its worst, the patient falls into a coma. To survive myxedema coma, patients need good supportive care in the hospital intensive care unit. Fortunately, myxedema is now rare in developed countries because most patients are treated before their hypothyroidism becomes severe.

Keeping Other People Informed

Tell Your Family

Because thyroid disease runs in families, you should explain your hypothyroidism to your blood relatives and encourage them to get a TSH test. If it is normal, they should be retested if they develop symptoms, or at least every 5 years.

Tell Your Other Doctors and Pharmacist

Keep your other doctors and your pharmacist informed about your hypothyroidism and about the drug and dose with which it is being treated. If you start seeing a new doctor, tell the doctor that you have hypothyroidism and you need your TSH tested every year. If you see an endocrinologist, ask that copies of your reports be sent to your primary care doctor.

You do not need to wear a medical alert bracelet, but it would be wise to keep a card in your wallet that lists:

* Your name and contact information

- Your doctor's name and contact information
- The name of your disease
- Your thyroxine brand name and dose

Partnership between Patient and Doctor

The more you and your doctor work as a team, the better you will do.

Your Jobs

Because you will probably have hypothyroidism for the rest of your life, you have to be your own main caretaker. You cannot depend on your doctor to do all the work for you. You have to fill your prescriptions and take your pills every day. You have to make and keep your appointments for blood tests and doctor visits. When you go for visits, you have to tell your doctor how you are feeling and be honest in saying how often you miss your pills. It is smart ahead of time to write a list of the things that you want to tell and ask the doctor.

Your Doctor's Jobs

Your doctor should explain your disease and its treatment, answer your questions, and listen to your concerns. The doctor should take your symptoms into account when adjusting your thyroxine dose. The doctor should give you your blood test results. The doctor should keep up to date about advances in the diagnosis and treatment of thyroid disease.

Your Emotional Needs

Many people get a diagnosis of hypothyroidism after years of feeling sick and believing or being told that their symptoms are: "all in your head, just stress, or a normal part of aging." Some people are so relieved finally to know what is wrong with them that all they want is to start treatment and then get on with their lives.

Other people are so exhausted and depressed that they do not feel that they have the physical or mental energy to work at getting better, and they may fear that they will never feel well again. There are lots of problems in our lives that we cannot do anything about. This is a problem that you can do something about.

You just have to be patient early in your treatment for hypothyroidism—patient with yourself, patient with the confusing changes happening in your body, and patient with your doctor and the people who are going through this with you. It can take weeks to start responding to thyroxine, and it can take months (for a few patients, longer than a year) before you and your doctor get the dose exactly right. But the effort is well worthwhile. Odds are that soon you will be feeling better than you have in years.

Living with Hypothyroidism

There is no cure for hypothyroidism, and most patients have it for life. There are exceptions: Many patients with viral thyroiditis have their thyroid function return to normal, as do some patients with thyroiditis after pregnancy. Rare patients with Hashimoto thyroiditis return to normal. Thyroid function may not return to normal after a person is treated with interferon alpha. Most hypothyroidism is permanent.

Hypothyroidism may become more or less severe, and your thyroxine dose may need to change over time. You have to make a lifetime commitment to treatment. You should never stop thyroxine treatment on your own. If you do, your hypothyroid symptoms will return.

If you take your pills every day and work with your doctor to get and keep your thyroxine dose right, you should be able to keep your hypothyroidism completely controlled throughout your life. Your symptoms should disappear and the serious effects of low thyroid hormone should stop getting worse and should actually improve. If you keep your hypothyroidism well-controlled, it will not shorten your life span.

Many questions about hypothyroidism remain mysteries, for example: Which genes increase people's risk for thyroid disease? What triggers the start of thyroid disease? Why does the immune system attack the thyroid? These are among the questions that researchers, including members of the American Thyroid Association, are working hard to answer.

Medical Terms in This Chapter

Addison's disease: Permanent loss of function of the adrenal glands, which make essential steroid hormones for the body.

Anemia: Too few of the red blood cells that deliver essential oxygen to the body's cells.

Antibodies: Proteins that the body's immune system makes to attack invaders like bacteria and viruses.

Anti-TPO antibodies: In autoimmune thyroid disease, proteins that mistakenly try to attack the thyroid peroxidase (TPO) enzymes that help the thyroid gland make hormone.

Autoimmune disease: Any disease in which the body's immune system, designed to protect the body from outside invaders like viruses and bacteria, mistakes a normal part of the body for an invader and tries to destroy it.

Autoimmune thyroiditis: Inflammation of the thyroid, caused by autoimmune disease.

Atrophic thyroiditis: A form of autoimmune thyroiditis in which the immune system's attack on the thyroid causes it to shrink and stop making thyroid hormone.

Coma: Unconsciousness from which a person cannot be awakened.

Congenital hypothyroidism: Hypothyroidism in a newborn baby.

Cretinism: Mental and physical retardation caused by severe congenital hypothyroidism.

Deficiency: A lack, too little.

Ectopic: In the wrong place; an ectopic thyroid gland is usually in the tongue and/or upper neck.

Endocrine gland: Any gland that produces and releases hormones directly into the blood, for example, the thyroid, pituitary, adrenals, and pancreas.

Endocrinologist: A medical doctor who specializes in endocrinology, the treatment of endocrine gland diseases like thyroid disease and diabetes.

Enzyme: Protein that helps chemical processes take place within the body but doesn't get used up in the process; the major enzymes in the thyroid gland are peroxidases.

Feedback loop: A system in which A affects B, which in turn affects A again.

Fetus: A developing baby inside the mother.

Free T4: The thyroid hormone T4 that circulates in the blood unattached to a protein, and that can be taken up by cells in tissues.

Free T4 index: An estimate of the amount of free T4 in the blood.

Gland: An organ or tissue that makes and sends out a hormone or other substance.

Goiter: An enlarged thyroid gland, which can cause swelling in the front of the neck.

Graves disease: Autoimmune hyperthyroidism, usually with goiter and eye symptoms.

Hashimoto thyroiditis: Autoimmune thyroiditis in which the immune system's attack on the thyroid causes a goiter (swelling), and sometimes, hypothyroidism.

Hormone: Substance made by an organ or tissue that affects the function of one or more other organs.

Hyperthyroidism: An overactive thyroid gland.

Hypothyroidism: An underactive thyroid gland.

I-131: One of several forms of radioactive iodine; low-dose I-131 is used for medical testing and to destroy an overactive thyroid gland.

Infiltrate: To deposit an abnormal substance in a tissue.

Immune system: The body's way of protecting itself from invaders like bacteria and viruses.

Inflammation: The body's response to injured cells.

Iodine: Chemical element that is an essential ingredient of thyroid hormone.

mcg: Unit of measure, abbreviation for micrograms; thyroxine doses may be measured in mcg (also written as µg); 50 mcg = .05 mg (milligrams).

Metabolism: All the processes by which the body makes and uses energy and builds tissues.

Mild hypothyroidism: Subclinical hypothyroidism.

mU/L: Unit of measure, abbreviation for milliunits per liter; TSH levels are measured in mU/L.

Myxedema: Severe hypothyroidism; the brain, heart, lungs, kidneys, and other organs slow to the point that they cannot keep up critical functions like maintaining temperature, heart rate, blood pressure, and breathing.

Myxedema coma: Often-fatal unconsciousness resulting from severe hypothyroidism.

Nodule: Small abnormal mass or lump; nodules in the thyroid are very common, but few are cancerous.

Paresthesia: Feeling of pins and needles in the hands and feet.

Pituitary (master) gland: From its position in the base of the brain, the pituitary monitors most basic body functions and sends out hormones that control those functions, for example, the rate at which the thyroid gland makes hormone.

Polyglandular autoimmune syndromes: Combinations of autoimmune diseases affecting both endocrine and non-endocrine organs and usually involving the thyroid.

Postpartum: After giving birth.

Premature ovarian failure: Before the normal age for menopause, the ovaries' loss of ability to produce estrogen and release eggs, leaving a woman unable to become pregnant.

Radioiodine: Iodine that has naturally or artificially been made radioactive; see I-131.

Secondary hypothyroidism: Hypothyroidism caused not by damage to the thyroid gland, but by damage to the pituitary gland, preventing it from being able to tell the thyroid to make hormone.

Set point: The body's preferred level or range for a function; for example, the pituitary gland knows the body's normal T4 range (set point) and works to keep the T4 within that range.

Silent: Not causing symptoms.

Subclinical (mild) hypothyroidism: A T4 in the normal range, but a slightly high TSH of 4.0 to 10.0 mU/L, causing few or no symptoms.

Supportive care: General medical care, such as nutrition and fluids, to help a patient recover when no targeted treatment can improve the person's condition.

Suppressive treatment: Thyroxine dose high enough to keep the TSH below normal.

Syndrome: A combination of symptoms.

Synthetic: Made in a laboratory.

T3: Triiodothyronine, a hormone with 3 iodine molecules, made in small amounts by the thyroid gland and in larger amounts from T4 in other body tissues.

T4: Thyroxine, the main hormone made by the thyroid gland, containing 4 iodine molecules.

Thyroid gland: An endocrine gland, normally in the lower front of the neck, that makes and sends out the hormones T4 and T3, which regulate the metabolism of every cell in the body.

Thyroid hormone: T4 and T3, the products of the thyroid gland.

Thyroiditis: Inflammation of the thyroid gland.

Thyroidologist: A medical doctor who specializes in the diagnosis and treatment of thyroid diseases.

Thyroid peroxidase (TPO) enzymes: Enzymes within the thyroid gland that help thyroid cells make hormone.

Thyroid-stimulating hormone (TSH): Hormone that the pituitary gland makes and sends into the blood to tell the thyroid gland how much T4 and T3 to make.

Thyroxine: T4, the main hormone made by the thyroid gland; also pills used to treat hypothyroidism by replacing the missing T4.

Trimester: Three months; the nine months of a pregnancy are broken into three trimesters.

TPO: Thyroid peroxidase.

TSH: Thyroid-stimulating hormone.

Section 24.2

Pregnancy-Related Issues

Hypothyroidism and Pregnancy

What are the normal changes in thyroid function associated with pregnancy?

Hormone Changes. A normal pregnancy results in a number of important physiological and hormonal changes that alter thyroid function. These changes mean that laboratory tests of thyroid function must be interpreted with caution during pregnancy. Thyroid function tests change during pregnancy due to the influence of two main hormones: human chorionic gonadotropin (hCG), the hormone that is measured in the pregnancy test and estrogen, the main female hormone. HCG can weakly turn on the thyroid and the high circulating hCG levels in the first trimester may result in a slightly low TSH. Typically, the TSH in the first trimester will be normal or slightly low and then remain normal throughout the duration of pregnancy (see Table 24.2). Estrogen increases the amount of thyroid hormone binding proteins in the serum which increases the total thyroid hormone levels in the blood since over 99% of the thyroid hormones in the blood are bound to these proteins. However, measurements of free hormone (that not bound to protein, representing the active form of the hormone) usually remain normal. The thyroid is functioning normally if the TSH, Free T4, and Free T3 are all normal throughout pregnancy.

Size Changes. The thyroid gland can increase in size during pregnancy (enlarged thyroid = goiter). However, pregnancy-associated goiters occur much more frequently in iodine-deficient areas of the world. It is relatively uncommon in the United States, which is thought to be relatively iodine sufficient. If very sensitive imaging techniques (ultrasound) are used, it is possible to detect an increase in thyroid volume in some women. This is usually only a 10–15% increase in size and is not typically apparent on physical examination by the physician. However, sometimes a significant goiter may develop and prompt the doctor to measure tests of thyroid function.

What is the interaction between the thyroid function of the mother and the baby?

For the first 10–12 weeks of pregnancy, the baby is completely dependent on the mother for the production of thyroid hormone. By the end of the first trimester, the baby's thyroid begins to produce thyroid hormone on its own. The baby, however, remains dependent on the mother for ingestion of adequate amounts of iodine, which is essential to make the thyroid hormones. The World Health Organization recommends iodine intake of 200 micrograms/day during pregnancy to maintain adequate thyroid hormone production. The normal diet in the United States contains sufficient iodine so additional iodine supplementation is rarely necessary.

What are the most common causes of hypothyroidism during pregnancy?

Overall, the most common cause of hypothyroidism is the autoimmune disorder known as Hashimoto thyroiditis. Hypothyroidism can occur during pregnancy due to the initial presentation of Hashimoto thyroiditis, inadequate treatment of a woman already known to have hypothyroidism from a variety of causes, or over-treatment of a hyperthyroid woman with antithyroid medications. Approximately, 2.5% of women will have a slightly elevated TSH of greater than 6 and 0.4% will have a TSH greater than 10 during pregnancy.

What are the risks of hypothyroidism to the mother?

Untreated, or inadequately treated, hypothyroidism has been associated with maternal anemia (low red blood cell count), myopathy (muscle pain, weakness), congestive heart failure, preeclampsia, placental abnormalities, low birth weight infants, and postpartum hemorrhage (bleeding). These complications are more likely to occur in women with severe hypothyroidism. Most women with mild hypothyroidism may have no symptoms or attribute symptoms they may have as due to the pregnancy.

What are the risks of maternal hypothyroidism to the baby?

Thyroid hormone is critical for brain development in the baby. Children born with congenital hypothyroidism (no thyroid function at birth) can have severe cognitive, neurological, and developmental abnormalities if the condition is not recognized and treated promptly. These developmental abnormalities can largely be prevented if the disease is recognized and treated immediately after birth. Consequently, all newborn babies in the United States are screened for congenital hypothyroidism so they can be treated with thyroid hormone replacement therapy as soon as possible.

The effect of maternal hypothyroidism on the baby's brain development is not as clear. Untreated severe hypothyroidism in the mother can lead to impaired brain development in the baby. This is mainly seen when the maternal hypothyroidism is due to iodine deficiency, which also affects the baby However, recent studies have suggested that mild brain developmental abnormalities may be present in children born to women who had mild untreated hypothyroidism during pregnancy. At this time there is no general consensus of opinion regarding screening all women for hypothyroidism during pregnancy. However, some physician groups recommend checking a woman's TSH value either before becoming pregnant (pre-pregnancy counseling) or

Table 24.2. Normal Thyroid Function during Pregnancy

	1st Trimester	2nd Trimester	3rd Trimester
TSH	Normal or Increased	Normal	Normal
Free T4	Normal	Normal	Normal
Free T3	Normal	Normal	Normal
Total T4	High	High	High
Total T3	High	High	High
T3 Resin Uptake (Inverse measure of protein binding)	Low	Low	Low
Free T4 Index (FT4I, FTI)	Normal	Normal	Normal

as soon as pregnancy is confirmed. This is especially true in women at high risk for thyroid disease, such as those with prior treatment for hyperthyroidism, a positive family history of thyroid disease and those with a goiter. Clearly, woman with established hypothyroidism should have a TSH test once pregnancy is confirmed, as thyroid hormone requirements increase during pregnancy, often leading to the need to increase the levothyroxine dose. If the TSH is normal, no further monitoring is typically required. This issue should be discussed further with your health care provider, particularly if you are contemplating pregnancy. Once hypothyroidism has been detected, the woman should be treated with levothyroxine to normalize her TSH and Free T4 values.

How should a woman with hypothyroidism be treated during pregnancy?

The treatment of hypothyroidism in a pregnant woman is the same as for a man or non-pregnant woman, namely, adequate replacement of thyroid hormone in the form of synthetic levothyroxine. It is important to note that levothyroxine requirements frequently increase during pregnancy, often times by 25 to 50 percent. Occasionally, the levothyroxine dose may double. Ideally, hypothyroid women should have their levothyroxine dose optimized prior to becoming pregnant. Women with known hypothyroidism should have their thyroid function tested as soon as pregnancy is detected and their dose adjusted by their physician as needed to maintain a TSH in the normal range. Thyroid function tests should be checked approximately every 6–8 weeks during pregnancy to ensure that the woman has normal thyroid function throughout pregnancy. If a change in levothyroxine dose is required, thyroid tests should be measured 4 weeks later. As soon as delivery of the child occurs, the woman may go back to her usual pre-pregnancy dose of levothyroxine. It is also important to recognize that prenatal vitamins contain iron that can impair the absorption of thyroid hormone from the gastrointestinal tract. Consequently, levothyroxine and prenatal vitamins should not be taken at the same time and should be separated by at least 2–3 hours.

Thyroid Problems During and After Pregnancy—Are You at Risk?

If you or a close relative have ever had an over- or underactive thyroid you should tell your obstetrician so you can be sure your thyroid function is checked before, during, and after pregnancy. Abnormal thyroid levels before pregnancy can make it more difficult to conceive. Your baby relies in part on your supplying thyroid hormone, especially before your baby's thyroid begins to develop at about the tenth week of pregnancy.

If you have ever had the form of hyperthyroidism known as Graves disease, your obstetrician should test your blood for thyroid stimulating immunoglobulins (TSIs), thyroid antibodies which caused your thyroid to become overactive and could have the same effect on your baby during pregnancy if your antibody levels are still increased. This could be your situation even though you feel completely well, even if you are taking thyroid hormone tablets once a day to treat an underactive thyroid.

There is another reason for re-testing your thyroid by means of a TSH test as pregnancy progresses. During pregnancy a mother's thyroid function gradually increases. If your thyroid is underactive, it cannot make more hormone during pregnancy. Therefore, your obstetrician will use TSH tests to tell whether your thyroid hormone dose needs to be increased as pregnancy progresses.

Thyroid Problems after Pregnancy

The birth of a baby is a joyous occasion. However, in the postpartum period you will experience many changes in your life. These may include physical problems of fatigue, anemia, pain (from an episiotomy or cesarean section), and breast soreness. Fatigue is especially common because of late night feedings and the continuous responsibilities of a new baby. The blues of postpartum depression are common.

These complications usually occur soon after the baby is born, and by the third month after delivery most women are feeling well again. Unfortunately, that is not always the case, and some women do not enjoy a rapid return to good health. For many of these mothers, the cause may be a change in thyroid function after delivery.

Why does it happen?

During pregnancy your immune system is suppressed as a protection for your baby. After delivery there is a marked rise in immune activity and sometimes a worsening of immune conditions such as rheumatoid arthritis and thyroid disease. Although thyroid dysfunction may occur anytime after pregnancy, it is most common about two to three months after delivery. By that time, your visits to your obstetrician may have ended if you had an uneventful pregnancy and delivery. Therefore, you may be more likely to visit your family physician or even the baby's pediatrician. Don't hesitate to discuss your thyroid condition with these caregivers.

How will I feel?

If your thyroid levels rise (hyperthyroidism), your whole system may feel speeded up. Your heart may race and you may feel nervous with shaking hands, increased sweating, insomnia, and anxiety. If your thyroid levels fall you could feel sluggish, tired, run down, depressed, and experience muscle cramps and constipation. In either instance your thyroid gland in the front of your neck may enlarge slightly and may feel mildly tender though extreme pain is uncommon.

Who should be tested?

Anyone with the symptoms of an overactive or underactive thyroid or postpartum depression should have a TSH test to tell whether thyroid levels are normal. Thyroid hormone levels do not need to be checked unless the TSH is high (indicating hypothyroidism) or low (indicating hyperthyroidism).

Since the symptoms of a change in thyroid function may be so mild as to be missed or mistaken for other health problems, your doctor may also choose to check your TSH level about two to four months after delivery if you or a close relative have ever had a thyroid problem. You may also have a TSH test after pregnancy if your doctor suspects that you are at increased risk for thyroid dysfunction. This could be your situation if you or close relatives have other disorders or physical traits suggesting an increased risk for thyroid problems. These include juvenile (Type I) diabetes, rheumatoid arthritis, pernicious anemia due to a lack of vitamin B12, colitis, and prematurely gray hair. There is even new research which suggests that if you or a close relative are either left-handed or ambidextrous you may have an increased risk for thyroid dysfunction and other immune problems.

If your close relatives have these thyroid or related conditions, your doctor may order a TSH test to be sure your thyroid is normal even if you feel well. This is because mild changes in thyroid function often do not appear to cause symptoms, but once treated you may find yourself healthier as symptoms you thought were due to other problems disappear. If you are found to have a thyroid problem, it is likely that you will recover and be able to stop treatment in a few months. However, not all patients get completely well. About one-third of the women who experience changes in thyroid function after pregnancy never fully recover and need thyroid treatment lifelong.

What about my next pregnancy?

If you have experienced a change in thyroid function in one pregnancy it is likely that your thyroid levels will change after subsequent pregnancies as well. In fact, your obstetrician is likely to order a TSH test to check your thyroid before and during your pregnancy, and after delivery too.

What about my baby?

Here the news is good. Most babies have completely normal thyroid function even if a mother has a thyroid problem during the pregnancy or after delivery. There is more good news. Every baby in the United States, Canada, and most developed countries is checked at birth to be sure thyroid function is normal. This is because babies with a thyroid problem may look normal for two to three months, and a delay in treatment of a baby born without a thyroid or with a poorly-functioning thyroid gland may have long-term effects on the baby's health and mental function. Be happy that your baby gets a check automatically. Above all, do not hesitate to talk with your obstetrician about your thyroid, especially if you or one of your relatives has a thyroid or related immune disorder.

Breastfeeding and Hypothyroidism

I may have hypothyroidism; can I still breastfeed my baby?

Hypothyroidism is the name given to the condition of having an underactive thyroid. Because the thyroid controls the body's metabolic process, it is a serious condition. Any mother with thyroid disease should be under the care of a doctor who is supportive of her desire to breastfeed.

Thyroid supplements—used to treat this condition—are not contraindicated while breastfeeding. They simply bring the mother's thyroid up to normal levels, making the mother feel better and increasing her milk supply.

Symptoms of hypothyroidism may include fatigue, poor appetite, depression, intolerance to cold, thinning hair, and dry skin. These symptoms, which are similar to those of anemia, may be wrongly attributed to normal postpartum fatigue, postpartum depression, or even breastfeeding.

Diagnosis of an underactive thyroid can usually be based on the mother's symptoms as well as a simple blood test. On occasion, radioactive testing is used to diagnose thyroid problems. If radioactive testing is recommended, the mother can ask her physician if the test could be postponed or another, non-radioactive test, be substituted.

If the radioactive test is used, temporary weaning is recommended. The length of time the mother needs to suspend breastfeeding will depend on the type and dosage of radioactive materials used for the test. Radioactivity of breast milk declines over time, and frequent milk expression will help the mother eliminate the radioactivity from her body more quickly. This milk must be discarded and not fed to the baby. (Frequent milk expression will not hasten the elimination of other drugs from breast milk.)

Additional Information

American Thyroid Association
6066 Leesburg Pike, Suite 550
Falls Church, VA 22041
Toll-Free: 800-THYROID (849-7643)
Phone: 703-998-8890
Fax: 703-998-8893
Website: http://www.thyroid.org
E-mail: admin@thyroid.org

La Leche League International
P.O. Box 4079
Schaumburg, IL 60168-4079
Phone: 847-519-7730
Fax: 847-519-0035
TTY: 847-592-7570
Website: http://www.lalecheleague.org

Thyroid Foundation of America
One Longfellow Place, Suite 1518
Boston, MA 02114
Toll-Free: 800-832-8321
Phone: 617-534-1500
Fax: 617-534-1515
Website: http://www.allthyroid.org
E-mail: info@allthyroid.org

Chapter 25

Hashimoto Thyroiditis

What Is Hashimoto Thyroiditis?

Hashimoto thyroiditis (also called autoimmune or chronic lympho-cytic thyroiditis) is the most common thyroid disease in the United States. It is an inherited condition that affects approximately 14 million Americans and is about 7 times more common in women than in men. Hashimoto thyroiditis is characterized by the production of immune cells and autoantibodies by the body's immune system, which can damage thyroid cells and compromise their ability to make thyroid hormone. Hypothyroidism occurs if the amount of thyroid hormone which can be produced is not enough for the body's needs. The thyroid gland may also enlarge in some patients, forming a goiter.

What Are the Symptoms of Hashimoto Thyroiditis?

Many patients with Hashimoto thyroiditis may have no symptoms for many years, and the diagnosis is made incidentally when an enlarged thyroid gland or abnormal blood tests are discovered as part of a routine examination. When symptoms do develop, they are either related to local pressure effects in the neck caused by the goiter itself, or to the low levels of thyroid hormone. The first sign of this disease may be painless swelling in the lower front of the neck. This enlargement may eventually become easily visible and may be associated with

"Hashimoto's Thyroiditis: Information for Patients," © 2004 American Association of Clinical Endocrinologists. Reprinted with permission.

an uncomfortable pressure sensation in the lower neck. Left untreated, a person may begin to have trouble swallowing or even breathing.

Although many of the symptoms associated with thyroid hormone deficiency occur commonly in patients without thyroid disease, patients with Hashimoto thyroiditis who develop hypothyroidism are more likely to experience the following:

- Fatigue
- Drowsiness
- Forgetfulness
- Difficulty with learning
- Dry, brittle hair, and nails
- Dry, itchy skin
- Puffy face
- Constipation
- Sore muscles
- Weight gain
- Heavy menstrual flow
- Increased frequency of miscarriages
- Increased sensitivity to many medications

The thyroid enlargement and/or hypothyroidism caused by Hashimoto thyroiditis tends to progress in many patients, causing a slow worsening of symptoms. Therefore, patients with any of these findings should be recognized and adequately treated with thyroid hormone. Optimal treatment with thyroid hormone will eliminate any symptoms due to thyroid hormone deficiency, usually prevent further thyroid enlargement, and may some times cause shrinkage of an enlarged thyroid gland.

What Is the Cause of Hashimoto Thyroiditis?

Hashimoto thyroiditis results from a malfunction in the immune system. When working properly, the immune system is designed to protect the body against invaders, such as bacteria, viruses, and other foreign substances. The immune system of someone with Hashimoto thyroiditis mistakenly recognizes normal thyroid cells as foreign tissue, and it produces antibodies that may destroy these cells. Although various environmental factors have been studied, none have been positively proven to be the cause of Hashimoto thyroiditis.

How Is Hashimoto Thyroiditis Diagnosed?

A physician experienced in the diagnosis and treatment of thyroid disease can detect a goiter due to Hashimoto thyroiditis by performing a physical examination and can recognize hypothyroidism by identifying characteristic symptoms, finding typical physical signs, and doing appropriate laboratory tests.

Antithyroid Antibodies

Increased antithyroid antibodies provide the most specific laboratory evidence of Hashimoto thyroiditis, but they are not present in all cases.

TSH (Thyroid-Stimulating Hormone or Thyrotropin) Test

Increased TSH level in the blood is the most accurate indicator of hypothyroidism. TSH is produced by another gland, the pituitary, which is located in the center of the head behind the nose. The level of TSH rises dramatically when the thyroid gland even slightly underproduces thyroid hormone, so a normal level of TSH reliably excludes hypothyroidism in patients with normal pituitary function.

Other Tests

- **Free T4 (thyroxine):** The active thyroid hormone in the blood. A low level of free T4 is consistent with thyroid hormone deficiency. However, free T4 values in the normal range may actually represent thyroid hormone deficiency in a particular patient, since a high level of TSH stimulation may keep the free T4 levels within normal limits for many years.
- **Fine-needle aspiration of the thyroid:** Usually not necessary for most patients with Hashimoto thyroiditis, but a good way to diagnose difficult cases and a necessary procedure if a thyroid nodule is also present.

How Is Hashimoto Thyroiditis Treated?

For patients with thyroid enlargement (goiter) or hypothyroidism, thyroid hormone therapy is clearly needed, since proper dosage corrects any symptoms due to thyroid hormone deficiency and may decrease the goiter's size. Treatment consists of taking a single daily tablet of levothyroxine. Older patients who may have underlying heart disease are usually started on a low dose and gradually increased, while younger healthy patients can be started on full replacement doses at once. Thyroid hormone acts very slowly in the body, so it may take several months after treatment is started to notice improvement in symptoms or goiter shrinkage. Because of the generally permanent and often progressive nature of Hashimoto thyroiditis, it is usually necessary to treat it throughout one's lifetime and to realize that medicine dose requirements may have to be adjusted from time to time.

Optimal adjustment of thyroid hormone dosage, based on laboratory tests rather than symptoms, is critical, since the body is very sensitive to even small changes in thyroid hormone levels. The tablets come in over 10 different strengths, and it is essential to take them in a consistent manner every day. If the dose is not adequate, the thyroid gland may continue to enlarge and symptoms of hypothyroidism will persist, and may be associated with increased serum cholesterol levels, which may increase the risk for atherosclerosis and heart disease. If the dose is too strong, it can cause symptoms of hyperthyroidism, creating excessive strain on the heart and an increased risk of developing osteoporosis.

Other Associated Disorders

As noted, Hashimoto thyroiditis is a common disorder of the immune system which affects the thyroid gland. However, much less often, the immune system can also mistakenly target virtually any other part of the body, causing it to malfunction, and this tendency runs in families. Although the majority of patients with Hashimoto thyroiditis and their genetic family members will never experience any other autoimmune condition, they do have a statistically increased risk of developing the following disorders:

- Type 1 diabetes mellitus (insulin-requiring)
- Graves disease (goiter and hyperthyroidism or overactive thyroid)
- Rheumatoid arthritis
- Pernicious anemia (inability to absorb vitamin B_{12}, potentially causing anemia and neurologic problems)
- Addison's disease (adrenal failure; the adrenal gland provides cortisone to handle stress and illness)
- Premature ovarian failure (early menopause)

- Vitiligo (patchy loss of skin pigmentation)
- Thrombocytopenic purpura (bleeding disorder due to inadequate platelets in the blood)
- Lupus erythematosus (autoimmune disease that involves skin, lymph glands, heart, lungs, kidneys)

Appropriate management of Hashimoto thyroiditis requires continued care by a physician who is experienced in the treatment of this disease.

Additional Information

American Association of Clinical Endocrinologists
1000 Riverside Ave, Suite 205
Jacksonville, FL 32204
Phone: 904-353-7878
Fax: 904-353-8185
Website: http://www.aace.com
E-mail: info@aace.com

Chapter 26

Subacute Thyroiditis

Alternative names: de Quervain's thyroiditis; Granulomatous giant cell thyroiditis

Definition: Subacute thyroiditis involves inflammation of the thyroid gland that usually follows an upper respiratory infection and then subsides.

Causes, Incidence, and Risk Factors

Subacute thyroiditis is an uncommon condition thought to be caused by viral infection of the thyroid gland. The condition often occurs after a viral infection of the upper respiratory tract. Mumps virus, influenza virus, and other respiratory viruses have been found to cause subacute thyroiditis.

The most prominent feature of subacute thyroiditis is gradual or sudden onset of pain in the region of the thyroid gland. Painful enlargement of the thyroid gland may persist for weeks or months. The condition is sometimes associated with fever. Hoarseness or difficulty swallowing may also develop.

Symptoms of thyroid hormone excess (hyperthyroidism) such as nervousness, rapid heart rate, and heat intolerance may be present early in the disease. Later, symptoms of too little thyroid hormone (hypothyroidism) such as fatigue, constipation, or cold intolerance may occur. Eventually, thyroid gland function returns to normal.

"Subacute Thyroiditis," © 2004 A.D.A.M., Inc. Reprinted with permission.

Subacute thyroiditis occurs most often in middle-aged women with recent symptoms of viral respiratory tract infection.

Symptoms

- pain in the front of the neck
- tenderness when gentle pressure is applied to the thyroid gland (palpation)
- fever
- weakness
- fatigue

Other symptoms may include:

- nervousness
- heat intolerance
- weight loss
- sweating
- diarrhea
- tremor
- palpitations

Signs and Tests

Laboratory tests in the early phase of disease may reveal:

- High serum thyroglobulin level
- Low radioactive iodine uptake
- Low serum thyroid stimulating hormone (TSH) level
- High serum free T4 (thyroid hormone, thyroxine) level
- High erythrocyte sedimentation rate (ESR)

Laboratory tests in the later phase of disease may show:

- High serum TSH level
- Low serum free T4

Anti-thyroid antibodies are either undetectable or present at low levels. Thyroid gland biopsy shows characteristic giant cell inflammation. Laboratory abnormalities return to normal as the condition resolves.

Treatment

The purpose of treatment is to reduce pain and inflammation and to treat any hyperthyroidism, if present. Anti-inflammatory medications such as aspirin or ibuprofen are used to control pain in mild cases of subacute thyroiditis.

More serious cases may require temporary treatment with steroids (for example, prednisone) to control inflammation. Symptoms of hyperthyroidism are treated with a class of medications called beta-blockers (for example, propranolol or atenolol).

Expectations (Prognosis)

Spontaneous improvement is the rule, but the illness may persist for months. Long-term or severe complications do not usually occur.

Complications

- Relapse of subacute thyroiditis

Calling Your Health Care Provider

Call your health care provider if symptoms of this disorder occur. Also call if you have thyroiditis and symptoms do not improve with treatment.

Prevention

MMR (measles, mumps, rubella) immunization (vaccine) or flu vaccine may be helpful to prevent these causes. Other causes may not be preventable.

Chapter 27

Congenital Hypothyroidism

A Note to Parents

You have just learned that your baby has congenital hypothyroidism. Suddenly, you have a lot of confusion and certainly may be frightened regarding the well being of your new infant. As a concerned parent, you probably wish to learn as much as you can about the condition, and what you and your health care professional can do to help your baby's condition as your child grows and develops.

Ask Questions

As you learn about congenital hypothyroidism, it is probable that you will have questions that may be specific to your child. Leave no questions unanswered, even if you think the questions are simple or silly. A greater understanding of this condition will allow you to provide optimal care for your child.

What Is Congenital Hypothyroidism?

This is a disorder that affects infants from birth (congenital), resulting from the loss of thyroid function (hypothyroidism), normally due to failure of the thyroid gland to develop correctly. Sometimes the thyroid gland is absent or ectopic (in an abnormal location). As a result, the thyroid gland does not produce enough thyroxine (T4) after birth. This may result in abnormal growth and development, as well as slower mental function.

What Is the Thyroid Gland?

The thyroid is a bow tie shaped gland located in the neck, below the Adam's apple. The thyroid gland is part of the endocrine system. This gland is responsible for secreting a hormone called thyroxine (T4) which plays a vital role in normal growth and development in children. This gland, like other glands in the endocrine system is controlled by the pituitary gland. It works very much like a thermostat. The brain senses the amount of T4 and then signals the thyroid with another hormone, thyroid-stimulating hormone (TSH) to produce more or less T4. When the thyroid gland produces enough T4, no extra stimulation is needed and the TSH level remains at a normal level. When there is not enough T4, the TSH rises. These characteristics of the T4 and TSH hormones allow for screening of newborns to assess whether or not they have hypothyroidism (an underactive thyroid gland).

Why Did My Child Develop Congenital Hypothyroidism?

In most hypothyroid babies, there is no specific reason why the thyroid gland did not develop normally, although some of these children have an inherited form of this disorder. Congenital hypothyroidism is present in about 1 out of 4,000 infants in North America. There are a small proportion of children who have temporary (transient) congenital hypothyroidism for a period of time after birth. It is impossible to distinguish these transient hypothyroid babies from those with true congenital hypothyroidism and so these infants will be treated as well. Often, after the age of 2 or 3, children for whom transient or temporary hypothyroidism is suspected, the medication can be gradually discontinued for a short amount of time on a trial basis. The child will be retested to see if they can remain off medicine. This is not the case for true congenital hypothyroidism, where L-thyroxine is necessary throughout your child's life.

Symptoms of Congenital Hypothyroidism

Often these babies appear perfectly normal at birth, which is why screening is so vital. However, some may have one or more of the following symptoms:

- Large, despite having poor feeding habits, increased birth weight.
- Puffy face, swollen tongue.
- Hoarse cry.
- Low muscle tone.
- Cold extremities.
- Persistent constipation, bloated, or full to the touch.
- Lack of energy, sleeps most of the time, appears tired even when awake.
- Little to no growth.

Children born with symptoms have a greater risk of developmental delay than children born without symptoms.

What Tests Are Used to Find Congenital Hypothyroidism?

The usual way to discover congenital hypothyroidism is by a screening process done on all newborns between 24 and 72 hours old. The reason this is done so early is that infants with congenital hypothyroidism usually appear normal at birth, and many do not show any of the signs or symptoms noted before. For the screening test, blood is obtained from your baby's heel and is placed on a filter paper. At a laboratory the T4 and/or TSH level is measured. If the T4 is low and/or the TSH is elevated, indicating hypothyroidism, your pediatrician is contacted immediately so treatment can begin without delay. It is likely that the blood test will be repeated to confirm the diagnosis. The physicians may also take an x-ray of the legs to look at the ends of the bones. In babies with hypothyroidism, the bones have an immature appearance which helps to confirm diagnosis of congenital hypothyroidism. A thyroid scan should be done to determine the location, or absence of the thyroid gland. These tests, bone age, and thyroid scan can be done at the time of diagnosis.

How Does One Treat Congenital Hypothyroidism?

Treatment for congenital hypothyroidism is replacement of the missing thyroid hormone in pill form. It is extremely important that these pills be taken daily for life because thyroxine (T4) is essential for all the body's functions. In general, the average starting dose for

L-thyroxine or Levothyroxine (synthetic T4) in a newborn is between 25 and 50 micrograms (mcg) per day or 10 milligrams (mg) to 15 mg/kilogram (kg) of body weight. This value increases dependent upon the individual needs of the child. The pill can be crushed, and then administered in a small amount of water or formula or breastmilk while your child is still an infant. Please be aware that L-thyroxine should not be mixed with soy formula as this product interferes with absorption. Blood tests will be done on a regular basis to ensure that the hormone levels are in a normal range. Thyroid hormone is necessary for normal brain and intellectual development and such development can be delayed when there is a lack of L-thyroxine. With early replacement of adequate thyroid hormone and proper follow-up and care, the outlook for most children with congenital hypothyroidism is excellent.

What Type of Medical Attention Should My Child Receive?

Generally, children are seen every 2–3 months, for the first three years, once normal levels have been established. The goal is to maintain the concentration of T4 in the mid to upper half of the normal range (10 mg/deciliter (dL) to 16 mg/dL) for the first years of life. The TSH level should be maintained within the normal reference range for infants. The treatment for hypothyroidism is safe, simple, and effective. Successful treatment, however, depends on lifelong daily medication with close follow-up of hormone levels. Making this procedure of taking medication on a routine basis needs to become a part of the lifestyle of you and your child in order to assure optimal growth and development.

Clinical Hypothyroidism

Recognizing Clinical Hypothyroidism

Hypothyroidism, or a deficiency in the secretion of the thyroid hormones, thyroxine (T4) and triiodothyronine (T3), by the thyroid gland may be difficult to recognize, but usually is very easy to treat. During childhood and adolescence the patient presents either with an enlarged thyroid gland, also known as a goiter, or diminution in the rate of growth in height. At the time of birth the symptoms and signs of hypothyroidism are minimal or absent, and the lack of adequate thyroid hormone from birth until approximately age 2 years is associated with varying degrees of permanent mental retardation. For these reasons most countries in the western world and every state in the United States routinely perform screening tests within the first week of life to detect congenital hypothyroidism so that prompt treatment can be initiated to prevent mental retardation.

Causes

Hypothyroidism usually is caused by an abnormality of the immune system that results in damage and destruction of the thyroid gland. This process results either in loss of thyroid tissue or an enlargement of the thyroid. The gland has the shape of a bow tie or butterfly, and is located just below the larynx, or Adam's apple, and in front of the trachea, or windpipe. In most instances there is no pain or tenderness associated with thyroid diseases, although patients occasionally complain of difficulty in swallowing as if there were a lump in their throat.

Signs

Often the only sign of hypothyroidism during childhood is an abnormal rate of linear growth. Actually the child may not be short compared to other children of the same age if he or she were above average in height before the disease occurred. Therefore, the most important feature of hypothyroidism is a decrease in the rate or velocity of growth in height. If the disease is recognized early and adequately treated, the child will grow at an accelerated rate until reaching the same growth percentile where the child measured prior to the onset of hypothyroidism. Hypothyroidism progresses very slowly and insidiously, making the diagnosis difficult for physicians. In the more advanced and long-standing the child may have other general symptoms of hypothyroidism, such as easy fatigue, mild weight gain in association with a reduction in appetite, constipation, an intolerance of cold weather, dry skin, and either delayed (usual) or early (rare) onset of sexual development at adolescence.

Other Possible Causes

Less often, hypothyroidism may be caused by a failure of the pituitary gland to secrete thyroid stimulating hormone, or TSH. This hormone is essential for stimulating the thyroid gland to make T4 and T3 in normal amounts. TSH may be deficient for several reasons:

1. The pituitary gland is diseased, a rare cause.

2. The area above the pituitary, called the hypothalamus that is necessary to stimulate the pituitary, is diseased.

3. There is a tumor, cyst, or other abnormal structure between the hypothalamus and pituitary gland that prevents the pituitary from receiving its stimulus to secrete TSH.

Usually patients with TSH deficiency also have deficient secretion of growth hormone, and may have deficient secretion of the gonadotropins, called LH and FSH, which stimulate puberty and reproduction, and adrenocorticotropic hormone (ACTH), which is necessary for cortisol and hydrocortisone secretion by the adrenal gland.

Treatment

The treatment of hypothyroidism, regardless of the cause, is easy and inexpensive. One or two tablets of the major thyroid hormone, thyroxine (trade names in the U.S. are Levothroid, Levoxyl, and Synthroid) once a day provides normal thyroid function and growth. The dose, depending upon the child's age, ranges between 50 micrograms (µg) (0.05 mg) and 200 µg (0.2 mg) although some infants require slightly lower doses. The blood levels of T4 and TSH should be monitored annually to assure that the dose remains adequate as the child grows. In most instances the treatment must be continued for life since the diseases that cause hypothyroidism are permanent rather than transient.

Every child that has a decrease in the rate of growth in height during childhood and adolescence should have blood tests to measure T4, free T4, and TSH in order to determine if the growth problem is caused by hypothyroidism.

Additional Information

Magic Foundation
6645 W. North Ave.
Oak Park, IL 60302
Phone: 708-383-0808
Fax: 708-383-0899
Website: http://www.magicfoundation.org

Chapter 28

Pendred Syndrome

What is Pendred syndrome?

Pendred syndrome is a genetic condition associated with deafness and goiter (an enlargement of the thyroid gland, which is a structure in the lower neck that produces hormones). Some people with Pendred syndrome also have malformations of the inner ear.

How common is Pendred syndrome?

This condition is one of the most common forms of syndromic deafness, or hearing loss associated with a genetic syndrome. Pendred syndrome accounts for at least 5 percent of cases of profound hearing loss.

What genes are related to Pendred syndrome?

Mutations in the *SLC26A4* gene cause Pendred syndrome. The protein made by the *SLC26A4* gene transports negatively charged particles (anions), particularly chloride and iodide, into and out of cells. The protein appears to be important for normal thyroid function and inner ear development. Mutations in the *SLC26A4* gene can

This chapter includes the following documents from Genetics Home Reference of the National Library of Medicine: "Pendred Syndrome," June 2004; "SLC26A4," June 2004; and "If a genetic disorder runs in my family, what are the chances that my children will have the condition?" August 2004.

lead to the signs of Pendred syndrome, such as hearing loss, structural changes in the inner ear, and goiter.

How do people inherit Pendred syndrome?

This condition is inherited in an autosomal recessive pattern, which means two copies of the gene must be altered for a person to be affected by the disorder. Most often, the parents of a child with an autosomal recessive disorder are not affected, but are carriers of one copy of the altered gene.

What other names do people use for Pendred syndrome?

- Autosomal Recessive Sensorineural Hearing Impairment and Goiter
- Deafness with goiter
- Goiter-deafness syndrome
- Pendred's syndrome

SLC26A4: *Solute Carrier Family 26, Member 4*

What is the normal function of the SLC26A4 gene?

The *SLC26A4* gene provides instructions to make a protein called pendrin, which transports negatively charged particles (anions), particularly chloride and iodide, across cell membranes. Pendrin is present in the kidneys, inner ear, and thyroid. The thyroid is a butterfly-shaped tissue in the lower neck that releases hormones to help regulate growth and the rate of chemical reactions in the body.

The specific function of pendrin in each of these organs and tissues is not fully understood; however, on the basis of cell experiments, researchers have proposed various roles for pendrin. In the thyroid, pendrin probably transports iodide out of cells to bind with a protein (thyroglobulin) that will form iodine-containing thyroid hormones. In the kidneys, pendrin probably assists with chloride transport and the regulation of acid levels. Pendrin's suggested role in the ear is to maintain the proper chloride balance, which affects the amount of fluid that bathes the inner ear. This fluid level appears to be particularly important during development of the ear, as it may influence the shape of the bony structures (such as cochlea and vestibular aqueduct) in the inner ear.

What conditions are related to the SLC26A4 gene?

Nonsyndromic deafness, autosomal recessive—caused by mutations in the SLC26A4 *gene*

Researchers have identified several *SLC26A4* mutations in individuals with nonsyndromic deafness (hearing loss without related signs and symptoms affecting other parts of the body). Most of these mutations change an amino acid (the building material of proteins) in the pendrin protein. A few mutations alter the *SLC26A4* gene by deleting or adding a small segment of DNA. These deletions or additions are predicted to introduce a stop signal that halts protein production prematurely, creating an abnormally short pendrin protein. *SLC26A4* mutations probably reduce pendrin activity, decreasing the transport of chloride, which upsets the fluid balance in the inner ear. Abnormal fluid levels presumably affect inner ear structures (such as the cochlea and vestibular aqueduct), causing hearing loss.

Pendred syndrome caused by mutations in the SLC26A4 *gene*

More than 70 *SLC26A4* mutations can cause Pendred syndrome, a condition characterized by hearing loss and an enlarged thyroid gland (goiter). Many of these mutations change an amino acid (the building material of proteins) in the pendrin protein. The most common substitutions are the replacement of threonine with proline at position 416 in the protein's chain of amino acids (also written as Thr416Pro) and the replacement of leucine with proline at position 236 (or Leu236Pro). Several mutations alter the *SLC26A4* gene by deleting or adding a small segment of DNA. These deletions or additions are predicted to introduce a stop signal that halts protein production prematurely, creating an abnormally short pendrin protein.

SLC26A4 mutations responsible for Pendred syndrome probably cause complete loss of pendrin function, disrupting the transport of chloride and iodide. In the thyroid, impaired transport means that iodide cannot bind effectively to thyroglobulin, a protein necessary for the production of thyroid hormones. The thyroid tissue may enlarge to compensate for the perceived lack of iodine. Disturbed chloride transport upsets the fluid balance in the inner ear, which presumably affects inner ear structures and causes hearing loss.

Where is the SLC26A4 gene located?

The *SLC26A4* gene is located on the long (q) arm of chromosome 7 at position 31 (7q31).

Inheriting Genetic Conditions

If a genetic disorder runs in my family, what are the chances that my children will have the condition?

When a genetic disorder is diagnosed in a family, family members often want to know the likelihood that they or their children will develop the condition. This can be difficult to predict in some cases because many factors influence a person's chances. One important factor is how the condition is inherited. For example:

- A person affected by an autosomal dominant disorder has a 50 percent chance of passing the mutated gene to each child. There is also a 50 percent chance that a child will not inherit the mutated gene.

- For an autosomal recessive disorder, two unaffected people who each carry one copy of the mutated gene (carriers) have a 25 percent chance with each pregnancy of having a child affected by the disorder. There is a 75 percent chance with each pregnancy that a child will be unaffected.

- The chance of passing on an X-linked dominant condition differs between men and women because men have one X and one Y chromosome, while women have two X chromosomes. A man passes on his Y chromosome to all of his sons and his X chromosome to all of his daughters. Therefore, the sons of a man with an X-linked dominant disorder will not be affected, and his daughters will all inherit the condition. A woman passes on one or the other of her X chromosomes to each child. Therefore, a woman with an X-linked dominant disorder has a 50 percent chance of having an affected daughter or son with each pregnancy.

- Because of the difference in sex chromosomes, the probability of passing on an X-linked recessive disorder also differs between men and women. The sons of a man with an X-linked recessive disorder will not be affected, and his daughters will carry one copy of the mutated gene. With each pregnancy, a woman who carries an X-linked recessive disorder has a 50 percent chance of having sons who are affected and a 50 percent chance of having daughters who carry one copy of the mutated gene.

It is important to note that the chance of passing on a genetic condition applies equally to each pregnancy. For example, if a couple has a child with an autosomal recessive disorder, the chance of having another child with the disorder is still 25 percent (or 1 in 4). Having one child with a disorder does not protect future children from inheriting the condition. Conversely, having a child without the condition does not mean that future children will definitely be affected.

Although the chances of inheriting a genetic condition appear straightforward, in some cases factors such as a person's family history and the results of genetic testing can modify those chances. In addition, some people with a disease-causing mutation never develop any health problems or may experience only mild symptoms of the disorder. If a disease that runs in a family does not have a clear inheritance pattern, predicting the likelihood that a person will develop the condition can be particularly difficult.

Because estimating the chance of developing or passing on a genetic disorder can be complex, genetics professionals can help people understand these chances and make informed decisions about their health.

Additional Information

Genetics Home Reference
Website: http://ghr.nlm.nih.gov

Part Five

Overactive Thyroid Gland Disorders

Chapter 29

Hyperthyroidism

Chapter Contents

Section 29.1

Overactive Thyroid: Overview

"Hyperthyroidism: Information for Patients," © 2004 American Association of Clinical Endocrinologists. Reprinted with permission.

Hyperthyroidism

Hyperthyroidism develops when the body is exposed to excessive
amounts of thyroid hormone. This disorder occurs in almost 1% of all
Americans and affects women 5 to 10 times more often than men. In
its mildest form, hyperthyroidism may not cause recognizable symptoms. More often, however, the symptoms are discomforting, disabling,
or even life threatening.

What Are the Symptoms of Hyperthyroidism?

When hyperthyroidism develops, a goiter (enlargement of the thyroid) is usually present and may be associated with some or many of
the following symptoms:

- Fast heart rate, often more than 100 beats per minute
- Nervousness, anxiety, or an irritable and quarrelsome feeling
- Trembling hands
- Weight loss, despite eating the same amount or even more than
  usual
- Intolerance of warm temperatures and increased likelihood to
  perspire
- Loss of scalp hair
- Rapid growth of fingernails and tendency of fingernails to sepa-
  rate from the nail bed
- Muscle weakness, especially of the upper arms and thighs
- Loose and frequent bowel movements
- Thin and delicate skin
- Change in menstrual pattern

- Increased likelihood for miscarriage
- Prominent stare of the eyes
- Protrusion of the eyes, with or without double vision (in patients with Graves disease)
- Irregular heart rhythm, especially in patients older than 60 years of age
- Accelerated loss of calcium from bones, which increases the risk of osteoporosis and fractures

What Are the Causes of Hyperthyroidism?

Graves Disease

Graves disease (named after Irish physician Robert Graves) is an autoimmune disorder that frequently results in thyroid enlargement and hyperthyroidism. In a minority of patients, swelling of the muscles and other tissues around the eyes may develop, causing eye prominence, discomfort, or double vision. Like other autoimmune diseases, this condition tends to affect multiple family members. It is much more common in women than in men, and tends to occur in younger patients.

Toxic Multinodular Goiter

Multiple nodules in the thyroid can produce excessive thyroid hormone, causing hyperthyroidism. Often diagnosed in patients over the age of 50, this disorder is more likely to affect heart rhythm. In many cases, the person has had the goiter for many years before it becomes overactive.

Toxic Nodule

A single nodule or lump in the thyroid can also produce more thyroid hormone than the body requires and lead to hyperthyroidism. This disorder is not familial.

Subacute Thyroiditis

This condition of unknown cause is characterized by painful thyroid gland enlargement and inflammation, which results in the release of large amounts of thyroid hormones into the blood. Fortunately, this condition usually resolves spontaneously. The thyroid usually heals itself over several months, but often not before a temporary period of low thyroid hormone production (hypothyroidism) occurs.

Postpartum Thyroiditis

5% to 10% of women develop mild to moderate hyperthyroidism within several months of giving birth. Hyperthyroidism in this condition usually lasts for approximately 1–2 months. It is often followed by several months of hypothyroidism, but most women will recover normal thyroid function eventually. In some cases, however, the thyroid gland does not heal, so the hypothyroidism becomes permanent and requires lifelong thyroid hormone replacement.

Silent Thyroiditis

Transient (temporary) hyperthyroidism can be caused by silent thyroiditis, a condition which appears to be the same as postpartum thyroiditis, but not related to pregnancy. It is not accompanied by a painful thyroid gland.

Excessive Iodine Ingestion

Various sources of high iodine concentrations, such as kelp tablets, some expectorants, amiodarone (Cordarone, Pacerone—a medication used to treat certain problems with heart rhythms), and x-ray dyes may occasionally cause hyperthyroidism in certain patients.

Overmedication with Thyroid Hormone

Patients who receive excessive thyroxine replacement treatment can develop hyperthyroidism. They should have their thyroid hormone dosage evaluated by a physician at least once each year and should never give themselves extra doses.

How Is Hyperthyroidism Diagnosed?

Characteristic symptoms and physical signs of hyperthyroidism can be detected by a physician. In addition, tests can be used to confirm the diagnosis and to determine the cause.

TSH (Thyroid-Stimulating Hormone or Thyrotropin) Test

A low TSH level in the blood is the most accurate indicator of hyperthyroidism. The body shuts off production of this pituitary hormone when the thyroid gland even slightly overproduces thyroid hormone. If the TSH level is low, it is very important to also check thyroid hormone levels to confirm the diagnosis of hyperthyroidism

Other Tests

- Free T4 (thyroxine) and Free T3 (triiodothyronine)—the active thyroid hormones in the blood. When hyperthyroidism develops, free T4 and T3 levels rise above previous values in that specific patient (although they may still fall within the normal range for the general population), and are often considerably elevated.

- TSI (thyroid-stimulating immunoglobulin)—a substance often found in the blood when Graves disease is the cause of hyperthyroidism. This test is ordered infrequently, since it rarely affects treatment decisions.

- Radioactive iodine uptake (RAIU; a measurement of how much iodine the thyroid gland can collect) and thyroid scan (a thyroid scan shows how the iodine is distributed throughout the thyroid gland). This information can be useful in determining the cause of hyperthyroidism and ultimately its treatment.

Sometimes a general physician can diagnose and treat the cause of hyperthyroidism, but assistance is often needed from an endocrinologist, a physician who specializes in managing thyroid disease.

How Is Hyperthyroidism Treated?

Before the development of current treatment options, the death rate from hyperthyroidism was as high as 50%. Now several effective treatments are available, and with proper management, death from hyperthyroidism is rare. Deciding which treatment is best depends on what caused the hyperthyroidism, its severity, and other conditions present. A physician who is experienced in the management of thyroid diseases can confidently diagnose the cause of hyperthyroidism and prescribe and manage the best treatment program for each patient.

Antithyroid Drugs

In the United States, 2 drugs are available for treating hyperthyroidism: propylthiouracil (PTU) and methimazole (Tapazole). These medications control hyperthyroidism by slowing thyroid hormone production, and are frequently used for several months after the initial diagnosis of hyperthyroidism to normalize the thyroid hormone levels. Some patients with hyperthyroidism caused by Graves disease experience a spontaneous or natural remission of hyperthyroidism after a 12 to 18 month course of treatment with these drugs, and may sometimes avoid permanent underactivity of the thyroid (hypothyroidism), which often occurs as a result of using the other methods of treating hyperthyroidism. Unfortunately, the remission is frequently only temporary, with the hyperthyroidism recurring after several months or years off medication and requiring additional treatment, so relatively few patients are treated solely with antithyroid medication in the United States.

Antithyroid drugs may cause an allergic reaction in about 5% of patients who use them. This usually occurs during the first 6 weeks of drug treatment. Such a reaction may include rash, hives, fever, or joint pain, but after discontinuing use of the drug the symptoms resolve within 1–2 weeks and there is no permanent damage.

A more serious effect, but occurring in only about 1 in 250–500 patients during the first 4 to 8 weeks of treatment, is a rapid decrease of white blood cells in the bloodstream. This could increase susceptibility to serious infection. Symptoms such as a sore throat, joint aches, infection, or fever should be reported promptly to your physician, and a blood cell count should be done immediately. In nearly every case, when a person stops using the medication, the white blood cell count returns to normal.

Very rarely, antithyroid drugs may cause liver problems, which can be detected by monitoring blood tests. Your physician should be contacted if there is yellowing of the skin (jaundice), fever, loss of appetite, or abdominal pain.

Radioactive Iodine Treatment

Iodine is an essential ingredient in the production of thyroid hormone. Each molecule of thyroid hormone contains either 4 (T4) or 3 (T3) molecules of iodine. Since most overactive thyroid glands are quite hungry for iodine, it was discovered in the 1940s that the thyroid could be tricked into destroying itself by simply feeding it radioactive iodine. The radioactive iodine is given by mouth, usually in capsule form, and is quickly absorbed from the bowel. It then enters the thyroid cells from the bloodstream and gradually destroys them. Maximal benefit is usually noted within 3 to 6 months.

It is not possible to reliably eliminate just the right amount of the diseased thyroid gland, since the effects of the radioiodine are slowly progressive on the thyroid cells. Therefore, most endocrinologists strive to completely destroy the diseased thyroid gland with a single dose of radioiodine. This results in the intentional development of an underactive thyroid state (hypothyroidism), which is easily, predictably, and inexpensively corrected by lifelong daily use of oral thyroid hormone replacement therapy. Although every effort is made to calculate the correct dose of radioiodine for each patient, not every treatment will successfully correct the hyperthyroidism, particularly if the goiter is quite large, and a second dose of radioactive iodine is occasionally needed.

In the 50+ years and hundreds of thousands of patients (including a former President of the United States and his wife) in which radioiodine has been used, no serious complications have been reported. Since the treatment appears to be extraordinarily safe, simple, and reliably effective, it is considered by most thyroid specialists in the United States to be the treatment of choice for those types of hyperthyroidism caused by overproduction of thyroid hormones.

Surgical Removal of the Thyroid

Although seldom used now as the preferred treatment for hyperthyroidism, operating to remove most of the thyroid gland may occasionally be recommended in certain situations, such as a pregnant woman with severe disease in whom radioiodine would not be safe for the baby, removal of a clinically suspicious thyroid nodule coexisting with hyperthyroidism, or for rare patients with Graves disease who have severe protrusion of their eyes. In such patients, permanent hypothyroidism usually results, and lifelong thyroxine replacement is required.

Other Treatments

A drug from the class of beta-adrenergic blocking agents (which decrease the effects of excess thyroid hormone) may be used temporarily to control hyperthyroid symptoms while one of the mentioned treatments becomes effective. In cases where hyperthyroidism is caused by thyroiditis or excessive ingestion of either iodine or thyroid hormone, this may be the only type of treatment required. Of course, taking too much of either substance should also be corrected.

Appropriate management of hyperthyroidism requires careful evaluation and ongoing care by a physician experienced in the treatment of this complex condition.

Additional Information

American Association of Clinical Endocrinologists (AACE)
1000 Riverside Ave., Suite 205
Jacksonville, FL 32204
Phone: 904-353-7878
Fax: 904-353-8185
Website: http://wwwaace.com
E-mail: info@aace.com

Section 29.2

Pregnancy-Related Issues

Excerpted with permission from *Thyroid Disease and Pregnancy*, Copyright © 2003 The American Thyroid Association. All rights reserved. Also, "FAQ: I may have a overactive thyroid, can I still breastfeed my baby?" © 2003 La Leche League International. All rights reserved. Reprinted with permission.

Hyperthyroidism and Pregnancy

What are the most common causes of hyperthyroidism during pregnancy?

Overall, the most common cause (80–85%) of maternal hyperthyroidism during pregnancy is Graves disease and occurs in 1 in 1500 pregnant patients. In addition to other usual causes of hyperthyroidism, very high levels of human chorionic gonadotropin (hCG), seen in severe forms of morning sickness (*hyperemesis gravidarum*), may cause transient hyperthyroidism. The diagnosis of hyperthyroidism can be somewhat difficult during pregnancy, as I-123 thyroid scanning is contraindicated during pregnancy due to the small amount of radioactivity, which can be concentrated by the baby's thyroid. Consequently, diagnosis is based on a careful history, physical exam, and laboratory testing.

What are the risks of Graves disease/hyperthyroidism to the mother?

Graves disease may present initially during the first trimester or may be exacerbated during this time in a woman known to have the disorder. In addition to the classic symptoms associated with hyperthyroidism, inadequately treated maternal hyperthyroidism can result in early labor and a serious complication known as pre-eclampsia. Additionally, women with active Graves disease during pregnancy are at higher risk of developing very severe hyperthyroidism known as thyroid storm. Graves disease often improves during the third trimester of pregnancy and may worsen during the postpartum period.

What are the risks of Graves disease/hyperthyroidism to the baby?

The risks to the baby from Graves disease are due to one of three possible mechanisms:

1. **Uncontrolled maternal hyperthyroidism:** Uncontrolled maternal hyperthyroidism has been associated with fetal tachycardia (fast heart rate), small for gestational age babies, prematurity, stillbirths, and possibly congenital malformations. This is another reason why it is important to treat hyperthyroidism in the mother.

2. **Extremely high levels of thyroid stimulating immunoglobulins (TSI):** Graves disease is an autoimmune disorder caused by the production of antibodies that stimulate thyroid gland referred to as thyroid stimulating immunoglobulins (TSI). These antibodies do cross the placenta and can interact with the baby's thyroid. Although uncommon (2–5% of cases of Graves disease in pregnancy), high levels of maternal TSIs, have been known to cause fetal or neonatal hyperthyroidism. Fortunately, this typically only occurs when the mother's TSI levels are very high (many times above normal). Measuring TSI in the mother with Graves disease is often done in the third trimester. In the mother with Graves disease requiring antithyroid drug therapy, fetal hyperthyroidism due to the mother's TSI is rare, since the antithyroid drugs also cross the placenta. Of potentially more concern to the baby is the mother with prior treatment for Graves disease (for example radioactive iodine or surgery) who no longer requires antithyroid drugs. It is very important

to tell your doctor if you have been treated for Graves disease in the past so proper monitoring can be done to ensure the baby remains healthy during the pregnancy.

3. **Anti-thyroid drug therapy (ATD):** Methimazole (Tapazole) or propylthiouracil (PTU) are the ATDs available in the United States for the treatment of hyperthyroidism. Both of these drugs cross the placenta and can potentially impair the baby's thyroid function and cause fetal goiter. Historically, PTU has been the drug of choice for treatment of maternal hyperthyroidism, possibly because transplacental passage may be less than with Tapazole. However, recent studies suggest that both drugs are safe to use during pregnancy. It is recommended that the lowest possible dose of ATD be used to control maternal hyperthyroidism to minimize the development of hypothyroidism in the baby or neonate. Neither drug appears to increase the general risk of birth defects. Overall, the benefits to the baby of treating a mother with hyperthyroidism during pregnancy outweigh the risks if therapy is carefully monitored.

What are the treatment options for a pregnant woman with Graves disease/hyperthyroidism?

Mild hyperthyroidism (slightly elevated thyroid hormone levels, minimal symptoms) often is monitored closely without therapy as long as both the mother and the baby are doing well. When hyperthyroidism is severe enough to require therapy, anti-thyroid medications are the treatment of choice, with PTU being the historical drug of choice. The goal of therapy is to keep the mother's free T4 and free T3 levels in the high normal range on the lowest dose of antithyroid medication. Targeting this range of free hormone levels will minimize the risk to the baby of developing hypothyroidism or goiter. Maternal hypothyroidism should be avoided. Therapy should be closely monitored during pregnancy. This is typically done by following thyroid function tests (TSH and thyroid hormone levels) monthly.

In patients who cannot be adequately treated with anti-thyroid medications (i.e., those who develop an allergic reaction to the drugs), surgery is an acceptable alternative. Surgical removal of the thyroid gland is only very rarely recommended in the pregnant woman due to the risks of both surgery and anesthesia to the mother and the baby.

Radioiodine is contraindicated to treat hyperthyroidism during pregnancy since it readily crosses the placenta and is taken up by the

baby's thyroid gland. This can cause destruction of the gland and result in permanent hypothyroidism.

Beta-blockers can be used during pregnancy to help treat significant palpitations and tremor due to hyperthyroidism. They should be
used sparingly due to reports of impaired fetal growth associated with
long-term use of these medications. Typically, these drugs are only
required until the hyperthyroidism is controlled with anti-thyroid
medications.

What is the natural history of Graves disease after delivery?

Graves disease typically worsens in the postpartum period, usually in the first 3 months after delivery. Higher doses of anti-thyroid
medications are frequently required during this time. At usual, close
monitoring of thyroid function tests is necessary.

Can the mother with Graves disease, who is being treated with anti-thyroid drugs, breastfeed her infant?

Yes. PTU is the drug of choice because it is highly protein bound.
Consequently, lower amounts of PTU cross into breastmilk compared
to Tapazole. It is important to note that the baby will require periodic assessment of his/her thyroid function to ensure maintenance of
normal thyroid status.

Breastfeeding Information from La Leche League International

I may have an overactive thyroid; can I still breastfeed my baby?

An overactive thyroid gland, also referred to as hyperthyroidism
or Graves disease, is an important health concern. Thyroid disease is
serious as the thyroid controls the body's metabolic processes. According to La Leche League International's *Breastfeeding Answer Book*
(*BAB*), any breastfeeding mother with thyroid disease should be under the care of a doctor who is supportive of her desire to breastfeed.

Diagnosis of an overactive thyroid can usually be based on the
mother's symptoms as well as a simple blood test. On occasion, radioactive testing is used to diagnose thyroid problems. If radioactive
testing is recommended, the mother can ask her physician if the test
could be postponed or another, non-radioactive test, be substituted.

If the radioactive test is used, temporary weaning is recommended. "The length of time the mother needs to suspend breastfeeding will depend on the type and dosage of radioactive materials used for the test" (*BAB*). Radioactivity of breast milk declines over time, and frequent milk expression will help the mother eliminate the radioactivity from her body more quickly. This milk must be discarded and not fed to the baby. (Frequent milk expression will not hasten the elimination of other drugs from breast milk.)

Some medications for overactive thyroid are not concentrated in human milk and result in minimal doses to the breastfed baby. If a mother is taking thyroid suppressants, she will need to tell her baby's doctor so the baby can be monitored for thyroid levels. Weaning is usually not necessary. If a doctor insists on weaning, the mother is encouraged to seek a second opinion before weaning. When temporary weaning is recommended, it is important to be sure the risks and benefits have been fully evaluated.

If radioactive compounds are used to treat an overactive thyroid, temporary weaning is necessary. The mother will need to pump and discard the milk during this time. Before a mother resumes breastfeeding, her milk must be checked for radioactivity. Your local La Leche League (LLL) Leader will be able to share more information and offer support. Contacting an LLL Leader in your area or attending a meeting will help you cope with this.

Additional Information

American Thyroid Association
6066 Leesburg Pike, Suite 550
Falls Church, VA 22041
Toll-Free: 800-THYROID (849-7643)
Phone: 703-998-8890
Fax: 703-998-8893
Website: http://www.thyroid.org
E-mail: admin@thyroid.org

La Leche League International
P.O. Box 4079
Schaumburg, IL 60168-4079
Phone: 847-519-7730
Fax: 847-519-0035
TTY: 847-592-7570
Website: http://www.lalecheleague.org

Section 29.3

Older Patients and Hyperthyroidism

What do the following patients over the age of 60 years have in common?

1. A 72 year old grandmother with fluttering of the heart and vague chest discomfort on climbing stairs;

2. An 80 year old man with severe constipation who falls asleep during Bingo;

3. A 63 year old retired grade school teacher who has lost strength in her legs, causing difficulty in climbing stairs and in carrying more than 3 books at a time; she has recently lost 15 pounds in spite of a very good appetite;

4. A 75 year old grandmother who has developed difficulty swallowing and a dry cough, accompanied by hoarseness, weight gain, and dry, itchy skin;

5. A 78 year old retired musician whose family complains because he turns the stereo volume up too high;

6. An 84 year old very energetic seamstress in whom a hand tremor has caused her to give up her favorite activity. She is so depressed that she will not eat, and she has lost 12 pounds in the last 4 months.

All of these patients have abnormal function of their thyroid glands. Patients 1, 3, and 6 have hyperthyroidism, that is, excessive production of thyroid hormone by their thyroid glands. Patients 2, 4, and 5 have hypothyroidism, or reduced production of thyroid hormone. While some of the symptoms of hyperthyroidism and hypothyroidism are similar to those in younger patients, it is not uncommon for both hyperthyroidism and hypothyroidism to be manifest in subtle ways in

271

older patients, often masquerading as diseases of the bowel or heart or a disorder of the nervous system. An important clue to the presence of thyroid disease in an elderly patient is a history of thyroid disease in another close family member such as a brother, sister, or child of the patient.

Hyperthyroidism in the Older Patient

As in all hyperthyroid patients, if there is too much thyroid hormone, every function of the body tends to speed up. However, while the younger patient often has multiple symptoms related to the overactive thyroid, the elderly patient may only have one or two symptoms. For example, patient number 1 experienced only a sensation of her heart fluttering, and some chest discomfort on climbing stairs. Other patients may also have few symptoms, such as patient number 6, whose main symptoms are depression and tremor. Such a patient may withdraw from interactions with friends and family.

Treatment of the Older Patient with Hyperthyroidism

As with younger patients, treatment of hyperthyroidism in the older patient includes antithyroid drugs and radioactive iodine. Surgery is rarely recommended due to increased operative risks in the older patient. While Graves disease is still a common cause of hyperthyroidism, toxic nodular goiter is seen more frequently in the older patient. During therapy, the effects of change in thyroid function on other body systems must be closely monitored, due to an increased likelihood of coexisting cardiac, central nervous system, and thyroid disease in older patients. Most often, thyroid function is brought under control first with antithyroid drugs (propylthiouracil or methimazole [Tapazole®]) before definitive treatment with radioactive iodine.

During the initial phase of treatment, doctors will observe cardiac function closely due to the effect of changing thyroid hormone levels on the heart. Symptoms of hyperthyroidism may be brought under control with adjunctive medications, such as beta-adrenergic blockers (propranolol [Inderal®], metoprolol [Lopressor®]), which are often given to slow a rapid heart rate, although they must be given with caution in the patient with coexisting congestive heart failure and the dose should be reduced once thyroid function is controlled in the normal range. Symptoms and signs of angina pectoris and heart failure must be treated in tandem with the treatment to bring thyroid function under control.

Once thyroid function is maintained in the normal range with oral medication, the doctor and patient can make a decision on definitive treatment with radioactive iodine together. In general, an attempt is made to render thyroid function either normal or low in an elderly patient treated with radioactive iodine. Treatment of an underactive thyroid condition (hypothyroidism) is usually more straightforward than the problem of recurrent hyperthyroidism in the older patient, because of the effect hyperthyroidism can have on the heart, as indicated previously.

Summary

Thyroid disorders have no age limits; indeed, hypothyroidism is clearly more common in older than in younger adults. Despite the increased frequency of thyroid problems in older individuals, physicians need a high index of suspicion to make the diagnosis since thyroid disorders often manifest as a disorder of another system in the body. Older patients with thyroid disorders require special attention to gradual and careful treatment, and, as always, require lifelong follow-up.

Additional Information

American Thyroid Association
6066 Leesburg Pike, Suite 550
Falls Church, VA 22041
Toll-Free: 800-THYROID (849-7643)
Phone: 703-998-8890
Fax: 703-998-8893
Website: http://www.thyroid.org
E-mail: admin@thyroid.org

Chapter 30

Graves Disease

Chapter Contents

Section 30.1

Frequently Asked Questions about Graves Disease

What Is Graves Disease?

The leading cause of hyperthyroidism, Graves disease, represents a basic defect in the autoimmune system, causing production of immunoglobulins (antibodies) which stimulate and attack the thyroid gland. This causes growth of the gland and overproduction of thyroid hormone. Similar antibodies may also attack the tissues in the eye muscles and in the pretibial skin (the skin on the front of the lower leg).

Facts

- Graves disease occurs in less than ¼ of 1% of the population.
- Graves disease is more prevalent among females than males.
- Graves disease usually occurs in middle age, but also occurs in children and adolescents.
- Graves disease is not curable, but is a completely treatable disease.

Symptoms

- Fatigue
- Weight loss
- Restlessness
- Tachycardia (rapid heart beat)
- Changes in libido (sex drive)
- Muscle weakness
- Heat intolerance

- Tremors
- Enlarged thyroid gland
- Heart palpitations
- Increased sweating
- Blurred or double vision
- Nervousness and irritability
- Eye complaints, such as redness and swelling
- Hair changes
- Restless sleep
- Erratic behavior
- Increased appetite

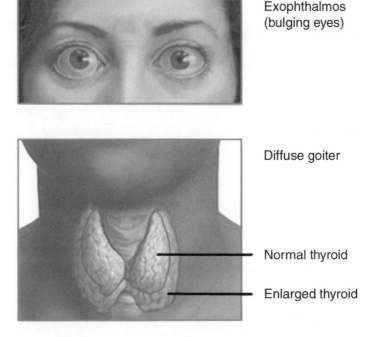

Exophthalmos (bulging eyes)

Diffuse goiter

Normal thyroid

Enlarged thyroid

Figure 30.1. Exophthalmos (Bulging Eyes) and Diffuse Goiter. Graves disease is thought to be an autoimmune disorder of the thyroid which causes over-production of thyroid hormones. Hallmarks of the condition are bulging eyes (exophthalmos), heat intolerance, increased energy, difficulty sleeping, diarrhea, and anxiety. (Source: "Graves Disease," © 2000 A.D.A.M., Inc. Reprinted with permission.)

- Distracted attention span
- Decrease in menstrual cycle
- Increased frequency of stools

Who Develops Graves Disease?

Although Graves disease most frequently occurs in women in the middle decades (8:1 more than men), it also occurs in children and in the elderly. There are several elements contributing to the development of Graves disease. There is a genetic predisposition to autoimmune disorders. Infections and stress play a part. Graves disease may have its onset after a severe external stressor. In other instances, it may follow a viral infection or pregnancy. Many times the exact cause of Graves is simply not known. It is not contagious, although it has been known to occur coincidentally between husbands and wives. Of research importance, the Graves gene in DNA has not yet been identified.

How Is Graves Disease Treated?

There are three standard ways of treating Graves disease. The choice of treatment varies to some degree from country to country and among particular physicians as well. The decision should be made with the full knowledge and informed consent of the patient, who is the primary member of the treatment team. The selection of treatment will include factors such as age, degree of illness, and personal preferences. Generally speaking, from least invasive to most invasive, the treatments include:

1. Anti-thyroid drugs that either block the production or the conversion of thyroid hormone into its active form in the body. They may be used exclusively or in combination with replacement hormone;

2. Radioactive iodine (I-131), which destroys part or all of the thyroid gland and renders it incapable of overproducing thyroid hormone; or

3. Subtotal thyroidectomy in which a surgeon removes most of the thyroid gland and renders it incapable of overproducing thyroid hormone.

The first treatment is about 30–50% effective and the latter two treatments result in about a 90–95% remission rate of the disease. In a few cases, the treatments must be repeated. In all cases, lifetime follow-up laboratory studies must be done, and in almost all cases, lifetime replacement thyroid hormone must be taken.

Are There Any Alternatives to These Treatments of Graves Disease?

There are a number of things you can do to assist your body in healing. However, the state of science as we know it indicates there is no natural way to cure Graves disease. For instance, although there are no specific foods that will change your thyroid function, the more healthy, nutritionally dense foods you eat, the better your body will be able to fight against infection and further insult. Equally, many treatments like acupuncture, exercise, meditation, and various mind-body therapies may provide comfort measures and relief, but are not a substitute for standard medical treatment. Be sure to consult and collaborate with your physician when embarking on additional therapies. There are many studies of other autoimmune disorders that indicate the more input and control a patient has in their care, the more rapid their recovery will be. It is of interest to all who are hopeful of more, effective additional treatment models in the future that the National Institutes of Health are trying to adequately research and evaluate the hard data of alternative therapies.

What Are the Complications?

Graves disease usually responds to treatment, and after the initial period of hyperthyroidism, is relatively easy to treat and manage. There are some exceptions to this, and for some, treatment and subsequent stabilization are much more challenging, both to the patient and the treating team of physicians. The more serious complications of prolonged, untreated, or improperly treated Graves disease includes the possibilities of weakened heart muscle leading to heart failure, osteoporosis, or possible severe emotional disorders.

Additional Information

National Graves' Disease Foundation (NGDF)
P.O. Box 8387
Fleming Island, FL 32006
Phone: 904-278-9488
Website: http://www.ngdf.org

The NGDF is a lay organization that provides patient education and support. Informational bulletins on topics that affect Graves patients and their families are available for a small fee.

The National Graves Disease Foundation seeks:

- To provide current medical information and referral and resource information to those with Graves disease.

- To provide social and psychological support for those with Graves disease by aiding in the development of locally based support groups.

- To provide public education through the distribution of literature, lectures, and presentations in the media and the community.

- To provide professional education through lectures and forums on the prevalence and treatment of Graves disease.

- To publish a periodic newsletter to share information with the membership.

- To establish liaison relationships with major schools, hospitals, and research institutions both nationally and internationally.

Section 30.2

Childhood and Adolescent Hyperthyroidism

Adapted with permission from: Stephen La Franchi, M.D. Hyperthyroidism in Childhood and Adolescence. In: UpToDate, Rose, BD (Ed), UpToDate, Wellesley, MA, 2004. Copyright 2004 UpToDate, Inc. For more information visit www.uptodate.com.

Note: This information has been written for trained healthcare professionals and assumes specialized knowledge. Reference to these materials is no substitute for medical advice based on individual patient assessment, and may not be applicable in all circumstances.

Hyperthyroidism in children and adolescents has unique effects on growth and development in addition to causing many of the same symptoms that it does in adults. The cause is nearly always Graves disease; Graves ophthalmopathy also may be present, but is less severe than in adults.

Incidence

Graves hyperthyroidism occurs in approximately 0.02 percent (1:5000) of children, mostly in the 11- to 15-year age group. Girls are affected more commonly than boys, at a ratio of about 5:1. The ratio is considerably lower among younger children, suggesting that estrogen secretion in some way affects the occurrence of Graves disease.

Pathogenesis

The proximate cause of Graves hyperthyroidism in children and adolescents, as in adults, is thyrotropin (TSH) receptor-stimulating antibodies (TSHR-Ab), which activate the TSH receptor. A population-based study of Danish twins suggested that approximately 80 percent of the risk of Graves disease is attributable to genetic factors. Graves ophthalmopathy may result from antibodies against a TSH receptor—like protein in retroorbital connective tissue.

Other autoimmune diseases—Many children and adolescents with Graves hyperthyroidism have a family history of autoimmune thyroid disease. The patients themselves may have an increased frequency of other autoimmune endocrine diseases such as diabetes mellitus, and primary adrenal insufficiency, and non-endocrine disorders such as vitiligo, systemic lupus erythematosus, rheumatoid arthritis, and pernicious anemia. Children with trisomy 21 (Down syndrome) have an increased risk for Graves hyperthyroidism.

Clinical Manifestations

The clinical features of hyperthyroidism in children and adolescents are similar to those in adults. There are also findings related to the effects of excess thyroid hormone on growth and pubertal development. Summarized briefly:

- Acceleration of growth accompanied by advancement of epiphyseal maturation, so that adult height is normal. The acceleration in growth is usually subtle and depends upon the duration of hyperthyroidism before diagnosis. In children who have hyperthyroidism for one to two years, for example, height may increase from the 50th to the 75th percentile.

- Failure to gain weight or weight loss, despite an increase in appetite, is common.

- Pubertal development tends to be delayed, and among those in whom it has begun, it slows until the hyperthyroidism is treated.

- Girls who have undergone menarche may develop secondary amenorrhea.

Section 30.3

Living with Graves Disease

"Living with Graves' Disease," by Nancy H. Patterson, Ph.D. © 1997 National Graves' Disease Foundation, Inc. Reprinted with permission. Reviewed in December 2004 by Dr. David A. Cooke, M.D., Diplomate, American Board of Internal Medicine.

Many people ask: "What can I do about my Graves disease?" When you feel helpless and powerless, a sense of hopelessness sets in. Although your Graves disease will not go away, there are many things you can do to have a greater sense of mastery in your life. What you eat, what you do, what you think, and what you know—all of these things can affect your life.

Medical Care

First and foremost, adequate health care is a must. Select your physician with care. Ask questions. Although your physician may not be able to spend hours with you, your questions deserve answers. If there are no answers (which in many instances there are none), you deserve that information, too—after all, this is a team effort, and you are the captain.

Your medication is essential. It is a replacement for the thyroid hormone that your body once manufactured. When your thyroid was overactive, there was too much of the hormone circulating. That was the cause of your symptoms of insomnia, anxiety, jitteriness, changes in libido (sex drive), heat intolerance, fatigue, heart racing, and weight loss. When your thyroid was surgically removed or deactivated by radioactive iodine treatments, your body's supply of thyroid hormone was instantly or progressively ended.

Your doctor will perform the blood tests to determine the level of thyroxine you need. If your blood level is too high, you will begin to experience similar symptoms as when you were hyperthyroid. If the blood level of the hormone is too low, you will experience hypothyroid symptoms. These are slow heart rate, hair and nail changes, dry skin, sensitivity to cold, joint pains, hoarseness, weight gain, loss of appetite, difficulty concentrating, depression, constipation, changes in libido (sex drive), muscle weakness or muscle cramps, and puffy eyes. If you begin to feel any of these symptoms, contact your doctor. A simple blood test will clarify if your medication needs adjusting. You are not bothering the doctor. If your blood levels are satisfactory, there may be other medications or therapies that will take care of the symptoms. The remainder of your care, however, is up to you.

Nutrition

There are a number of nutritional concepts with which you need to become familiar and keep in mind when you plan your meals. Weight control is usually important to people with Graves disease. Your thyroid controls metabolism, and you may now have a tendency to gain weight. Eating to reduce caloric intake while maintaining high nutrition requires more effort than you may have expended in the past.

- Focus on fresh fruits and vegetables. These will give you the most vitamins and minerals for your efforts and offer the balance you need.

- The preservatives (sodium) in canned and frozen foods may contribute to edema. Swelling is frequently a problem for Graves patients. You may now need to be more aware of your total salt intake.

- People with Graves disease sometimes develop problems with elevated total cholesterol.

- You may have to become aware of your fat intake. Fish and chicken will be better for you rather than excessive amounts of pork and beef. Limit rich sauces and cheeses.

Learn about nutrition. There are many resources. Both the American Heart Association and the American Diabetes Association have excellent, nutritional food plans, as does Weight Watchers, your local hospital dietitians, and registered dietitian consultants. Fad diets are not healthy—avoid them.

Exercise

You will feel better if you develop a regular exercise program. No one expects you to be an Olympic athlete. Exercises that strengthen your heart and improve circulation and muscle tone are needed to keep your cardiovascular system functioning well and keep you physically fit. The emphasis on exercise for Graves patients needs to be on weight-bearing exercise. This type of exercise has the most benefit to maintaining bone density. Studies show that exercise reduces appetite and increases your energy level. Concentrate on activities you already know how to do, as well as learning new ones. Have a variety of physical activities to avoid boredom, as well as the limitations of weather. Walking continues to be the most overall beneficial physical activity, and it is available to everyone. If you can't walk, bike, or swim—rock! Vigorous rocking in a stable rocking chair uses all the muscles in the body.

Relaxation

Learning to relax refers to reducing the muscular tension in order to increase effective circulation, as well as mental calmness. It is not only an attitude, but a learnable skill. Relaxation is more than just getting away. It is a positive and satisfying experience that gives peace of mind. It is well documented that Graves disease is also a stress-related and stress-mediated illness. The stress is often simply a result of the fast-paced, action-packed lifestyle we lead. Relaxation may take many forms: learning new things, exercising, gardening, walking in the woods, creative activities, soft lighting, soft music, a bubble bath, a good book. Whatever is totally absorbing.

If you are interested in some of the mental exercises to create peace of mind and relaxed bodies, there are many to choose from. You might prefer the systematic tension and letting go of specific muscle groups, known as progressive muscle relaxation (PMR), or you might like imagining beautiful scenes. There is considerable research being done on the effectiveness of mental imagery (visualization) and its effect on the immune system. Yoga, Tai Chi, self-hypnosis, and meditation are all ways to practice relaxation and visualization.

Relaxation exercises must be practiced daily. When you discover your favorite activities, plan to devote at least one half hour each day. You have to make a personal commitment to yourself. The National Institute of Mental Health says: "Remember, finding effective techniques for relaxation is not merely a pastime for the idle rich. It is essential for everyone's physical and mental well-being."

Another phase of relaxation is developing the ability to pace yourself. As a rule, people with Graves are the type that are intense, fast-paced, and accustomed to doing many things at once, and at full speed ahead. This is not conducive to maintaining a balance. There is the tendency that when one is having a good day to try to finish up everything that has been left unattended. The result is utter exhaustion the next day. This can be avoided by pacing your activities to make every day a productive day.

Support System

A support system may be defined as those caring and available people in your life who will listen, who will tell it like it is, and who allow you to reciprocate that caring, sharing dialogue. It is important that people in your support system be available, that is, live near you. Long-distance friends are good to have, but do not substitute for a support system near at hand. Listening is important. Many times you do not need advice. You just need to say what you are thinking and feeling out loud, and have those thoughts and feelings acknowledged. You need to discuss things; not necessarily have problems solved.

One of the purposes of the National Graves Disease Foundation is to establish support groups in as many places as possible. In that way, those with Graves disease can talk with others who understand. There is significant evidence that support groups are one of the most powerful institutions for specific groups. Support groups provide the essential ingredient that is needed for everyone who has to live with a disorder—hope and a sense of humor!

Additional Information

National Graves' Disease Foundation (NGDF)
P.O. Box 8387
Fleming Island, FL 32006
Phone: 904-278-9488
Website: http://www.ngdf.org

The NGDF is a lay organization that provides patient education and support. Informational bulletins on topics that affect Graves patients and their families are available for a small fee.

Chapter 31

Toxic Nodular Goiter

Alternative names: Toxic adenoma; Toxic multinodular goiter; Plummer's disease

Definition: Toxic nodular goiter involves an enlarged thyroid gland that contains a small rounded mass or masses called nodules, which produce too much thyroid hormone.

Causes, Incidence, and Risk Factors

Toxic nodular goiter arises from a long-standing simple goiter and occurs most often in the elderly. Symptoms are those of hyperthyroidism, but the protruding eyeballs seen in Graves disease do not occur. Risk factors include being female and over 60 years old. This disorder is never seen in children.

Symptoms

- weight loss
- increased appetite
- nervousness
- restlessness
- heat intolerance

"Toxic Nodular Goiter," © 2004 A.D.A.M., Inc. Reprinted with permission.

- increased sweating
- fatigue
- muscle cramps
- frequent bowel movements
- menstrual irregularities (in women)

Signs and Tests

A physical examination reveals single or multiple nodules in the thyroid. There may be a rapid heart rate.

- A thyroid scan shows elevated radioactive iodine uptake in the nodules.
- Serum TSH (thyroid stimulating hormone) is decreased.
- Serum thyroid hormone levels (T3, T4) are elevated.

Treatment

Radioactive iodine, surgery, or antithyroid drugs (propylthiouracil, methimazole) are the treatments used for toxic nodular goiter.

Beta-blockers, such as propranolol, can control some of the symptoms of hyperthyroidism until thyroid hormone levels in the body are under control.

Expectations (Prognosis)

Since toxic nodular goiter is primarily a disease of the elderly, other chronic health problems may influence the outcome of this condition. The elderly person may be less able to tolerate the effect of hyperthyroidism on the heart.

Complications

Cardiac complications include rapid heart rate, congestive heart failure, and atrial fibrillation (a rapid and irregular heart rhythm). Another complication of hyperthyroidism is bone loss leading to osteoporosis.

Thyroid crisis or storm is an acute worsening of the symptoms of hyperthyroidism, which may occur with infection or stress. Fever, decreased mental alertness, and abdominal pain may occur, and immediate hospitalization is necessary.

Calling Your Health Care Provider

Call your health care provider if symptoms of this disorder occur. Follow the health care provider's recommendations for follow-up visits.

Prevention

To prevent toxic nodular goiter, treat hyperthyroidism and simple goiter as your health care provider recommends.

Note: This information provided should not be used during any medical emergency or for the diagnosis or treatment of any medical condition. A licensed physician should be consulted for diagnosis and treatment of any and all medical conditions. Call 911 for all medical emergencies.

Chapter 32

Thyrotoxic Periodic Paralysis

Alternative names: Periodic paralysis–thyrotoxic

Definition: Thyrotoxic periodic paralysis a syndrome character-ized by intermittent episodes of muscle weakness that occurs in people with high levels of thyroid hormone (thyrotoxicosis, hyperthyroidism).

Causes, Incidence, and Risk Factors

Thyrotoxic periodic paralysis is a rare condition that occurs only in people with thyrotoxicosis (high thyroid hormone levels). It is seen most commonly in Asian men. There is a similar disorder, hypokale-mic periodic paralysis (familial periodic paralysis), that is an inher-ited condition and is not associated with high thyroid levels.

Thyrotoxic periodic paralysis involves attacks of muscle weakness or paralysis alternating with periods of normal muscle function. At-tacks usually begin after symptoms of hyperthyroidism have devel-oped. The frequency of attacks varies from daily to yearly. Episodes of muscle weakness may last for a few hours or may persist for sev-eral days.

During an attack, there is a low level of potassium in the blood-stream (serum). Serum potassium levels are normal between attacks. There is no decrease in total body potassium, however.

"Thyrotoxic Periodic Paralysis," © 2004 A.D.A.M., Inc. Reprinted with per-mission.

Normally, potassium flows from the bloodstream into muscle cells. When levels of potassium are low (hypokalemia), there may not be enough for proper muscle function. Insulin levels may affect the disorder because insulin increases the flow of potassium into cells.

Weakness most commonly affects the muscles of the arms and legs. It may occasionally affect the muscles of the eyes. The muscles involved in breathing and swallowing can sometimes be affected and this can be fatal.

Heart arrhythmias can also occur during attacks because of the drop in potassium levels. Although muscle strength is initially normal between attacks, repeated attacks may eventually cause progressive and persistent muscle weakness.

Risk factors include a family history of periodic paralysis and hyperthyroidism. Attacks may be triggered by eating high-carbohydrate or high-salt meals. Rest after vigorous exercise can also trigger an attack.

Symptoms

- weakness/paralysis
  - most common in shoulders and hips
  - more common in legs than arms
  - intermittent occurrences
  - triggered by rest after exercise
  - triggered by heavy, high-carbohydrate, high-salt meals
  - lasting for up to several days
- spontaneous recovery of normal strength between attacks
- vision changes (rare)
- swallowing difficulty (rare)
- speech difficulty (rare)
- difficulty breathing (rare)
- alert during attacks

Symptoms of hyperthyroidism:

- increased appetite
- weight loss
- skin changes: moist, warm, thin, pale (occasionally)

- tremors
- fast heart rate
- sensation of feeling the heart beat (palpitations)
- headache
- excessive sweating (diaphoresis)
- insomnia
- heat intolerance
- fatigue

Signs and Tests

The health care provider may suspect thyrotoxic periodic paralysis based on a family history of the disorder, the episodic nature of symptoms, low potassium levels during attacks, abnormal thyroid hormone levels, and elimination of other disorders associated with low potassium as the cause of symptoms.

Between attacks, examination is normal, or there may be signs of hyperthyroidism, such as an enlarged thyroid. During an attack, reflexes may be decreased or absent. Weakness is constant rather than spastic (spasmodic) and is greater in muscle groups near the body (such as shoulders and hips) than muscle groups farther away from the body (such as arms, hands, legs, or feet). The health care provider may attempt to trigger an attack by administering insulin and glucose (which reduces potassium levels) or thyroid hormone.

Hyperthyroidism is confirmed by abnormal results of:

- low serum TSH (thyroid stimulating hormone) levels
- high thyroid hormone levels (T3 or T4)

Serum potassium is low during attacks, but is normal between attacks, confirming the diagnosis. An ECG (electrocardiogram) may be abnormal during attacks. An EMG (electromyogram) is normal between attacks. During an attack EMG is abnormal, showing electrical silence. A muscle biopsy may occasionally show abnormalities.

Treatment

The best treatment is rapid reduction in thyroid hormone levels. Potassium should also be given during the attack. It is preferred that potassium be given by mouth, but if weakness is severe, intravenous potassium may be necessary. (Note: intravenous potassium should be given only if kidney function is adequate and if the person is monitored in the hospital.)

Weakness that involves the muscles used for breathing or swallowing is an emergency and patients must be taken to a hospital. Dangerous heart arrhythmias may also occur during attacks.

A diet that is low in carbohydrates and salt may be recommended to prevent attacks. In addition, medications called beta-blockers may reduce the number and severity of attacks while hyperthyroidism is brought under control.

Acetazolamide, a medication that is effective in attack prevention with familial periodic paralysis, is usually not effective with thyrotoxic periodic paralysis.

Expectations (Prognosis)

Chronic attacks will eventually result in progressive muscle weakness that is present even between attacks. Thyrotoxic periodic paralysis responds well to treatment. Treatment of hyperthyroidism will prevent attacks and may even reverse progressive muscle weakness.

Complications

- heart arrhythmias during attacks
- difficulty breathing, speaking, or swallowing during attacks (rare)
- progressive muscle weakness

Calling Your Health Care Provider

Go to the emergency room or call the local emergency number (such as 911) if intermittent muscle weakness occurs, particularly if there is a family history of periodic paralysis or thyroid disorders.

Fainting and difficulty breathing, speaking, or swallowing are among the emergency symptoms.

Prevention

Genetic counseling may be advised. Treatment of the underlying thyroid disorder prevents attacks of weakness.

Note: The information provided herein should not be used during any medical emergency or for the diagnosis or treatment of any medical condition. A licensed physician should be consulted for diagnosis and treatment of any and all medical conditions. Call 911 for all medical emergencies.

Additional Information

National Institute of Diabetes and Digestive and Kidney Diseases (NIDDK)
NIH Building 31, Room 9A04
Bethesda, MD 20892
Phone: 301-496-3583
Website: http://www.niddk.nih.gov

Muscular Dystrophy Association
3300 E. Sunrise Dr.
Tucson, AZ 85718-3208
Toll-Free: 800-572-1717
Phone: 520-529-2000
Fax: 520-529-5300
Website: http://www.mdausa.org
E-mail: mda@mdausa.org

Chapter 33

Thyroid-Stimulating Hormone (TSH) Producing Pituitary Gland Tumors

TSH-Producing Tumors

These pituitary tumors produce too much thyroid-stimulating hormone (TSH, also called thyrotrophin), causing the thyroid gland to become overactive (hyperthyroidism). They are among the least common types of pituitary tumors.

Symptoms

TSH-producing tumors may cause the following signs and symptoms:

- rapid heart rate
- tremors
- unexplained weight loss
- increased appetite
- feeling too warm or hot
- trouble falling asleep
- anxiety
- frequent bowel movements

- a lump in the front of the neck (due to an enlarged thyroid gland)

Diagnosis

If your doctor suspects a TSH-producing tumor, a blood test may be ordered to measure your level of TSH and thyroid hormones. MRI may also be used to visualize the tumor.

Treatment

Surgery to remove the tumor is the primary therapy for TSH-secreting tumors. Surgery for pituitary tumors is often performed through a minimally invasive approach called transsphenoidal hypophysectomy, whereby the surgeon removes the tumor through an incision in the nasal passage. In cases where the tumor is too large to be removed through this approach, the surgeon performs a craniotomy, removing the tumor through an incision in the front of the skull.

If surgery alone is not curative, you may also have radiation therapy. Some patients receive injections of octreotide acetate (Sandostatin). Given just once a month, this long-acting medication works by suppressing TSH production.

Follow-Up

Your doctor will see you periodically and perform certain tests to ensure that your pituitary tumor has not returned. If medication is part of your treatment, you may need to take it for the rest of your life to prevent tumor recurrence.

Pituitary Tumors in Children

The pituitary gland is a peanut-shaped gland in the brain, behind and between the eyes. Childhood pituitary tumors, although rare, do occur. Such tumors are usually benign, that is, non-cancerous. However, because the pituitary gland is very important in helping to regulate the hormones of the body, even a small disruption can have serious effects on mood, on the ability to focus and concentrate, as well as on growth and overall maturation. Pituitary tumors can also cause symptoms due to pressure on other parts of the brain and may cause headaches, dizziness, or problems with vision.

New diagnostic techniques and chemical assays or tests for specific hormones, as well as computerized imaging tools such as magnetic resonance tomography (MR) and computerized tomography (CT) are used to locate and diagnose pituitary tumors. Then microsurgery, radiation therapy, hormones, and/or drugs are used to treat pituitary tumors in children. The effects of some tumors can also often be improved by hormone replacement therapies. Scientists at the National Institutes of Health and others around the world are improving the diagnosis and therapy of pituitary tumors and learning about the molecular mechanisms that cause these tumors. There is also a constant search for genetic patterns and an on-going effort to develop new gene-based therapies to prevent or treat pituitary tumors.

The Pituitary Gland

The pituitary gland is called a master gland, one that coordinates signals for hormone production from the brain, the hypothalamus, and from other parts of the body This gland secretes a number of hormones that help control and respond to stress, affect brain functions, such as the ability to focus and pay attention, and to govern growth and sexual development, energy metabolism, and the body's ability to defend itself.

Classification of Pituitary Tumors

Pituitary tumors that secrete hormones take the name of the hormone they secrete and the ending "oma." For instance, a tumor that secretes prolactin is called prolactinoma. Other pituitary tumors secreting corticotropin are termed corticotropinomas, and so on. Each of these tumors produces a characteristic syndrome in patients because of excessive hormone secretion. Tumors that do not secrete hormones can cause problems by interfering with the functioning of the pituitary gland and by causing pressure on other parts of the brain.

Symptoms

In general, the symptoms seen with pituitary tumors are related to a disturbance in production of a specific hormone or group of hormones and relate to the role the hormones play in maintaining health and development. The symptoms of pituitary tumors vary depending on the size and location of the tumor and whether the tumor presses on other organs or affects the secretion of hormones. For instance, pituitary tumors may press on the optic nerve, causing problems with vision.

The symptoms of a pituitary tumor can range from simple common complaints such as listlessness or restlessness to more severe symptoms such as headaches, vomiting, or dizziness. One problem in determining whether or not a tumor is present is that every child has minor and relatively unimportant symptoms such as restlessness or headaches from time to time. Of course, when more distressing signs or multiple symptoms are seen, parents and doctors search for an explanation and more precise tests are recommended.

In older children or adolescents, other signs may be seen including problems with normal growth and development. For instance, sometimes young girls or boys, under age 9, experience a very early puberty, referred to as precocious puberty. This is caused by tumors that secrete luteinizing hormone (LH). Girls may develop breasts, have pubic hair, and begin menstruation. Boys may find their genitals enlarging and facial and pubic hair beginning to grow. Tumors that secrete follicle stimulating hormone (FSH), in contrast, can retard sexual development in both sexes and stunt growth.

If the tumor limits the secretion of gonadotropin, it can affect the development and functioning of the ovaries and testes. Adolescent boys may fail to enter puberty or may lose facial or pubic hair and notice an effect on their genital size. Adolescent girls may also fail to enter puberty or may find their breasts smaller, some loss of pubic hair, and perhaps an interruption of menstruation.

Where secretion of adrenocorticotropic hormone (ACTH) is low, the child can experience low blood sugar, fatigue, and low blood pressure which can cause dizziness when standing. On the other hand, with pituitary tumors that secrete ACTH, a variety of problems can result. These include stunted growth, delayed or stopped puberty, weight gain, acne, purple streaks in the skin, a round red face, and a bulge of fat on the back of or below the neck. These tumors can also cause weakness, depression, or forgetfulness, and trigger a sudden complete or partial loss of vision.

Some pituitary tumors can disrupt the function of the thyroid gland by secreting thyroid stimulating hormone (TSH). This in turn enlarges the thyroid, causing a visibly large lump in the neck known as a goiter. These tumors also cause nervousness, a rapid pulse, weight loss, excess eating and sweating, and a sensitivity to heat.

Pituitary tumors that limit the secretion of TSH can also affect a child in many ways, including making it harder to concentrate, tiredness, constipation, dry skin, and a sensitivity to cold. It may also cause girls to have irregular periods or not to menstruate at all.

Some pituitary tumors decrease the secretion of vasopressin, the hormone that triggers the kidney's reabsorption of water from urine. A lack of vasopressin can cause a great thirst, excess urination, voracious appetite accompanied by emaciation, loss of strength, and fainting.

Other pituitary tumors secrete an excess of the hormone prolactin. In girls who have gone through puberty, tumors that secrete the hormone prolactin can cause the production of breast milk and stop menstruation, while in post-pubertal boys they can cause impotence. An excess of prolactin can also delay or stop puberty in both sexes.

A pituitary tumor that limits the secretion of growth hormone (GH) can stunt the growth of children and cause low blood sugar, which can induce fainting, dizziness, anxiety, and intense hunger. Growth hormone secreting tumors in growing children can boost growth excessively so that, if not treated, the children can grow unusually tall.

In adolescent children who have gone through puberty, and whose bones have stopped growing, excess GH can cause enlargement of their feet, hands, lips, nose, and jaw, a condition referred to as acromegaly It also can foster excess perspiration and fatigue, a widening of the spaces between the teeth, furrows in the forehead, and weakness in the hands.

The most common type of pituitary tumor in children is due to growth of embryonic remnants in the area of the pituitary gland and is called craniopharyngioma. This tumor often disrupts vision by pressing on the optic nerve. Craniopharyngiomas also cause a lack of most pituitary hormones, prompting a combination of some of the symptoms previously described for tumors that induce a deficiency of single pituitary hormones.

Diagnosis and Testing

Doctors can detect larger pituitary tumors on an x-ray, computerized tomography scan, or magnetic resonance scan. Many pituitary tumors, however, are too small to be seen on these images of the pituitary region of the brain. To diagnose these tumors, doctors try to detect the hormonal abnormalities with various tests. Often blood or urine levels of specific hormones are measured within a few hours of giving the patient compounds known to stimulate or suppress production of the hormones.

For instance, sometimes patients are given a glucose tolerance test. After fasting overnight, the patient drinks a sugar solution, then has blood samples taken in which sugar or growth hormone levels are measured. Sometimes, in order to locate a very small tumor in the pituitary gland, an invasive procedure is required. This procedure is called inferior petrosal sinus sampling. A radiologist inserts special catheters from the groin veins into the vessels that drain the pituitary gland at the top of the neck and draws blood for measurement of the hormone that the tumor secretes.

Treatment

Doctors can successfully treat most pituitary tumors with microsurgery performed under the magnification of a surgical microscope, radiation therapy, surgery, drugs, or a combination of these treatments. Surgery is the treatment of choice for tumors that enlarge rapidly and threaten vision. The treatment plan for other pituitary tumors varies according to the type and size of the tumor.

Depending on each individual diagnosis, a physician can prescribe a wide variety of treatments. Sometimes treatments stimulate or compensate for missing hormones, others reduce the production of hormones. In some cases, drugs must be taken on a daily basis.

The National Institute of Child Health and Human Development supports an abundance of research aimed at developing better ways to diagnose and treat children with pituitary tumors.

Chapter 34

Factitious Hyperthyroidism

Alternative names: Factitious thyrotoxicosis; Thyrotoxicosis factitia; Thyrotoxicosis medicamentosa

Definition: Factitious hyperthyroidism involves high levels of thyroid activity caused by ingestion of excessive amounts of thyroid hormone.

Causes, Incidence, and Risk Factors

The thyroid gland produces the hormones thyroxine (T4) and tri-iodothyronine (T3). Hyperthyroidism is the clinical condition which results from excessive levels of these hormones, which can be caused in a number of ways.

In the vast majority of cases, hyperthyroidism is caused by over-production of thyroid hormones by the thyroid gland itself. In some other cases, the pituitary gland produces too much thyroid-stimulating hormone (TSH).

Thyroid hormone preparations have been available as medications since 1891 and are used to treat hypothyroidism. Ingesting too much thyroid hormone medication can also cause hyperthyroidism. Hyper-thyroidism caused by taking too much of this hormone is called facti-tious hyperthyroidism.

Factitious hyperthyroidism may occur when thyroid hormone is prescribed to treat hypothyroidism and the prescribed dose is too high.

It can also occur when a person intentionally takes an excessive amount of thyroid hormone; people with psychiatric disorders such as Munchausen syndrome deliberately (and usually secretively) take these hormones.

Patients attempting to lose weight and individuals fraudulently seeking to receive insurance compensation also sometimes misuse thyroid hormone and induce this condition. Children may occasionally require treatment for accidental ingestion of thyroid hormone pills.

In rare cases, factitious hyperthyroidism has been found to be caused by ingestion of meat contaminated with thyroid gland tissue.

Symptoms

Symptoms of factitious hyperthyroidism are identical to the symptoms of hyperthyroidism caused by the thyroid gland, with the following exceptions:

- There is no goiter. The thyroid gland is usually small.
- The eyes do not protrude, as in ophthalmopathy of Graves disease.
- Thickening of the skin does not occur, as it occasionally does with Graves disease.

Signs and Tests

- TSH (low)
- Total T4 (high)
- Free T4 (high)
- Total T3 (high)
- Radioactive iodine uptake (low)

Treatment

Ingestion of thyroid hormone is stopped. If thyroid hormone supplementation is medically necessary, the dosage must be reduced.

Patients need to be re-evaluated in 2 to 4 weeks to be sure that signs and symptoms of hyperthyroidism have resolved. This also helps to confirm the diagnosis.

Expectations (Prognosis)

Factitious hyperthyroidism will clear up on its own when thyroid hormone ingestion is stopped or the prescribed dose is lowered.

Complications

If factitious hyperthyroidism is long-standing, patients are at risk for the same complications as those of hyperthyroidism caused by the thyroid gland that is not properly treated. These complications include the following:

- Irregular heart rhythm
- Atrial fibrillation
- Chest pain (angina)
- Heart attack
- Loss of bone mass (if severe, osteoporosis)
- Weight loss

Calling Your Health Care Provider

Contact your health care provider if symptoms of hyperthyroidism occur.

Prevention

Thyroid hormone should be taken only by prescription and under the supervision of a licensed physician.

Note: The information provided herein should not be used during any medical emergency or for the diagnosis or treatment of any medical condition. A licensed physician should be consulted for diagnosis and treatment of any and all medical conditions. Call 911 for all medical emergencies.

Part Six

Parathyroid Gland Disorders

Chapter 35

Hyperparathyroidism

Primary Hyperparathyroidism

Primary hyperparathyroidism is a hormonal problem due to one or more parathyroid glands producing too much parathyroid hormone. Parathyroid glands, four small glands located in the neck near the thyroid gland, keep blood calcium from falling below normal. Rarely, there are more than four of these glands, and they may be in other parts of the neck or in the chest. In 80 to 85 percent of patients with primary hyperparathyroidism, a single gland is affected. In 15 to 20 percent of patients, two or more glands are affected. The affected gland(s) enlarge and produce too much parathyroid hormone. As a result, blood calcium becomes high, bones may lose calcium, and kidneys may excrete too much calcium.

Who Is Affected?

In the United States, 28 out of 100,000 people develop primary hyperparathyroidism each year. Women outnumber men 3 to 1, and frequency increases with age. In most cases, the cause is unknown. Previous exposure to radiation in the facial or neck area and certain medications

This chapter begins with text excerpted from "Primary Hyperparathyroidism," Osteoporosis and Related Bone Diseases–National Resource Center, July 2000. Text under the heading "Questions and Answers about Primary Hyperparathyroidism" is from "Primary Hyperparathyroidism Q and A," © The Paget Foundation. Reprinted with permission. For additional information visit The Paget Foundation website at http://www.paget.org.

(including thiazide diuretics and lithium) may cause primary hyperparathyroidism. In some families, the disease may be inherited. Parathyroid cancer is an extremely rare cause of primary hyperparathyroidism.

Symptoms

Even in patients who have no symptoms, primary hyperparathyroidism can cause bones to become less dense and can also lead to kidney stones. When the blood calcium exceeds the routine elevations seen in primary hyperparathyroidism, symptoms can include:

- loss of appetite
- thirst
- frequent urination
- lethargy
- fatigue
- muscle weakness
- joint pain
- constipation

When the blood calcium becomes very high, more severe symptoms include:

- nausea
- vomiting
- abdominal pain
- memory loss
- depression

Diagnosis

Primary hyperparathyroidism is usually diagnosed through a routine blood test. Once suspected, the following additional tests are done:

- **Blood test:** For calcium, phosphorus, alkaline phosphatase, 25-hydroxyvitamin D, 1,25-dihydroxy-vitamin D, and parathyroid hormone to determine the activity of the disease.

- **Urine test:** For calcium, kidney function, and bone markers that indicate whether a patient is likely to be losing bone calcium.

- **Urinalyses and kidney x-rays:** In some cases these are needed to check on kidney stone formation.

- **Bone density test:** This test is the only way to measure bone density.

Surgery

At present, the only known cure for primary hyperparathyroidism is surgical removal of the affected gland(s). Experts have developed guidelines to help determine who should have surgery. The decision requires careful evaluation and individual assessment.

Alternatives to Surgery

- **Monitoring:** Asymptomatic patients are not always recommended for surgery. If surgery is not to be performed, these patients should be monitored regularly with blood testing for calcium every 6 months. Every year these patients should undergo a urinary calcium test and a bone density test. Most patients do not get worse over years of follow-up care.
- **Estrogen therapy:** This treatment may reduce some effects of the disease in postmenopausal women, but will not directly control glandular overactivity.
- **Bisphosphonates:** These drugs, used to treat osteoporosis and Paget's disease of bone, are currently being evaluated in primary hyperparathyroidism.
- **Experimental drugs:** Some drugs that control serum calcium are being investigated. These drugs are not yet approved or available.

Prognosis

Removing the affected gland(s) cures the condition. Kidney stones do not tend to recur. In patients with reduced bone density, major improvements are seen over 1 to 4 years. However, nonspecific symptoms such as weakness and easy fatigability are not always eliminated.

Questions and Answers about Primary Hyperparathyroidism

What are the parathyroid glands?

They are four small glands located in the neck, close to the thyroid gland. Rarely there are more than four, and they may be located in other parts of the neck, or even in the chest.

What is their purpose?

The glands produce parathyroid hormone which plays a critical role in maintaining normal blood calcium levels.

How do these small glands maintain normal calcium levels in the blood?

Parathyroid hormone, released by these glands, keeps the amount of calcium in the blood from falling below normal:

- By conserving calcium at the kidneys
- By releasing calcium from the bones
- By increasing absorption of calcium from food

What goes wrong in primary hyperparathyroidism?

One or more of the glands becomes enlarged and overactive, producing too much parathyroid hormone. This leads to a rise in the blood calcium. In most patients (80–85%), a single parathyroid gland becomes enlarged and develops into a benign tumor, known as an adenoma. In nearly all other patients (15–20%), two or more glands enlarge, again in a benign fashion, a condition called hyperplasia. Parathyroid cancer is an extremely rare cause of primary hyperparathyroidism.

What are the harmful effects of primary hyperparathyroidism?

The most common symptoms of too much calcium in the blood are loss of appetite, thirst, frequent urination, lethargy, fatigue, muscle weakness, joint pains and constipation. More severe symptoms include nausea and vomiting, abdominal pain, memory loss and depression. These signs are not generally present unless the blood calcium is very high. Most patients with primary hyperparathyroidism in the United States do not have blood calcium levels in the range where these signs typically occur. In fact, many patients with primary hyperparathyroidism have no signs or symptoms at all. Primary hyperparathyroidism, even when patients are completely asymptomatic, can cause bones to become weak from loss of calcium. Skeletal weakening is one of the classical effects of primary hyperparathyroidism. Primary hyperparathyroidism can also lead to kidney stones.

Do all patients with primary hyperparathyroidism have symptoms?

No. Most patients are discovered to have primary hyperparathyroidism incidentally, in the course of a routine blood test.

Do all patients with primary hyperparathyroidism develop complications including bone loss, kidney stones, weakness, fatigability, etc.?

Many patients do not develop obvious complications, but bone loss is not uncommon.

How does the physician know who will develop complications?

The physician cannot predict, but complete evaluation will identify the more serious complications at early stages.

What is a complete evaluation?

Blood is tested for calcium, phosphorus, alkaline phosphatase, 25-hydroxyvitamin D, 1,25-dihydroxyvitamin D, and parathyroid hormone to determine the activity of the disease. A urine test (24-hour collection) is obtained to measure urinary calcium, kidney function and bone markers that indicate whether a patient is likely to be losing bone calcium. In some cases, urinalyses and kidney x-rays are needed to evaluation kidney stone formation. All patients should have a bone density test. This test is important because it is much more sensitive than routine x-rays and detects early bone loss, if it is present. Although it is advisable to measure all three sites (back, hip, and forearm), the most sensitive area to measure in primary hyperparathyroidism is the forearm.

What causes primary hyperparathyroidism?

In most cases the cause is unknown. Previous exposure to radiation in the facial or neck area is thought to be a cause in some patients as are certain medications (thiazide diuretics, lithium). Some families inherit the tendency to develop primary hyperparathyroidism. A careful family history and special tests of blood and urine can usually exclude these rare conditions. A great majority of individuals with primary hyperparathyroidism do not have any relatives with this disorder.

How common is primary hyperparathyroidism?

In the United States, 28 out of every 100,000 people can be expected to develop primary hyperparathyroidism each year. Women outnumber men by three to one, and the frequency of the condition increases with age.

Is there a cure for primary hyperparathyroidism?

Yes. Surgery to remove the affected gland(s) cures the condition. When performed by an experienced parathyroid surgeon, the operation is successful in over 95% of cases. Serious surgical complications are uncommon. The surgery usually leaves a thin, faint horizontal scar about three inches long in the lower neck.

Should all patients with primary hyperparathyroidism undergo surgery?

Not necessarily. Although surgery is considered an appropriate treatment even in patients without signs or symptoms (i.e., asymptomatic), patients with asymptomatic primary hyperparathyroidism are not always operated upon. Most, but not all, patients who are monitored without surgery do not get worse over years of follow-up care. If surgery is not to be performed, these patients should be monitored regularly with blood testing for calcium every six months and with urinary calcium and bone density yearly. This will allow the physician to identify those who show signs of progression at an early stage.

Who should have surgery?

Experts have developed guidelines to help determine who should have surgery. In each case, the decision about surgery requires careful evaluation and individual assessment.

What is the standard surgical procedure?

The traditional approach is to perform the operation under general anesthesia. All four parathyroid glands are identified. Any enlarged glands, usually one, are removed.

Is there a way to locate the enlarged parathyroid gland(s) before surgery is performed?

In most cases, patients do not require any special imaging studies to locate the affected parathyroid gland prior to surgery. An experienced surgeon who performs many parathyroid operations yearly is generally not helped by a preoperative localization test. There are exceptions to this rule, however. Patients who have had previous neck surgery represent a special situation. A second parathyroid operation should not be undertaken without first attempting to locate the missing parathyroid gland.

What preoperative localization tests are available?

There are a number of non-invasive imaging tests to locate abnormal parathyroid glands. They include ultrasound, computerized tomography (CT), magnetic resonance imaging (MRI), positron emission tomography (PET), and the sestamibi scan. Sestamibi is a chemical that localizes in the abnormal parathyroid gland. The sestamibi scan, especially when it is performed with computerized tomography (SPECT) is the most sensitive and specific test available. In some cases, the quest to find the parathyroid gland advances to invasive tests (arteriography and blood sampling of veins in the neck for parathyroid hormone) that require great expertise and are more difficult. Patients who are considering minimally invasive parathyroid surgery require preoperative sestamibi imaging to localize the abnormal parathyroid glands.

Are there alternatives to this standard approach?

Yes. Recently three techniques have been developed. They go under the term minimally invasive parathyroidectomy. These include preoperative localization with a sestamibi scan. The minimal operation is performed under local anesthesia with removal of the single gland visualized by the parathyroid scan. This operation is usually combined with the use of the intraoperative parathyroid hormone measurement, which can be done literally in minutes. If the blood parathyroid hormone falls to normal, the operation has succeeded in removing the culprit parathyroid gland. A second new approach calls for the sestamibi scan to be done literally a few hours before the surgery. At the time of surgery, a detector is passed over the area of the operation to identify the gland(s) that are overactive. After the gland is identified and removed, the detector no longer picks up any signals of abnormal residual overactivity in the neck. A third approach is endoscopy to remove the parathyroid gland. These three approaches are performed only in select centers by expert surgeons with great experience in parathyroid surgery.

Can the standard parathyroid operation be performed under local anesthesia?

Yes. Parathyroid surgery can be performed under general, regional, or local anesthesia. In some centers, local anesthetic techniques have become the most common and the procedure of choice. The use of local anesthesia does not prevent the surgeon from identifying all parathyroid glands before the operation is concluded. In all cases, an experienced surgeon is strongly recommended.

Is there a role for parathyroid autotransplantation?

Yes, in certain situations. Parathyroid autotransplantation is reserved for those patients who undergo a repeat parathyroid operation when there is concern that when the parathyroid gland is removed the patient will be left without any parathyroid tissue resulting in hypoparathyroidism. This is also a concern in the multiple gland hyperplasia syndromes in which all four parathyroid glands are involved. All parathyroid tissue in the neck is removed and a small amount is transplanted to the forearm. In this way, the patient is left with some functioning parathyroid tissue. If the forearm parathyroid enlarges over time, the transplanted tissue can be readily reduced by a simple, local office procedure. Parathyroid autotransplantation should be performed only in medical centers and by surgeons with experience in this technique.

What are the results of successful surgery?

Successful removal of the parathyroid gland(s) leads to normal calcium and parathyroid hormone levels. In patients who have had kidney stones, they do not tend to recur. In patients with reduced bone density, major improvements are seen typically over a period of 1–4 years. Non-specific symptoms such as weakness and easy fatigability are not always affected with some feeling better and others not noticing any difference after surgery.

Are there alternatives to surgery?

There are no other cures besides surgery for primary hyperparathyroidism. Estrogen therapy may reduce some effects of the disease in postmenopausal women, but this will not directly control the glandular overactivity. There are also some experimental drugs that are being investigated to control the serum calcium, including a calcimimetic (a drug that suppresses the release of parathyroid hormone from the parathyroid glands). These drugs are not yet approved or available. Bisphosphonates, a group of drugs used to treat osteoporosis and Paget's disease of bone, are currently being evaluated in primary hyperparathyroidism.

Are there general measures patients with primary hyperparathyroidism should follow?

Yes. Patients should drink enough fluids to avoid becoming dehydrated. (Dehydration will lead to an increase in the blood calcium). Similarly, to avoid worsening calcium levels, immobilization should be avoided. Calcium-containing foods should not be avoided, nor should the diet be deficient in calcium because this could actually stimulate the parathyroid glands further. On the other hand, it is not advisable for patients to take too much calcium. The calcium content in the diet should be normal (approximately 1200 milligrams).

Which types of physicians are specialists in treating primary hyperparathyroidism?

Endocrinologists (medical specialists who specialize in hormonal disorders); metabolic bone disease specialists; and surgeons who specialize in endocrine surgery. Upon request, The Paget Foundation will supply a list of medical specialists.

Additional Information

The Paget Foundation
120 Wall Street, Suite 1602
New York, NY 10005-4001
Toll-Free: 800-23-PAGET (72438)
Phone: 212-509-5335
Fax: 212-509-8492
Website: http://www.paget.org
E-mail: PagetFdn@aol.com

Chapter 36

Multiple Endocrine Neoplasia

Chapter Contents

Section 36.1

Multiple Endocrine Neoplasia Type 1 (MEN-1)

"Multiple Endocrine Neoplasia Type 1," National Institute of Diabetes
and Digestive and Kidney Diseases (NIDDK), NIH Publication
No. 02-3048, June 2002.

Multiple endocrine neoplasia type 1 (MEN-1) is an inherited disorder that affects the endocrine glands. It is sometimes called multiple endocrine adenomatosis or Wermer's syndrome, after one of the first doctors to recognize it. MEN-1 is quite rare, occurring in about 3 to 20 persons out of 100,000. It affects both sexes equally and shows no geographical, racial, or ethnic preferences.

Endocrine glands are different from other organs in the body because they release hormones into the bloodstream. Hormones are powerful chemicals that travel through the blood, controlling and instructing the functions of various organs. Normally, the hormones released by endocrine glands are carefully balanced to meet the body's needs.

In patients with MEN-1, sometimes more than one group of endocrine glands, such as the parathyroid, the pancreas, and the pituitary become overactive at the same time. Most people who develop overactivity of only one endocrine gland do not have MEN-1.

How Does MEN-1 Affect the Endocrine Glands?

The Parathyroid Glands

The parathyroids are the endocrine glands earliest and most often affected by MEN-1. The human body normally has four parathyroid glands, which are located close to the thyroid gland in the front of the neck. The parathyroids release into the bloodstream a chemical called parathyroid hormone, which helps maintain a normal supply of calcium in the blood, bones, and urine.

In MEN-1, all four parathyroid glands tend to be overactive. They release too much parathyroid hormone, leading to excess calcium in the blood. High blood calcium, known as hypercalcemia, can exist for many years before it is found by accident or by family screening. Unrecognized hypercalcemia can cause excess calcium to spill into the urine, leading to kidney stones or kidney damage.

Nearly everyone who inherits a susceptibility to MEN-1 (a carrier) will develop overactive parathyroid glands (hyperparathyroidism) by age 50, but the disorder can often be detected before age 20. Hyperparathyroidism may cause no problems for many years or it may cause problems such as tiredness, weakness, muscle or bone pain, constipation, indigestion, kidney stones, or thinning of bones.

Treatment of Hyperparathyroidism

It is sometimes difficult to decide whether hyperparathyroidism in MEN-1 is severe enough to need treatment, especially in a person who has no symptoms. The usual treatment is an operation to remove the three largest parathyroid glands and all but a small part of the fourth. After parathyroid surgery, regular testing of blood calcium should continue, since the small piece of remaining parathyroid tissue can grow larger and cause recurrent hyperparathyroidism. People whose parathyroid glands have been completely removed by surgery must take daily supplements of calcium and vitamin D to prevent hypocalcemia (low blood calcium).

The Pancreas

The pancreas gland, located behind the stomach, releases digestive juices into the intestines and releases key hormones into the bloodstream. Some hormones produced in the islet cells of the pancreas and their effects are:

- insulin—lowers blood sugar
- glucagon—raises blood sugar
- somatostatin—inhibits many cells

Gastrin is another hormone that can be over-secreted in people with MEN-1. The gastrin comes from one or more tumors in the pancreas and small intestine. Gastrin normally circulates in the blood, causing the stomach to secrete enough acid needed for digestion. If exposed to too much gastrin, the stomach releases excess acid, leading to the formation of severe ulcers in the stomach and small intestine. Too much gastrin can also cause serious diarrhea.

About one in three patients with MEN-1 has gastrin-releasing tumors, called gastrinomas. (The illness associated with these tumors is sometimes called Zollinger-Ellison syndrome.) The ulcers caused by gastrinomas are much more dangerous than typical stomach or intestinal ulcers; left untreated, they can cause rupture of the stomach or intestine and even death.

Treatment of Gastrinomas

The gastrinomas associated with MEN-1 are difficult to cure by surgery, because it is difficult to find the multiple small gastrinomas in the pancreas and small intestine. In the past, the standard treatment for gastrinomas was the surgical removal of the entire stomach to prevent acid production. Now the mainstay of treatment is very powerful medicines that block stomach acid release, called acid pump inhibitors. Taken by mouth, these have proven effective in controlling most cases of Zollinger-Ellison syndrome.

The Pituitary Gland

The pituitary is a small gland inside the head, behind the bridge of the nose. Though small, it produces many important hormones that regulate basic body functions. The major pituitary hormones and their effects are:

- Prolactin—controls formation of breast milk, influences fertility, and influences bone strength.
- Growth hormone—regulates body growth, especially during adolescence.
- Adrenocorticotropic hormone (ACTH)—stimulates the adrenal glands to produce cortisol.
- Thyrotropin (TSH)—stimulates the thyroid gland to produce thyroid hormones.
- Luteinizing hormone (LH)—stimulates the ovaries or testes to produce sex hormones that determine many features of maleness or femaleness.
- Follicle stimulating hormone (FSH)—regulates fertility in men through sperm production and in women through ovulation.

The pituitary gland becomes overactive in about one of four persons with MEN-1. This overactivity can usually be traced to a very small, benign tumor in the gland that releases too much prolactin, called a prolactinoma. High prolactin can cause excessive production of breast milk or it can interfere with fertility in women or with sex drive and fertility in men.

Treatment of Prolactinomas

Most prolactinomas are small, and treatment may not be needed. If treatment is needed, a very effective type of medicine known as a dopamine agonist can lower the production of prolactin and shrink the prolactinoma. Occasionally, prolactinomas do not respond well to this medication. In such cases, surgery, radiation, or both may be needed.

Rare Complications of MEN-1

Occasionally, a person who has MEN-1 develops islet tumors of the pancreas that secrete high levels of pancreatic hormones other than gastrin. Insulinomas, for example, produce too much insulin, causing serious low blood sugar, or hypoglycemia. Pancreatic tumors that secrete too much glucagon or somatostatin can cause diabetes, and too much vasoactive intestinal peptide can cause diarrhea.

Other rare complications arise from pituitary tumors that release high amounts of ACTH, which in turn stimulates the adrenal glands to produce excess cortisol. Pituitary tumors that produce growth hormone cause excessive bone growth or disfigurement.

Another rare complication is an endocrine tumor inside the chest or in the stomach, known as a carcinoid. In general, surgery is the mainstay of treatment for all of these rare types of tumors, except for gastric carcinoids which usually require no treatment.

Are the Tumors Associated with MEN-1 Cancerous?

The overactive endocrine glands associated with MEN-1 may contain benign tumors, but usually they do not have any signs of cancer. Benign tumors can disrupt normal function by releasing hormones or by crowding nearby tissue. For example, a prolactinoma may become quite large in someone with MEN-1. As it grows, the tumor can press against and damage the normal part of the pituitary gland or the nerves that carry vision from the eyes. Sometimes impaired vision is the first sign of a pituitary tumor in MEN-1.

Another type of benign tumor often seen in people with MEN-1 is a plum-size, fatty tumor called a lipoma, which grows under the skin. Lipomas cause no health problems and can be removed by simple cosmetic surgery if desired. These tumors are also fairly common in the general population.

Benign tumors do not spread to or invade other parts of the body. Cancer cells, by contrast, break away from the primary tumor and spread, or metastasize, to other parts of the body through the bloodstream or lymphatic system.

The pancreatic islet cell tumors associated with MEN-1 tend to be numerous and small, but most are benign and do not release active hormones into the blood. Eventually, about half of MEN-1 cases will develop a cancerous pancreatic tumor.

Treatment of Pancreatic Endocrine Cancer in MEN-1

Since the type of pancreatic endocrine cancer associated with MEN-1 can be difficult to recognize, difficult to treat, and very slow to progress, doctors have different views about the value of surgery in managing these tumors.

One approach is to watch and wait, using medical or nonsurgical treatments. According to this school of thought, pancreatic surgery has serious complications, so it should not be attempted unless it will cure a tumor that is secreting too much hormone.

Another school advocates early surgery, perhaps when a tumor grows to a certain size, to remove pancreatic endocrine cancer in MEN-1 (even if it does not over secrete a hormone) before it spreads and becomes dangerous. There is no clear evidence however, that aggressive surgery to prevent pancreatic endocrine cancer from spreading actually leads to longer survival for patients with MEN-1.

Doctors agree that excessive release of certain hormones (such as gastrin) from pancreatic endocrine cancer in MEN-1 needs to be treated, and medications are often effective in blocking the effects of these hormones. Some tumors, such as insulin-producing tumors of the pancreas, are usually benign and single and are curable by pancreatic surgery. Such surgery needs to be considered carefully in each patient's case.

Is MEN-1 the Same in Everyone?

Although MEN-1 tends to follow certain patterns, it can affect a person's health in many different ways. Not only do the features of MEN-1 vary among members of the same family, but some families with MEN-1 tend to have a higher rate of prolactin-secreting pituitary tumors and a much lower frequency of gastrin-secreting tumors.

In addition, the age at which MEN-1 can begin to cause endocrine gland over-function can differ strikingly from one family member to another. One person may have only mild hyperparathyroidism beginning at age 50, while a relative may develop complications from tumors of the parathyroid, pancreas, and pituitary by age 20.

Sometimes a patient with MEN-1 knows of no other case of MEN-1 among relatives. The commonest explanations are that knowledge about the family is incomplete or that the patient carries a new MEN-1 gene mutation.

Can MEN-1 Be Cured?

There is no cure for MEN-1 itself, but most of the health problems caused by MEN-1 can be recognized at an early stage and controlled or treated before they become serious problems.

If you have been diagnosed with MEN-l, it is important to get periodic checkups because MEN-1 can affect different glands, and even after treatment, residual tissue can grow back. Careful monitoring enables your doctor to adjust your treatment as needed and to check for any new disturbances caused by MEN-1. Most people with MEN-1 will have long and productive lives.

How Is MEN-1 Detected?

Each of us has millions of genes in each of our cells, which determine how our cells and bodies function. In people with MEN-1, there is a mutation, or mistake, in one gene of every cell. A carrier is a person who has the MEN-1 gene mutation. The MEN-1 gene mutation is transmitted directly to a child from a parent carrying the gene mutation.

The MEN-1 gene was very recently identified. As of 2001, a small number of centers around the world have begun to offer MEN-1 gene testing on a research or commercial basis. The likelihood of finding a mutation in an MEN-1 family has varied from 60 percent to 94 percent depending on methods. When a mutation is found, further testing in other relatives can become much easier. Many relatives can be tested once and be found without the known MEN-1 mutation in their family, and then they can be freed from uncertainty and from any further testing ever for MEN-1. When a mutation is not found in a family or isolated case, it does not prove that no MEN-1 mutation is present. Depending on the clinical and laboratory information, it may still be very likely that a mutation is present but undetected.

In the meantime, though, screening of close relatives of persons with MEN-1, who are at high risk, generally involves testing for hyperparathyroidism, the most common and usually the earliest sign of MEN-1. Any doctor can screen for hyperparathyroidism by testing the blood for total calcium and sometimes one or two other substances such as ionized calcium and parathyroid hormone. An abnormal result indicates that the person probably has MEN-1, but normal findings cannot rule out the chance that he or she will develop hyperparathyroidism at a later time. Blood testing can usually show signs of early hyperparathyroidism many years before symptoms of hyperparathyroidism occur.

What is the Role for Genetic Counseling with MEN-1 Gene Testing?

Genetic counseling, which should accompany the gene testing, can assist family member(s) to address how the test results affect them individually and as a family. In genetic counseling, there can be a review and discussion of issues about the psychosocial benefits and risks of the genetic testing results. Genetic testing results can affect self-image, self-esteem, and individual and family identity. In genetic counseling, issues related to how and with whom genetic test results will be shared and their possible effect on important matters such as health and life insurance coverage can be reviewed and discussed. The times for these discussions can be when a family member is deciding whether or not to go ahead with the gene testing and again later when the gene testing results are available. The person, who provides the genetic counseling to the family member(s), may be a professional from the disciplines of genetics, nursing, or medicine.

MEN-1 Screening

Who Should Consider MEN-1 Screening by Gene Testing?

Screening may be offered to persons with MEN-1 or with features resembling it. Affected relatives of persons with MEN-1 can be tested. Asymptomatic offspring, brothers, or sisters of a person with MEN-1 were born with a 50 percent chance of having inherited the gene; they too can be offered gene testing. While gene testing for certain genes can be definitive at any age, it is usually not offered to children below age 18 unless the test outcome would have an important effect on their medical treatment. Since treatable tumors occasionally begin by age 5 in MEN-1, gene testing and tumor surveillance can begin at age 5.

Who Should Consider MEN-1 Screening by Laboratory Tests?

MEN-1 screening by gene testing will be the most definitive test, when it is available. However, it is not yet widely available, and when no gene mutation is found in a MEN-1 family, then it may be necessary to rely upon laboratory tests for diagnosis. Hyperparathyroidism, most often the first sign of MEN-1, can usually be detected by blood tests between the ages of 15 and 50. Periodic testing should begin around age 10 and be repeated every year. There is no age at which periodic testing should stop, since doctors cannot rule out the chance that a person has inherited the MEN-1 gene mutation. However, a person with normal testing beyond age 50 is very unlikely to have inherited the MEN-1 gene mutation.

Why Screen for MEN-1 Tumors?

MEN-1 is not an infectious or contagious disease, nor is it caused by environmental factors. Because MEN-1 is a genetic disorder inherited from one parent, and its transmission pattern is well understood, family members at high risk for the disorder can be easily identified.

Testing can detect the problems caused by MEN-1 tumors many years before their later complications develop. Finding these tumors early enables your doctor to begin preventive treatment, reducing the chances that MEN-1 will cause problems later.

Should a Person Who Has MEN-1 Avoid Having Children?

A person who has MEN-1 or who has a positive MEN-1 gene mutation may have a hard time deciding whether to have a child. No one can make this decision for anyone else, but some of the important facts can be summarized as follows:

- A man or a woman with MEN-1 has a 50-50 risk with each pregnancy of having a child with MEN-1.

- MEN-1 tends to fit a broad pattern within a given family, but the severity of the disorder varies widely from one family member to another. In particular, a parent's experience with MEN-1 cannot be used to predict the severity of MEN-1 in a child.

- MEN-1 is a problem that does not usually develop until adulthood. Treatment may require regular monitoring and considerable expense, but the disease usually does not prevent an active, productive adulthood.

- Prolactin-releasing tumors in a man or woman with MEN-1 may inhibit fertility and make it difficult to conceive. Also, hyperparathyroidism in a woman during pregnancy may raise the risks of complications for mother and child.

Genetic counseling can help individuals and couples through the decision-making process with family planning. Genetic counselors will provide information to help with the decision-making process, but they will not tell individuals or couples what decision to make or how to make it.

Additional Reading

The following articles about MEN-1 can be found in medical libraries, some college and university libraries, and through interlibrary loan in most public libraries.

Chandrasekharappa, S.C., Guru, S.C., Manickam, P., Olufemi, S., Collins, F.S. Emmert-Buck, M.R., Debelenko, L.V., Zhuang, Z., Lubensky, I.A., Liotta, L.A., Crabtree, J.S., Wang, Y., Roe, B.A., Weisemann, J., Boguski, M.S., Agarwal, S.K., Kester, M.B., Kim, Y.S., Heppner, C., Dong, Q., Spiegel, A.M., Burns, A.L., Marx, S.J., "Positional cloning of the gene for multiple endocrine neoplasia-type 1," *Science* 276:404-407, 1997.

Marx SJ. Multiple endocrine neoplasia type 1. In: *Metabolic Basis of Inherited Diseases, 8th Ed.* ed. Scriver CS, et al. McGraw Hill, NY, 2001. pp 943-966.

Schussheim DH, Skarulis MC, Agarwal SK, Simonds WF, Burns AL, Spiegel AM, Marx SJ. MEN-1: New clinical and basic findings. *Trends Endocrinol Metab* 12: 173-178, 2001.

Additional Information

Pituitary Network Association
P.O. Box 1958
Thousand Oaks, CA 91358
Phone: 805-499-9973
Fax: 805-480-0633
Website: http://www.pituitary.org

National Institute of Diabetes and Digestive and Kidney Diseases
Building 31, Room 9A04
Center Drive, MSC 2560
Bethesda, MD 20892
Phone: 301-496-3583
Website: http://niddk.nih.gov

March of Dimes/Birth Defects Foundation
1275 Mamaroneck Avenue
White Plains, NY 10605
Phone: 914-428-7100
Website: http://www.modimes.org

Alliance of Genetic Support Groups
4301 Connecticut Ave., N.W., Suite 404
Washington, DC 20008-2304
Toll-Free Help Line: 800-336-GENE (4363)
Phone: 202-966-5557
Fax: 202-966-8553
Website: http://www.geneticalliance.org
E-mail: info@geneticalliance.org

Section 36.2

Multiple Endocrine Neoplasia Type 2 (MEN-2)

"Multiple Endocrine Neoplasia (MEN) II," © 2003 A.D.A.M., Inc.
Reprinted with permission.

Alternative names: Sipple's syndrome

Definition: Multiple Endocrine Neoplasia II (MEN-2) is a hereditary disorder in which patients develop a type of thyroid cancer accompanied by recurring cancer of the adrenal glands. One type of this
disease (MEN-2a) is also associated with overgrowth (hyperplasia) of
the parathyroid gland.

Causes, Incidence, and Risk Factors

The cause of MEN-2 is genetic—a mutation in a gene called *RET*.
Multiple tumors may appear in the same person, but not necessarily
at the same time. The adrenal tumor is a pheochromocytoma and the
thyroid tumor is a medullary carcinoma of the thyroid.

The disorder may occur at any age, and affects men and women
equally. The main risk factor is a family history of MEN-2.

Symptoms

- severe headache
- palpitations
- rapid heart rate
- sweating
- chest pain
- abdominal pain
- nervousness
- irritability

- loss of weight
- diarrhea
- cough
- cough with blood
- fatigue
- back pain
- increased urine output

- increased thirst
- loss of appetite
- nausea
- muscular weak-ness
- depression
- personality changes

Note: The symptoms may vary, but are consistent with those of pheochromocytoma, medullary carcinoma of the thyroid, and sometimes
hyperparathyroidism.

Signs and Tests

Diagnosis depends on identification of mutation of the *RET* gene. This can be done with a blood test.

A physical examination may reveal enlarged cervical lymph nodes. An examination of the thyroid may reveal a single or multiple thyroid nodules. The patient may have high blood pressure (sustained or episodic), rapid heart rate, and elevated temperature.

In MEN-2b, mucosal neuromas (benign tumors of the mucosa) may be present, as well as puffy lips, and a prominent jaw.

Diagnostic tests are also used to evaluate the function of each endocrine gland. These tests help confirm the diagnosis:

- adrenal biopsy showing pheochromocytoma
- MIBG (iodine-131-meta-iodobenzylguanidine) scintiscan showing tumor
- MRI (magnetic resonance image) of abdomen showing adrenal mass
- Abdominal CT (computed tomography) scan showing mass
- elevated urine metanephrine
- elevated urine catecholamines
- thyroid biopsy showing medullary carcinoma cells
- ultrasound of the thyroid revealing nodule
- thyroid scan showing cold nodule
- elevated calcitonin
- parathyroid biopsy showing tumor or hyperplasia
- radioimmune assay of parathyroid hormone showing increased level
- increased serum calcium
- decreased serum phosphorus
- possibly increased serum alkaline phosphatase
- imaging of the kidneys or ureters showing calcification or obstruction
- ECG (electrocardiogram) possibly showing abnormalities

Treatment

Surgery is needed to remove both the medullary carcinoma of the thyroid and the pheochromocytoma. Medullary carcinoma of the thyroid must be treated with total removal of the thyroid gland and removal of surrounding lymph nodes. Hormone replacement therapy is given after surgery.

Family members should be screened for the *RET* gene mutation.

Expectations (Prognosis)

Pheochromocytoma is usually benign (not cancer), but the accompanying medullary carcinoma of the thyroid that characterizes this condition is a very aggressive and potentially fatal cancer. Nonetheless, early diagnosis and surgery can often lead to cure.

Complications

A complication is the metastasis of cancerous cells.

Calling Your Health Care Provider

Call your health care provide if you notice symptoms of MEN-2.

Prevention

Screening of close relatives of a person with MEN-2 may lead to early detection.

Additional Information

National Cancer Institute
6115 Executive Blvd., MSC 8322
Bethesda, MD 20892-8322
Toll-Free: 800-4-CANCER (22-6237)
Toll-Free TTY: 800-332-8615
Website: http://www.cancer.gov/
E-mail: cancergovstaff@mail.nih.gov

National Institute of Diabetes and Digestive and Kidney Diseases
Building 31, Room 9A04
Center Drive, MSC 2560
Bethesda, MD 20892-2560
Phone: 301-496-3583
Website: http://niddk.nih.gov

Chapter 37

Hypoparathyroidism

- **Definition:** Too little parathyroid hormone production

Hypoparathyroidism is the combination of symptoms due to inadequate parathyroid hormone production. This is a very rare condition, and most commonly occurs because of damage or removal of parathyroid glands at the time of parathyroid or thyroid surgery. Hyperparathyroidism (too much parathyroid hormone) is much more common than hypoparathyroidism.

Hypoparathyroidism is the state of decreased secretion or activity of parathyroid hormone (PTH). This leads to decreased blood levels of calcium (hypocalcemia) and increased levels of blood phosphorus (hyperphosphatemia). Symptoms can range from quite mild (tingling in the hands, fingers, and around the mouth), to more severe forms of muscle cramps, leading all the way to tetany (severe muscle cramping of the entire body), and convulsions (this is very rare).

Parathyroid gland insufficiency is quite rare, but it can occur in several well defined ways. The most common cause of hypoparathyroidism is the loss of active parathyroid tissue following thyroid or parathyroid surgery. Rarer is a defect present at birth (congenital) where a person is born without parathyroid glands. Occasionally, the specific cause of hypoparathyroidism cannot be determined.

"Hypoparathyroidism," by James Norman, M.D., Norman Endocrine Surgery Clinic, Tampa, Florida. © 2004 Norman Endocrine Surgery Clinic. Reprinted with permission.

Three Categories of Hypoparathyroidism

Deficient Parathyroid Hormone Secretion

This type of hypoparathyroidism is the easiest to understand. A patient afflicted with this condition simply has too little (or a complete absence of) parathyroid tissue therefore, inadequate PTH is produced. There are two major causes of this problem:

Post Surgical. The first (and most common) mechanism by which inadequate parathyroid hormone is produced is due to the removal of parathyroid glands at the time of surgery. The operations which are typically associated with this problem are operations designed to remove parathyroid glands for hyperparathyroidism. The goal of this operation is to remove those parathyroid glands which are overproducing PTH, however, occasionally, (less than 1%) too much parathyroid tissue is removed. The second operation which is associated with postoperative hypoparathyroidism is total thyroidectomy. This operation is performed for a number of reasons, but because of the close relationship that the thyroid and parathyroid have to one another (including sharing the same blood supply) the parathyroid glands can be injured or removed. This is very rare and occurs in much less than 1% of thyroid operations. In many patients, the inadequate secretion of PTH is transient following surgery on the thyroid or parathyroid glands, so this diagnosis cannot be made immediately following surgery.

Idiopathic. Deficient PTH secretion without a defined cause (e.g., surgical injury) is termed Idiopathic hypoparathyroidism. This disease is rare and can be congenital or acquired later in life.

- **Congenital.** Patients in this category are born without parathyroid tissues. Most patients with congenital hypoparathyroidism have no family history of the disease. Those who do may have any one of a number of congenital causes. The pattern of inheritance is as varied as the kinds of genetic abnormalities that cause the disease. The children in some families are at a 50% risk for disease (dominant gene defect) while others are at a risk of 25% or less (recessive gene defect). In some families only the boys suffer from disease. This sex-linked inheritance pattern indicates the presence of a genetic defect on the X chromosome. The inherited forms tend to arise from abnormal genes that either:

1. encode abnormal forms of PTH or its receptor,

2. prevent normal conduction of cell signals from the PTH receptor to the nucleus, or

3. prevent normal gland development before birth.

Hypoparathyroidism with onset during the first few months of life can be permanent or temporary. The cause is usually unknown and if spontaneous, resolution occurs. If it does not, it will usually become manifest by 24 months of age. Finally, mothers who have overactive parathyroid glands may have high calcium levels. The excess ionized calcium can enter the baby and suppress the baby's parathyroid gland function. If suppression of the gland is not released quickly enough after birth, low calcium levels can be a temporary problem for the baby. This will not result in permanent parathyroid gland dysfunction in the child.

- **Acquired.** The acquired form of this disease typically arises because the immune system has developed antibodies against parathyroid tissues in an attempt to reject what it sees as a foreign tissue, much as it would a transplanted organ. This disease can affect the parathyroid glands in isolation or can be part of a syndrome that involves many organs. An antibody that binds to the calcium sensor in the parathyroid gland has been discovered in the blood of patients with autoimmune hypoparathyroidism. It has been proposed that such binding tricks the parathyroid gland into believing that the blood level of ionized calcium is high. Responding to this signal, the parathyroid stops making PTH.

Hypomagnesemia. The element magnesium is closely related to the action of calcium in the body. When magnesium levels are too low, calcium levels may also fall. It appears that magnesium is important for parathyroid cells to make PTH normally. Once recognized, this is usually very easy to fix. Chronic alcoholism is a frequent cause of low calcium and magnesium levels.

Secretion of Biologically Inactive Parathyroid Hormone

There have only been a few cases of this syndrome ever reported, but one can see that if the PTH which is produced is actually a defective hormone, it would not have the same biologic strength as its normal counterpart.

Resistance to Parathyroid Hormone (Pseudo-Hypoparathyroidism)

This disease is also very rare. Like all patients with hypoparathyroidism, this disease is characterized by hypocalcemia (too low calcium levels), or hyperphosphatemia (too high phosphorus levels), and they are distinguished by the fact that they produce PTH, but their bones and kidneys do not respond to it. Even if PTH is given to them in their veins, they do not respond to it. Therefore, these rare individuals have plenty of PTH, but their organs do not behave appropriately to it (so they look to be hypoparathyroid but they are not—thus the name pseudo-hypoparathyroid).

Treatment of Hypoparathyroidism

Vitamin D and calcium supplements are the primary treatments for this disease regardless of the cause. The only exception is when the inactivity of PTH is due to hypomagnesemia which is readily treated with magnesium supplementation. At this time, a replacement form of PTH is not available.

Additional Information

Norman Endocrine Surgery Clinic
505 South Boulevard
Tampa, FL 33606
Phone: 813-991-6922
Fax: 813-991-6918
Website: http://www.endocrineweb.com

Chapter 38

Pseudohypoparathyroidism

Alternative Names: Albright's hereditary osteodystrophy; Types 1a and 1b pseudohypoparathyroidism

Definition: Pseudohypoparathyroidism is a genetic disorder that resembles hypoparathyroidism (lowered levels of parathyroid hormone), but is caused by a lack of response to parathyroid hormone rather than a deficiency in the hormone itself.

Causes, Incidence, and Risk Factors

Parathyroid hormone (PTH) is a hormone produced by the parathyroid glands that helps regulate calcium and phophate levels in the blood. The effects of PTH are seen in several body systems including the skeletal, gastrointestinal, renal (kidney), muscular, and central nervous system.

In pseudohypoparathyroidism, there is an adequate amount of PTH, but the body cannot respond to it. The body is resistant to the effects of PTH. As a result, a picture very similar to hypoparathyroidism develops with low calcium levels in the blood and high phosphate levels. This results in the characteristic symptoms which are generally first seen in childhood.

There are two different types of pseudohypoparathyroidism, both of which are caused by abnormal genes.

- Type 1 can be further divided into two sub-types:
  - Type 1a is caused by a one-gene abnormality inherited in an autosomal dominant manner (only one parent needs to have the gene for the child to inherit it). This defect also causes short stature, round face, and short hand bones, and is also called Albright's hereditary osteodystrophy.
  - Type 1b is characterized by resistance to PTH confined to the kidney. As a result, the calcium and phosphate problems are seen, but not the rest of the syndrome. The genetic and molecular features of 1b are less clear.
- Type 2 is very similar to type 1 in its clinical features, but the underlying mechanism in the kidney is different.

When Albright's hereditary osteodystrophy occurs without hypocalcemia (low levels of calcium in the blood), it is known as pseudopseudohypoparathyroidism.

All forms of pseudohypoparathyroidism are very rare.

Symptoms

Symptoms are related to low levels of calcium and include sensations of numbness and seizures.

Signs and Tests

Signs related to Albright's hereditary osteodystrophy include:

- short stature
- round face and short neck
- brachydactyly (short hand bones, especially the bone below the 4th finger)
- subcutaneous calcification
- dimples can replace knuckles on affected digits

Signs of hypocalcemia include:

- seizures
- tetany
- cataracts
- dental abnormalities

Hypocalcemia typically begins in childhood. Tests may show:

- low serum calcium
- elevated serum phosphorus
- elevated intact PTH
- abnormal urinary cAMP (cyclic adenosine monophosphate) response to PTH challenge (Type 1a and 1b)
- abnormal gene testing
- head MRI (magnetic resonance image) or CT (computed tomography) scan of the brain showing calcification of basal ganglia

Treatment

Treatment consists of calcium and vitamin D supplementation to maintain high calcium levels without the aid of PTH.

Expectations (Prognosis)

Hypocalcemia in pseudohypoparathyroidism is usually milder than in other forms of hypoparathyroidism.

Complications

Patients with type 1a pseudohypoparathyroidism have an increased incidence of other endocrine abnormalities (such as hypothyroidism and hypogonadism).

Complications of hypocalcemia associated with pseudohypoparathyroidism may include seizures and other endocrine problems leading to lowered sexual drive and development, lowered energy levels, and increased weight.

Calling Your Health Care Provider

Call your health care provider if you or your child have any symptoms of hypocalcemia or features of this disorder.

The information provided herein should not be used during any medical emergency or for the diagnosis or treatment of any medical condition. A licensed physician should be consulted for diagnosis and treatment of any and all medical conditions. Call 911 for all medical emergencies.

Part Seven

Thyroid and Parathyroid Cancer

Chapter 39

What You Need to Know about Thyroid Cancer

Chapter Contents

Section 39.1

Understanding Cancer

Excerpted from "What You Need to Know about Thyroid Cancer," National Cancer Institute (NCI), NIH Publication No. 01-4994, September 2002.

Each year in the United States, thyroid cancer is diagnosed in 14,900 women and 4,600 men. Research is increasing what we know about thyroid cancer. Scientists are studying its causes. They are also looking for better ways to detect, diagnose, and treat this disease. Because of research, people with thyroid cancer can look forward to a better quality of life and less chance of dying from the disease.

The Thyroid

The thyroid is a gland in the neck. It has two kinds of cells that make hormones. Follicular cells make thyroid hormone, which affects heart rate, body temperature, and energy level. C cells make calcitonin, a hormone that helps control the level of calcium in the blood.

The thyroid is shaped like a butterfly and lies at the front of the neck, beneath the voice box (larynx). It has two parts, or lobes. The two lobes are separated by a thin section called the isthmus.

A healthy thyroid is a little larger than a quarter. It usually cannot be felt through the skin. A swollen lobe might look or feel like a lump in the front of the neck. A swollen thyroid is called a goiter. Most goiters are caused by not enough iodine in the diet. Iodine is a substance found in shellfish and iodized salt.

Cancer

Cancer is a group of many related diseases. All cancers begin in cells, the body's basic unit of life. Cells make up tissues, and tissues make up the organs of the body. Normally, cells grow and divide to form new cells as the body needs them. When cells grow old and die, new cells take their place.

Sometimes this orderly process goes wrong. New cells form when the body does not need them, and old cells do not die when they should.

These extra cells can form a mass of tissue called a growth or tumor. Growths on the thyroid are usually called nodules.

Thyroid nodules can be benign or malignant:

- **Benign** nodules are not cancer. Cells from benign nodules do not spread to other parts of the body. They are usually not a threat to life. Most thyroid nodules (more than 90 percent) are benign.

- **Malignant** nodules are cancer. They are generally more serious and may sometimes be life threatening. Cancer cells can invade and damage nearby tissues and organs. Also, cancer cells can break away from a malignant nodule and enter the bloodstream or the lymphatic system. That is how cancer spreads from the original cancer (primary tumor) to form new tumors in other organs. The spread of cancer is called metastasis.

The following are the major types of thyroid cancer:

- **Papillary and follicular thyroid cancers** account for 80 to 90 percent of all thyroid cancers. Both types begin in the follicular cells of the thyroid. Most papillary and follicular thyroid

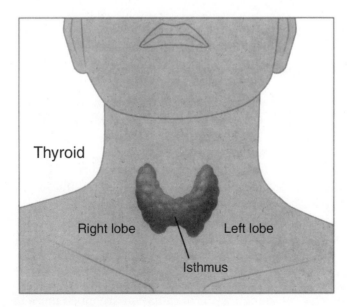

Figure 39.1. *Thyroid Gland*

cancers tend to grow slowly. If they are detected early, most can be treated successfully.

- **Medullary thyroid cancer** accounts for 5 to 10 percent of thyroid cancer cases. It arises in C cells, not follicular cells. Medullary thyroid cancer is easier to control if it is found and treated before it spreads to other parts of the body.

- **Anaplastic thyroid cancer** is the least common type of thyroid cancer (only 1 to 2 percent of cases). It arises in the follicular cells. The cancer cells are highly abnormal and difficult to recognize. This type of cancer is usually very hard to control because the cancer cells tend to grow and spread very quickly.

If thyroid cancer spreads (metastasizes) outside the thyroid, cancer cells are often found in nearby lymph nodes, nerves, or blood vessels. If the cancer has reached these lymph nodes, cancer cells may have also spread to other lymph nodes or to other organs, such as the lungs or bones.

When cancer spreads from its original place to another part of the body, the new tumor has the same kind of abnormal cells and the same name as the primary tumor. For example, if thyroid cancer spreads to the lungs, the cancer cells in the lungs are thyroid cancer cells. The disease is metastatic thyroid cancer, not lung cancer. It is treated as thyroid cancer, not as lung cancer. Doctors sometimes call the new tumor distant or metastatic disease.

Thyroid Cancer: Who's at Risk?

No one knows the exact causes of thyroid cancer. Doctors can seldom explain why one person gets this disease and another does not. However, it is clear that thyroid cancer is not contagious. No one can catch cancer from another person.

Research has shown that people with certain risk factors are more likely than others to develop thyroid cancer. A risk factor is anything that increases a person's chance of developing a disease.

The following risk factors are associated with an increased chance of developing thyroid cancer:

Radiation

People exposed to high levels of radiation are much more likely than others to develop papillary or follicular thyroid cancer. One important source of radiation exposure is treatment with x-rays. Between the 1920s and the 1950s, doctors used high-dose x-rays to treat children who had enlarged tonsils, acne, and other problems affecting the head and neck. Later, scientists found that some people who had received this kind of treatment developed thyroid cancer. (Routine diagnostic x-rays—such as dental x-rays or chest x-rays—use very small doses of radiation. Their benefits nearly always outweigh their risks. However, repeated exposure could be harmful, so it is a good idea for people to talk with their dentist and doctor about the need for each x-ray and to ask about the use of shields to protect other parts of the body.)

Another source of radiation is radioactive fallout. This includes fallout from atomic weapons testing (such as the testing in the United States and elsewhere in the world, mainly in the 1950s and 1960s), nuclear power plant accidents (such as the Chernobyl accident in 1986), and releases from atomic weapons production plants (such as the Hanford facility in Washington state in the late 1940s). Such radioactive fallout contains radioactive iodine (I-131). People who were exposed to one or more sources of I-131, especially if they were children at the time of their exposure, may have an increased risk for thyroid diseases.

People who are concerned about their exposure to radiation from medical treatments or radioactive fallout may wish to review chapter 41 "Thyroid Cancer Information for People Exposed to Radioactive Iodine (I-131)."

Family History

Medullary thyroid cancer can be caused by a change, or alteration, in a gene called *RET*. The altered *RET* gene can be passed from parent to child. Nearly everyone with the altered *RET* gene will develop medullary thyroid cancer. A blood test can detect an altered *RET* gene. If the abnormal gene is found in a person with medullary thyroid cancer, the doctor may suggest that family members be tested. For those found to carry the altered *RET* gene, the doctor may recommend frequent lab tests or surgery to remove the thyroid before cancer develops. When medullary thyroid cancer runs in a family, the doctor may call this familial medullary thyroid cancer or multiple endocrine neoplasia (MEN) syndrome. People with the MEN syndrome tend to develop certain other types of cancer. A small number of people with a family history of goiter or certain precancerous polyps in the colon are at risk for developing papillary thyroid cancer.

Being Female

In the United States, women are two to three times more likely than men to develop thyroid cancer.

Age

Most patients with thyroid cancer are more than 40 years old. People with anaplastic thyroid cancer are usually more than 65 years old.

Race

In the United States, white people are more likely than African Americans to be diagnosed with thyroid cancer.

Not Enough Iodine in the Diet

The thyroid needs iodine to make thyroid hormone. In the United States, iodine is added to salt to protect people from thyroid problems. Thyroid cancer seems to be less common in the United States than in countries where iodine is not part of the diet.

Most people who have known risk factors do not get thyroid cancer. On the other hand, many who do get the disease have none of these risk factors. People who think they may be at risk for thyroid cancer should discuss this concern with their doctor. The doctor may suggest ways to reduce the risk and can plan an appropriate schedule for checkups.

Symptoms

Early thyroid cancer often does not cause symptoms. But as the cancer grows, symptoms may include:

- A lump, or nodule, in the front of the neck near the Adam's apple
- Hoarseness or difficulty speaking in a normal voice
- Swollen lymph nodes, especially in the neck
- Difficulty swallowing or breathing
- Pain in the throat or neck

These symptoms are not sure signs of thyroid cancer. An infection, a benign goiter, or another problem also could cause these symptoms. Anyone with these symptoms should see a doctor as soon as possible. Only a doctor can diagnose and treat the problem.

Section 39.2

Diagnosing Thyroid Cancer

This chapter begins with text excerpted from "What You Need to Know about Thyroid Cancer," National Cancer Institute (NCI), NIH Publication No. 01-4994, September 2002. Also included is, "PET Scans Can Uncover Difficult-to-Find Thyroid Cancer and Predict Survival Once Metastases Are Found," September 18, 2003. Copyright The American Thyroid Association. Reprinted with permission.

Diagnosis

If a person has symptoms that suggest thyroid cancer, the doctor may perform a physical exam and ask about the patient's personal and family medical history. The doctor also may order laboratory tests and imaging tests to produce pictures of the thyroid and other areas. The exams and tests may include the following:

- **Physical exam:** The doctor will feel the neck, thyroid, voice box, and lymph nodes in the neck for unusual growths (nodules) or swelling.

- **Blood tests:** The doctor may test for abnormal levels (too low or too high) of thyroid-stimulating hormone (TSH) in the blood. TSH is made by the pituitary gland in the brain. It stimulates the release of thyroid hormone. TSH also controls how fast thyroid follicular cells grow. If medullary thyroid cancer is suspected, the doctor may check for abnormally high levels of calcium in the blood. The doctor also may order blood tests to detect an altered *RET* gene or to look for a high level of calcitonin.

- **Ultrasonography:** The ultrasound device uses sound waves that people cannot hear. The waves bounce off the thyroid, and a computer uses the echoes to create a picture called a sonogram. From the picture, the doctor can see how many nodules are present, how big they are, and whether they are solid or filled with fluid.

- **Radionuclide scanning:** The doctor may order a nuclear medicine scan that uses a very small amount of radioactive material to make thyroid nodules show up on a picture. Nodules that absorb

349

less radioactive material than the surrounding thyroid tissue are called cold nodules. Cold nodules may be benign or malignant. Hot nodules take up more radioactive material than surrounding thyroid tissue and are usually benign.

- **Biopsy:** The removal of tissue to look for cancer cells is called a biopsy. A biopsy can show cancer, tissue changes that may lead to cancer, and other conditions. A biopsy is the only sure way to know whether a nodule is cancerous. The doctor may remove tissue through a needle or during surgery:

  - **Fine-needle aspiration:** For most patients, the doctor removes a sample of tissue from a thyroid nodule with a thin needle. A pathologist looks at the cells under a microscope to check for cancer. Sometimes, the doctor uses an ultrasound device to guide the needle through the nodule.

  - **Surgical biopsy:** If a diagnosis cannot be made from the fine-needle aspiration, the doctor may operate to remove the nodule. A pathologist then checks the tissue for cancer cells.

A person who needs a biopsy may want to ask the doctor the following questions:

- What kind of biopsy will I have?
- How long will the procedure take?
- Will I be awake?
- Will it hurt?
- Will I have a scar on my neck after the biopsy?
- How soon will you have the results?
- Who will explain the results to me?
- If I do have cancer, who will talk to me about treatment? When?

Staging

If the diagnosis is thyroid cancer, the doctor needs to know the stage, or extent, of the disease to plan the best treatment. Staging is a careful attempt to learn whether the cancer has spread and, if so, to what parts of the body.

The doctor may use ultrasonography, magnetic resonance imaging (MRI), or computed tomography (CT) to find out whether the cancer has spread to the lymph nodes or other areas within the neck. The doctor may use a nuclear medicine scan of the entire body, such as a radionuclide scan known as the diagnostic I-131 whole body scan, or other imaging tests to learn whether thyroid cancer has spread to distant sites.

PET Scans Can Uncover Difficult-to-Find Thyroid Cancer and Predict Survival Once Metastases Are Found

A noninvasive imaging test, known as a positron emission tomography (PET) scan, can find metastatic thyroid cancer cells—thyroid cancer that has spread to other parts of the body—that are invisible by radioactive iodine scans, and it can also predict the patient's prognosis, according to a study presented September 18, 2003 at the 75th Annual Meeting of the American Thyroid Association.

There are approximately 23,000 new cases of thyroid cancer each year in the United States and 1,500 deaths, which amounts to nearly 300,000 thyroid cancer survivors who should be under observation. Some patients with lung metastases, for example, can live for 20–30 years without an obvious progression of the disease, while in others the cancer will steadily progress over just two to three years.

Radioactive iodine scans are the most commonly used method of treating and monitoring thyroid cancer. Thyroid cancer cells absorb radioactive iodine (I-131) similar to how regular thyroid cells naturally absorb potassium iodide. Cancer cell deposits that absorb I-131 are called radioactive iodine (RAI) positive. An I-131 scan can reveal areas of uptake outside the region of the neck that may indicate metastases of thyroid cancer. This may prompt further investigation with other radiographic tests or further treatment with I-131, which kills cancer cells.

Differentiated thyroid cancer cells may transform over time and lose some or all of the ability to take up and retain I-131. However, these cells may still be able to absorb a different radioactive tracer called 18-fluorodeoxyglucose (FDG), a form of sugar that can be detected by the positron emission tomography (PET) scan, which produces three-dimensional images of the body at work. After a patient receives a dose of FDG, the images produced by the PET scan can reveal abnormal areas of increased uptake, called FDG positive, suggestive of thyroid cancer cells.

Due to the difficult nature of predicting the outcome of patients who develop metastases from thyroid cancer, researchers at Memorial Sloan-Kettering Cancer Center (MSKCC) in New York City reviewed the records of thyroid cancer patients who underwent comprehensive diagnostic testing during 1996–2002 to find out the prognostic value of the PET scan.

Patients were followed for one to seven years. Those with medullary thyroid cancer and other active cancers were excluded. Of the 403 patients included in the analysis, 57 percent were women, 61.5 percent were RAI positive, and 55 percent were FDG positive. Their average age was 54 years old.

The researchers found that age, uptake, and the number of FDG deposits, or lesions, were significantly associated with survival. Each 10-year increase in age at PET increased the risk of death by 28 percent. Each additional FDG lesion increased the risk of death by 9 percent. A positive FDG scan, by itself, was associated with an eight-fold increased risk of death.

The researchers found that patients who had a negative PET scan have excellent short- and medium-term prognoses, regardless of any other clinical characteristic. Only three deaths, two of which were from other causes, occurred in the 179 patients who had a negative FDG scan, making it unlikely that a person would die in the next five years of thyroid cancer if they had a negative FDG-PET scan.

Patients who have a positive PET scan may need more aggressive therapy. "The positivity of the scan, however, does not directly tell the clinician how to treat the patient," said Richard Robbins, M.D., lead author of the study and chief of the Endocrine Service at MSKCC and professor of medicine at Weill Medical College of Cornell University. "However, we have found that FDG positive lesions are somewhat resistant to therapy with radioactive iodine."

"There is no perfect test to find residual thyroid cancer," added Dr. Robbins. "A negative FDG-PET scan result does not mean that the patient is cured. It only means that there is no rapidly growing, aggressive, site of metastatic thyroid cancer. Small slow growing or dormant lesions may be missed by a PET scan."

Additional Information

American Thyroid Association
6066 Leesburg Pike, Suite 550
Falls Church, VA 22041
Toll-Free: 800-THYROID (849-7643)
Phone: 703-998-8890
Fax: 703-998-8893
Website: http://www.thyroid.org
E-mail: admin@thyroid.org

Section 39.3

Treatment Overview

Excerpted from "What You Need to Know about Thyroid Cancer,"
National Cancer Institute (NCI), NIH Publication No. 01-4994,
September 2002.

Treatment

People with thyroid cancer often want to take an active part in making decisions about their medical care. They want to learn all they can about their disease and their treatment choices. However, the shock and stress that people may feel after a diagnosis of cancer can make it hard for them to think of everything they want to ask the doctor. It often helps to make a list of questions before an appointment. To help remember what the doctor says, patients may take notes or ask whether they may use a tape recorder. Some also want to have a family member or friend with them when they talk to the doctor— to take part in the discussion, to take notes, or just to listen.

The doctor may refer patients to doctors (oncologists) who specialize in treating cancer, or patients may ask for a referral. Specialists who treat thyroid cancer include surgeons, endocrinologists (some of whom are called thyroidologists because they specialize in thyroid diseases), medical oncologists, and radiation oncologists. Treatment generally begins within a few weeks after the diagnosis. There will be time for patients to talk with the doctor about treatment choices, get a second opinion, and learn more about thyroid cancer.

Getting a Second Opinion

Before starting treatment, the patient might want a second opinion about the diagnosis and the treatment plan. Some insurance companies require a second opinion; others may cover a second opinion if the patient or doctor requests it. Gathering medical records and arranging to see another doctor may take a little time. In most cases, a brief delay does not make treatment less effective.

There are a number of ways to find a doctor for a second opinion:

- The patient's doctor may refer the patient to one or more specialists. At cancer centers, several specialists often work together as a team.

- The Cancer Information Service, at 1-800-4-CANCER, can tell callers about treatment facilities, including cancer centers and other programs supported by the National Cancer Institute.

- A local medical society, a nearby hospital, or a medical school can usually provide the name of specialists.

- The American Board of Medical Specialties (ABMS) has a list of doctors who have met certain education and training requirements and have passed specialty examinations. The Official ABMS Directory of Board Certified Medical Specialists lists doctors' names along with their specialty and their educational background. The directory is available in most public libraries. Also, ABMS offers this information on the Internet at http://www.abms.org (click on Who's Certified).

Preparing for Treatment

The doctor can describe treatment choices and discuss the results expected with each treatment option. The doctor and patient can work together to develop a treatment plan that fits the patient's needs.

Treatment depends on a number of factors, including the type of thyroid cancer, the size of the nodule, the patient's age, and whether the cancer has spread.

These are some questions a person may want to ask the doctor before treatment begins:

- What type of thyroid cancer do I have?

- Has the cancer spread? What is the stage of the disease?

- Do I need any more tests to check for spread of the disease?

- What are my treatment choices? Which do you recommend for me? Why?

- What are the benefits of each kind of treatment?

- What are the risks and possible side effects of each treatment?

- What is the treatment likely to cost?

- How will the treatment affect my normal activities?

- Would a clinical trial (research study) be appropriate for me? Can you help me find one?

People do not need to ask all of their questions or understand all of the answers at one time. They will have other chances to ask the doctor to explain things that are not clear and to ask for more information.

Methods of Treatment

People with thyroid cancer have many treatment options. Depending on the type and stage, thyroid cancer may be treated with surgery, radioactive iodine, hormone treatment, external radiation, or chemotherapy. Some patients receive a combination of treatments.

The doctor is the best person to describe the treatment choices and discuss the expected results. A patient may want to talk to the doctor about taking part in a clinical trial, a research study of new treatment methods. Chapter 52—Clinical Trials: Researching New Treatments has more information about clinical trials.

Surgery

Surgery is the most common treatment for thyroid cancer. The surgeon may remove all or part of the thyroid. The type of surgery depends on the type and stage of thyroid cancer, the size of the nodule, and the patient's age.

- **Total thyroidectomy:** Surgery to remove the entire thyroid is called a total thyroidectomy. The surgeon removes the thyroid through an incision in the neck. Nearby lymph nodes are sometimes removed, too. If the pathologist finds cancer cells in the lymph nodes, it means that the disease could spread to other parts of the body. In a small number of cases, the surgeon removes other tissues in the neck that have been affected by the cancer. Some patients who have a total thyroidectomy also receive radioactive iodine or external radiation therapy.

- **Lobectomy:** Some patients with papillary or follicular thyroid cancer may be treated with lobectomy. The lobe with the cancerous nodule is removed. The surgeon also may remove part of the remaining thyroid tissue or nearby lymph nodes. Some patients who have a lobectomy receive radioactive iodine therapy or additional surgery to remove remaining thyroid tissue.

Nearly all patients who have part or all of the thyroid removed will take thyroid hormone pills to replace the natural hormone. After the initial surgery, the doctor may need to operate on the neck again for thyroid cancer that has spread. Patients who have this surgery also may receive I-131 therapy or external radiation therapy to treat thyroid cancer that has spread.

These are some questions a person may want to ask the doctor before having surgery:

- What kind of operation will I have?
- How will I feel after the operation?
- What will you do for me if I have pain?
- How long will I be in the hospital?
- Will I have any long-term effects?
- When can I get back to my normal activities?
- What will my scar look like?
- What is my chance of a full recovery?
- Will I need to take thyroid hormone pills?
- How often will I need checkups?

Radioactive Iodine Therapy

Radioactive iodine therapy (also called radioiodine therapy) uses radioactive iodine (I-131) to destroy thyroid cancer cells anywhere in the body. The therapy usually is given by mouth (liquid or capsules) in a small dose that causes no problems for people who are allergic to iodine. The intestine absorbs the I-131, which flows through the bloodstream and collects in thyroid cells. Thyroid cancer cells remaining in the neck and those that have spread to other parts of the body are killed when they absorb I-131.

If the dose of I-131 is low enough, the patient usually receives I-131 as an outpatient. If the dose is high, the doctor may protect others from radiation exposure by isolating the patient in the hospital during the treatment. Most radiation is gone in a few days. Within 3 weeks, only traces of radioactive iodine remain in the body.

Patients with medullary thyroid cancer or anaplastic thyroid cancer generally do not receive I-131 treatment. These types of thyroid cancer rarely respond to I-131 therapy.

Hormone Treatment

Hormone treatment after surgery is usually part of the treatment plan for papillary and follicular cancer. When a patient takes thyroid hormone pills, the growth of any remaining thyroid cancer cells slows down, which lowers the chance that the disease will return.

After surgery or I-131 therapy (which removes or destroys thyroid tissue), people with thyroid cancer may need to take thyroid hormone pills to replace the natural thyroid hormone.

People may want to ask these questions about radioactive iodine (I-131) therapy or hormone therapy:

- Why do I need this treatment?
- What will it do?
- Will I need to stay in the hospital for this treatment?
- Will it cause side effects? What can I do about them?
- How long will I be on this treatment?
- How often will I need checkups?

External Radiation Therapy

External radiation therapy (also called radiotherapy) uses high-energy rays to kill cancer cells. A large machine directs radiation at the neck or at parts of the body where the cancer has spread.

External radiation therapy is local therapy. It affects cancer cells only in the treated area. External radiation therapy is used mainly to treat people with advanced thyroid cancer that does not respond to radioactive iodine therapy. For external radiation therapy, patients go to the hospital or clinic, usually 5 days a week for several weeks. External radiation may also be used to relieve pain or other problems.

Questions a person may want to ask the doctor before having external radiation therapy:

- Why do I need this treatment?
- When will the treatments begin? When will they end?
- How will I feel during therapy? Are there side effects?
- What can I do to take care of myself during therapy?
- How will we know if the radiation is working?
- Will I be able to continue my normal activities during treatment?
- How often will I need checkups?

Chemotherapy

Chemotherapy, the use of drugs to kill cancer cells, is sometimes used to treat thyroid cancer. Chemotherapy is known as systemic therapy because the drugs enter the bloodstream and travel throughout the body. For some patients, chemotherapy may be combined with external radiation therapy.

Patients may want to ask these questions about chemotherapy:

- Why do I need this treatment?
- What will it do?
- Will I have side effects? What can I do about them?
- How long will I be on this treatment?
- How often will I need checkups?

Side Effects of Cancer Treatment

Because cancer treatment may damage healthy cells and tissues, unwanted side effects sometimes occur. These side effects depend on many factors, including the type and extent of the treatment. Side effects may not be the same for each person, and they may even change from one treatment session to the next. Before treatment starts, the health care team will explain possible side effects and suggest ways to help the patient manage them.

Surgery

Patients are often uncomfortable for the first few days after surgery. However, medicine can usually control their pain. Patients should feel free to discuss pain relief with the doctor or nurse. It is also common for patients to feel tired or weak. The length of time it takes to recover from an operation varies for each patient.

After surgery to remove the thyroid and nearby tissues or organs, such as the parathyroid glands, patients may need to take medicine (thyroid hormone) or vitamin and mineral supplements (vitamin D and calcium) to replace the lost functions of these organs. In a few cases, certain nerves or muscles may be damaged or removed during surgery. If this happens, the patient may have voice problems or one shoulder may be lower than the other.

Radioactive Iodine (I-131) Therapy

Some patients have nausea and vomiting on the first day of I-131 therapy. Thyroid tissue remaining in the neck after surgery may become swollen and painful. If the thyroid cancer has spread to other parts of the body, the I-131 that collects there may cause pain and swelling.

Other I-131 therapy side effects include:

- Patients may have a dry mouth or lose their sense of taste or smell for a short time after I-131 therapy. Chewing sugar-free gum or sucking on sugar-free hard candy may help.
- During treatment, patients are encouraged to drink lots of water and other fluids. Because fluids help I-131 pass out of the body more quickly, the bladder's exposure to I-131 is reduced.
- Because radioactive iodine therapy destroys the cells that make thyroid hormone, patients may need to take thyroid hormone pills to replace the natural hormone.
- A rare side effect in men who received large doses of I-131 is loss of fertility. In women, I-131 may not cause loss of fertility, but some doctors suggest that women avoid pregnancy for one year after I-131 therapy.
- Researchers have reported that a very small number of patients may develop leukemia years after treatment with high doses of I-131.

Hormone Treatment

Thyroid hormone pills seldom cause side effects. However, a few patients may get a rash or lose some of their hair during the first months of treatment.

The doctor will closely monitor the level of thyroid hormone in the blood during follow-up visits. Too much thyroid hormone may cause patients to lose weight and to feel hot and sweaty. It also may cause chest pain, cramps, and diarrhea. (The doctor may call this condition hyperthyroidism.) If the thyroid hormone level is too low, the patient may gain weight, feel cold, and have dry skin and hair. (The doctor may call this condition hypothyroidism.) If necessary, the doctor will adjust the dose so that the patient takes the right amount.

External Radiation Therapy

External radiation therapy may cause patients to become very tired as treatment continues. Resting is important, but doctors usually advise patients to try to stay as active as they can. In addition, when patients receive external radiation therapy, it is common for their skin to become red, dry, and tender in the treated area. When the neck is treated with external radiation therapy, patients may feel hoarse or have trouble swallowing. Other side effects depend on the area of the body that is treated. If chemotherapy is given at the same time, the side effects may worsen. The doctor can suggest ways to ease these problems.

Chemotherapy

The side effects of chemotherapy depend mainly on the specific drugs that are used. The most common side effects include nausea and vomiting, mouth sores, loss of appetite, and hair loss. Some side effects may be relieved with medicine.

Section 39.4

Follow-Up Care

This section begins with text excerpted from "What You Need to Know about Thyroid Cancer," National Cancer Institute (NCI), NIH Publication No. 01-4994, September 2002. "Thyroid Cancer Study Simplifies Follow-Up Exams," March 30, 2004, is reprinted with permission from the Washington University in St. Louis Office of Medical Public Affairs.

Follow-up care after treatment for thyroid cancer is an important part of the overall treatment plan. Regular checkups ensure that any changes in health are noted. Problems can be found and treated as soon as possible. Checkups may include a careful physical exam, x-rays and other imaging tests (such as a nuclear medicine scan), and laboratory tests (such as a blood test for calcitonin). The doctor can explain the follow-up plan—how often the patient must visit the doctor and which types of tests are needed.

An important test after thyroid cancer treatment measures the level of thyroglobulin in the blood. Thyroid hormone is stored in the thyroid as thyroglobulin. If the thyroid has been removed, there should be very little or no thyroglobulin in the blood. A high level of thyroglobulin may mean that thyroid cancer cells have returned.

For six weeks before the thyroglobulin test, patients must stop taking their usual thyroid hormone pill. For part of this time, some patients may take a different, shorter-lasting thyroid hormone pill. But all patients must stop taking any type of thyroid hormone pill for the last two weeks right before the test. Without adequate levels of thyroid hormone, patients are likely to feel uncomfortable. They may gain weight and feel very tired. It may be helpful to talk with the doctor or nurse about ways to cope with such problems. After the test, patients go back to their usual treatment with thyroid hormone pills.

The doctor may request an I-131 scan of the entire body. This may be called a diagnostic I-131 whole body scan. For a short time (usually six weeks) before this scan, the patient stops taking thyroid hormone pills. Thyroid cancer cells anywhere in the body will show up on the scan. After the test, the doctor will tell the patient when to start taking thyroid hormone pills again.

Support for People with Thyroid Cancer

Living with a serious disease such as cancer is not easy. Some people find they need help coping with the emotional and practical aspects of their disease. Support groups can help. In these groups, patients or their family members get together to share what they have learned about coping with the disease and the effects of treatment. Patients may want to talk with a member of their health care team about finding a support group. Groups may offer support in person, over the telephone, or on the Internet.

People living with cancer may worry about caring for their families, keeping their jobs, or continuing daily activities. Concerns about treatments and managing side effect, hospital stays, and medical bills are also common. Doctors, nurses, and other members of the health care team can answer questions about treatment, working, or other activities. Meeting with a social worker, counselor, or member of the clergy can be helpful to those who want to talk about their feelings or discuss their concerns. Often, a social worker can suggest resources for financial aid, transportation, home care, or emotional support.

The Cancer Information Service of the National Cancer Institute can provide information to help patients and their families locate programs, services, and publications.

The Promise of Cancer Research

Doctors all over the country are conducting many types of clinical trials. These are research studies in which people take part voluntarily. Studies include new ways to treat thyroid cancer. Research already has led to advances, and researchers continue to search for more effective approaches.

Patients who join these studies have the first chance to benefit from treatments that have shown promise in earlier research. They also make an important contribution to medical science by helping doctors learn more about the disease. Although clinical trials may pose some risks, researchers take very careful steps to protect their patients.

Patients who are interested in being part of a clinical trial should talk with their doctor. They may also want to read Chapter 52—Clinical Trials: Researching New Treatments.

Thyroid Cancer Study Simplifies Follow-Up Exams

An unpleasant postoperative procedure for thyroid cancer patients who have had their thyroid glands surgically removed may be unnecessary for most patients, according to Washington University researchers at Siteman Cancer Center and Barnes-Jewish Hospital in St. Louis.

Physicians have long assumed that early follow-up scans for residual or recurrent thyroid cancer are only possible when patients have been through six weeks of a weaker thyroid medication and two to three weeks of no thyroid medication.

Withdrawal from medication leads patients' bodies to produce their own thyroid-stimulating hormone (TSH), and exposure to sufficiently high levels of TSH creates an increased thirst for iodine in any remaining thyroid cells. Scientists can then give patients small doses of radioactive iodine that will be taken up by the cells. A weaker dose lets scientists detect the cells; a stronger dose kills them.

In a study published in the April 2004 issue of *The Journal of Nuclear Medicine*, Washington University School of Medicine scientists report that simply taking patients off thyroid medication for two weeks prior to the scan produces the desired changes in nearly 90 percent of patients.

"When patients are taken off thyroid medication, they get tired, gain weight, and just generally don't feel very good," says lead investigator Perry W. Grigsby, M.D., professor of radiology and of radiation oncology. "We don't want patients to feel bad, so we want them to be off medication for as short a time as possible."

Physicians diagnose an estimated 14,000 new cases of thyroid cancer per year, with women developing the cancer at rates two to three times those of men. Located in the neck, the thyroid gland regulates metabolism through the production of thyroid hormone, which affects cell activity levels throughout the body.

Treatment of a cancerous thyroid generally begins with surgical removal of the gland. To compensate, patients take thyroid medication for the rest of their lives.

In early postoperative scans, increased risk of recurrent or residual tumors limits physicians' options for preparing patients for those scans, according to Grigsby. "The classic procedure is to put the patient on a weaker thyroid medication for six weeks and then take them off medication entirely for two to three weeks," Grigsby explains.

For the study, Grigsby and colleagues closely monitored the TSH levels in nearly 300 thyroid cancer patients whose thyroids had been removed and who were not taking medication. Some of the patients were just out of surgery and had not yet started taking the hormone; others were taken off the hormone without the standard six-week period on the weaker form of the drug. Researchers found that 89 percent of the group had achieved the TSH level needed for postoperative imaging in one to two weeks. By the third week, 96 percent were at or beyond the desired level.

"We don't seem to need six weeks on the less effective medication," Grigsby says. "That approach appears to have originated as someone's best guess as to what we needed to do to prepare patients for scans, and no one ever questioned it. But now we know we can do it in a way that is simpler, quicker, and above all easier on patients."

Grigsby notes that the introduction of recombinant human thyroid-stimulating hormone (rhTSH) five years ago greatly reduced the need to take patients off thyroid medication for later follow-up scans. The body responds to rhTSH in the same way it responds to cessation of thyroid medication, making it possible for scientists to scan for cancer cells. However, rhTSH can also complicate and delay treatment of tumors, so physicians generally do not use it in the earliest postoperative scans, when odds of finding tumors again are highest.

Reference

Grigsby PW, Siegel BA, Bekker S, Clutter WE, Moley JF. Preparation of Patients with Thyroid Cancer for 131I Scintigraphy or Therapy by 1–3 Weeks of Thyroxine Discontinuation. *Journal of Nuclear Medicine*, April 2004.

Additional Information

Society of Nuclear Medicine
1850 Samuel Morse Drive
Reston, VA 20190-5316
Phone: 703-708-9000
Fax: 703-708-9015
Website: http://www.snm.org

National Cancer Institute
6116 Executive Blvd., MSC 8322
Bethesda, MD 20892-8322
Toll-Free: 800-4-CANCER (800-422-6237)
Toll-Free TTY: 800-332-8615
Website: http://www.cancer.gov
E-mail: cancergovstaff@mail.nih.gov

Chapter 40

Thyroid Cancer Statistics

Death Caused by Thyroid Cancer in the U.S. 1997–2001

Information about Table 40.1

- Standard population = 2000 U.S.
- Site = Thyroid
- Year of death = 1997–2001
- Age at death = All ages

Thyroid Cancer Diagnosed in the U.S. from 1997–2001

Information about Table 40.2

- Standard population = 2000 U.S.
- Site = Thyroid
- Year of diagnosis = 1997–2001
- Age at diagnosis = All ages

"SEER Incidence–U.S. Mortality (by State) AA Rates for White/Black/Other, 1969-2001," Surveillance, Epidemiology, and End Results (SEER) Program, National Cancer Institute, 2004. And "SEER Incidence–AA Rates for Additional Races/Registries, 1992–2001," Surveillance, Epidemiology, and End Results (SEER) Program, National Cancer Institute, 2004.

Table 40.1. U.S. Thyroid Cancer Mortality 1997–2001 By State: All Ages, Cases Per 100,000. (continued on next page)

State	Race	Male and Female	Male	Female
Total U.S.	All races	0.4621	0.4438	0.4683
	White	0.4557	0.4515	0.4500
	Black	0.4769	0.3591	0.5479
Alabama	All races	0.4238	0.4824	0.3793
	White	0.3947	0.4722	0.3275
	Black	0.5357	***	0.5788
Alaska	All races	***	***	***
	White	***	***	***
	Black	***	***	***
Arizona	All races	0.3956	0.4817	0.3192
	White	0.4054	0.5128	0.3102
	Black	***	***	***
Arkansas	All races	0.4134	0.4936	0.3419
	White	0.3756	0.4830	0.2892
	Black	0.7799	***	***
California	All races	0.5081	0.4694	0.5313
	White	0.4864	0.4771	0.4859
	Black	0.3722	***	0.4450
Colorado	All races	0.5074	0.5077	0.5105
	White	0.5061	0.5188	0.5016
	Black	***	***	***
Connecticut	All races	0.4898	0.5495	0.4512
	White	0.4964	0.5735	0.4455
	Black	***	***	***
Delaware	All races	0.3914	***	0.4405
	White	0.3867	***	***
	Black	***	***	***
Washington DC	All races	0.5735	***	***
	White	***	***	***
	Black	0.7231	***	***
Florida	All races	0.4293	0.4158	0.4365
	White	0.4271	0.4293	0.4214
	Black	0.4600	***	0.5749

Table 40.1. (continued) U.S. Thyroid Cancer Mortality 1997–2001 By State: All Ages, Cases Per 100,000. (continued on next page)

State	Race	Male and Female	Male	Female
Georgia	All races	0.4104	0.3927	0.4084
	White	0.4102	0.4373	0.3720
	Black	0.3510	***	0.4166
Hawaii	All races	0.6140	0.6017	0.6411
	White	***	***	***
	Black	***	***	***
Idaho	All races	0.3458	***	0.3653
	White	0.3516	***	0.3708
	Black	***	***	***
Illinois	All races	0.4394	0.4302	0.4391
	White	0.4405	0.4637	0.4155
	Black	0.4579	***	0.6052
Indiana	All races	0.5156	0.4850	0.5275
	White	0.5154	0.5048	0.5095
	Black	***	***	***
Iowa	All races	0.4260	0.4458	0.3940
	White	0.4251	0.4386	0.3993
	Black	***	***	***
Kansas	All races	0.5184	0.6486	0.4278
	White	0.5366	0.6624	0.4497
	Black	***	***	***
Kentucky	All races	0.5658	0.5014	0.5887
	White	0.5529	0.4862	0.5792
	Black	***	***	***
Louisiana	All races	0.5402	0.4625	0.5848
	White	0.5131	0.4719	0.5374
	Black	0.6470	***	0.7485
Maine	All races	0.5000	0.5557	0.4698
	White	0.5038	0.5592	0.4739
	Black	***	***	***
Maryland	All races	0.3728	0.3114	0.4078
	White	0.3465	0.2629	0.3930
	Black	0.4080	***	0.4035

Table 40.1. (continued) U.S. Thyroid Cancer Mortality 1997–2001 By State: All Ages, Cases Per 100,000. (continued on next page)

State	Race	Male and Female	Male	Female
Massachusetts	All races	0.4663	0.5014	0.4289
	White	0.4530	0.4791	0.4247
	Black	***	***	***
Michigan	All races	0.4801	0.4167	0.5248
	White	0.4899	0.4321	0.5320
	Black	0.3586	***	0.3985
Minnesota	All races	0.5121	0.5042	0.5091
	White	0.5038	0.4989	0.4985
	Black	***	***	***
Mississippi	All races	0.4720	0.4061	0.5161
	White	0.4407	0.4328	0.4360
	Black	0.4888	***	0.6599
Missouri	All races	0.4364	0.4961	0.3809
	White	0.4380	0.5177	0.3642
	Black	***	***	***
Montana	All races	0.4197	0.4842	***
	White	0.4117	0.5014	***
	Black	***	***	***
Nebraska	All races	0.4373	0.4480	0.4360
	White	0.4387	0.4361	0.4507
	Black	***	***	***
Nevada	All races	0.3616	0.4378	0.3071
	White	0.3708	0.4509	0.3151
	Black	***	***	***
New Hampshire	All races	0.4445	***	0.4969
	White	0.4485	***	0.5013
	Black	***	***	***
New Jersey	All races	0.5229	0.4793	0.5490
	White	0.5326	0.4921	0.5562
	Black	0.4128	***	0.4397
New Mexico	All races	0.5746	0.4885	0.6261
	White	0.5603	0.4511	0.6332
	Black	***	***	***

Table 40.1. (continued) U.S. Thyroid Cancer Mortality 1997–2001
By State: All Ages, Cases Per 100,000. (continued on next page)

State	Race	Male and Female	Male	Female
New York	All races	0.4970	0.4221	0.5365
	White	0.4913	0.4354	0.5149
	Black	0.5468	0.3489	0.6537
North Carolina	All races	0.4117	0.4939	0.3546
	White	0.3967	0.5013	0.3166
	Black	0.4618	***	0.4691
North Dakota	All races	0.3368	***	***
	White	0.3410	***	***
	Black	***	***	***
Ohio	All races	0.4423	0.4908	0.4006
	White	0.4484	0.5035	0.4037
	Black	0.3989	***	0.4108
Oklahoma	All races	0.3651	0.3975	0.3356
	White	0.3747	0.3978	0.3523
	Black	***	***	***
Oregon	All races	0.4419	0.2949	0.5425
	White	0.4403	0.2798	0.5549
	Black	***	***	***
Pennsylvania	All races	0.4765	0.4228	0.5052
	White	0.4678	0.4302	0.4815
	Black	0.5885	***	0.7660
Rhode Island	All races	0.4853	0.5642	0.3944
	White	0.4695	0.5923	0.3425
	Black	***	***	***
South Carolina	All races	0.4063	0.4205	0.3782
	White	0.3331	0.4122	0.2577
	Black	0.6398	***	0.7555
South Dakota	All races	0.4327	***	***
	White	0.3924	***	***
	Black	***	***	***
Tennessee	All races	0.4015	0.3362	0.4308
	White	0.4125	0.3720	0.4196
	Black	0.2952	***	***

Table 40.1. (continued) U.S. Thyroid Cancer Mortality 1997–2001 By State: All Ages, Cases Per 100,000.

State	Race	Male and Female	Male	Female
Texas	All races	0.4524	0.4123	0.4808
	White	0.4588	0.4296	0.4793
	Black	0.4246	***	0.5041
Utah	All races	0.5317	0.4988	0.5514
	White	0.4926	0.4573	0.5170
	Black	***	***	***
Vermont	All races	0.5546	***	***
	White	0.5259	***	***
	Black	***	***	***
Virginia	All races	0.4207	0.3026	0.4844
	White	0.3998	0.2809	0.4591
	Black	0.5370	***	0.6095
Washington	All races	0.3999	0.3726	0.4133
	White	0.4012	0.3631	0.4212
	Black	***	***	***
West Virginia	All races	0.4879	0.5472	0.4420
	White	0.4939	0.5627	0.4401
	Black	***	***	***
Wisconsin	All races	0.4987	0.4681	0.5127
	White	0.5008	0.4756	0.5116
	Black	***	***	***
Wyoming	All races	0.5125	***	***
	White	0.5221	***	***
	Black	***	***	***

Notes:

• Rates are expressed as cases per 100,000.

• Statistics were generated from data provided by the U.S. National Center for Health Statistics.

• Statistics are provided by the SEER Program for research purposes only.

*** When upper value for the 95% confidence interval (CI) of the age adjusted rate was more than four times the lower value, the figure is not shown. For additional statistical information, visit http://www.seer.cancer.gov.

Table 40.2. U.S. Thyroid Cancer Diagnosed from 1997–2001 for All Ages, Rates Per 100,000 by Race and Regional Registry. (continued on next page)

SEER Registry and Race/Ethnicity	Male and Female	Male	Female
Total (registries depend on race/ethnicity)			
All races	7.1910	3.8229	10.4491
White	7.4775	4.0155	10.9454
Black	4.1490	2.1873	5.7484
American Indian/Alaska Native	4.0164	1.5305	6.3008
Asian or Pacific Islander	8.0647	3.8726	11.7956
Hispanic	6.4863	2.8844	9.9250
San Francisco-Oakland Standard Metropolitan Statistical Area			
All races	5.8345	3.1310	8.4921
White	5.7396	3.3497	8.2730
Black	2.9292	1.3417	4.3318
American Indian/Alaska Native	*	*	*
Asian or Pacific Islander	7.0618	2.7133	10.7659
Hispanic	5.3979	3.1742	7.8491
Connecticut			
All races	7.8476	4.5331	10.9870
White	8.1457	4.8270	11.3409
Black	3.8578	*	6.0139
American Indian/Alaska Native	*	*	*
Asian or Pacific Islander	13.4014	*	22.1717
Hispanic	9.0213	*	13.1414
Detroit (Metropolitan)			
All races	7.5568	4.1660	10.7398
White	8.2665	4.5091	12.0150
Black	5.2384	2.8540	7.1001
American Indian/Alaska Native	*	*	*
Asian or Pacific Islander	9.6298	*	13.9188
Hispanic			
Hawaii			
All races	8.7258	4.4510	13.0247
White	6.7344	3.9027	9.9859
Black	*	*	*
American Indian/Alaska Native	*	*	*
Asian or Pacific Islander	9.4905	4.6220	14.0675
Hispanic			

Table 40.2. (continued) U.S. Thyroid Cancer Diagnosed from 1997–2001 for All Ages, Rates Per 100,000 by Race and Regional Registry. (continued on next page)

SEER Registry and Race/Ethnicity	Male and Female	Male	Female
Iowa			
All races	7.2617	3.6446	10.8051
White	7.2009	3.5654	10.7535
Black	5.3647	*	*
American Indian/Alaska Native	*	*	*
Asian or Pacific Islander	17.7351	*	*
Hispanic	*	*	*
New Mexico			
All races	8.4191	4.4293	12.2152
White	8.9295	4.7393	12.9548
Black	*	*	*
American Indian/Alaska Native	4.8921	*	8.0807
Asian or Pacific Islander	*	*	*
Hispanic	8.2554	4.3672	11.8658
Seattle (Puget Sound)			
All races	7.5455	3.9278	11.1373
White	7.5764	3.9766	11.1989
Black	4.7831	*	6.1107
American Indian/Alaska Native	8.2260	*	*
Asian or Pacific Islander	8.2151	3.1831	12.2850
Hispanic	8.1656	*	12.0129
Utah			
All races	8.4280	4.0357	12.7893
White	8.5615	4.0719	13.0125
Black	*	*	*
American Indian/Alaska Native	*	*	*
Asian or Pacific Islander	6.5978	*	*
Hispanic	9.3505	*	15.0453
Atlanta (Metropolitan)			
All races	6.0214	3.2806	8.5575
White	7.1602	4.0978	10.3136
Black	3.5743	0.9078	5.5339
American Indian/Alaska Native	*	*	*
Asian or Pacific Islander	7.3577	*	9.7210
Hispanic	6.9706	*	11.0274

Table 40.2. (continued) U.S. Thyroid Cancer Diagnosed from 1997–2001 for All Ages, Rates Per 100,000 by Race and Regional Registry. (continued on next page)

SEER Registry and Race/Ethnicity	Male and Female	Male	Female
San Jose-Monterey			
All races	6.7064	3.7741	9.7819
White	6.7039	3.8172	9.8324
Black	*	*	*
American Indian/Alaska Native	*	*	*
Asian or Pacific Islander	6.9515	3.6105	10.1207
Hispanic	5.5733	2.3867	9.0109
Los Angeles			
All races	7.0728	3.7150	10.2517
White	7.4256	3.8451	10.9581
Black	3.9067	2.4299	5.0296
American Indian/Alaska Native	*	*	*
Asian or Pacific Islander	7.9784	4.0856	11.3498
Hispanic	6.0803	2.3725	9.4350
Alaska Natives			
All races	6.6672	*	11.7637
White			
Black			
American Indian/Alaska Native	6.6672	*	11.7637
Asian or Pacific Islander			
Hispanic			

Notes:

- Statistics were generated from malignant cases only.
- Rates are expressed as cases per 100,000.
- Statistics are provided by the SEER Program for research purposes only.
- Hispanic and Non-Hispanic are not mutually exclusive from White, Black, American Indian/Alaska Native, and Asian or Pacific Islander.
- Statistics for Hispanics and Non-Hispanics do not include cases from the Detroit, Hawaii, and Alaska Natives registries.
- * When upper value for the 95% confidence interval (CI) of the age adjusted rate was more than four times the lower value, the figure is not shown. For additional statistical information, visit http://www.seer.cancer.gov.

Chapter 41

Thyroid Cancer Information for People Exposed to Radioactive Iodine (I-131)

Chapter Contents

Section 41.1

Fallout from I-131 Affected Most of the U.S. between 1951 and 1963

"Radfacts: A Quick-Reference Guide to Radiation Terms and Concepts," Environmental Protection Agency (EPA), August 13, 2004. Also, excerpts from "Making Choices: Screening for Thyroid Disease," National Cancer Institute (NCI), September 2002.

This information is for you if:

• You lived in the United States between 1951 and 1963.

• You are concerned that exposure to I-131 from the Nevada nuclear weapons tests may have affected your thyroid gland.

• You want to consider options for thyroid screening.

Radiation Facts from the Environmental Protection Agency

What is radiation?

Radiation is a form of energy. The radiation of concern here is called ionizing radiation. Atoms release radiation as they change from unstable, energized forms to more stable forms.

What is a radionuclide?

All matter is composed of elements, and elements that are radioactive are generally referred to as radionuclides. Each element can take many different forms (called isotopes). Some of these isotopes are unstable and emit radiation; these unstable isotopes are known as radioisotopes or radionuclides. Stable isotopes do not undergo radioactive decay and therefore do not emit radiation.

What are the types of radiation?

Alpha particles can travel only a few inches in the air and lose their energy almost as soon as they collide with anything. They are easily shielded by a sheet of paper or the outer layer of a person's skin. Alpha particles are hazardous only when they are inhaled or swallowed. Beta particles can travel in the air for a distance of a few feet.

Beta particles can pass through a sheet of paper, but can be stopped by a sheet of aluminum foil or glass. Beta particles can damage skin, but are most hazardous when swallowed or inhaled.

Gamma rays are waves of pure energy and are similar to x-rays. They travel at the speed of light through air or open spaces. Concrete, lead, or steel must be used to block gamma rays. Gamma rays can present an extreme external hazard.

Neutrons are small particles that have no electrical charge. They can travel long distances in air and are released during nuclear fission. Water or concrete offer the best shielding against neutrons. Like gamma rays, neutrons can present an extreme external hazard.

What terms are used for radiation measurements?

Radiation is measured in different ways. Measurements used in the United States include the following (the internationally used equivalent unit of measurement follows in parenthesis):

- Rad (radiation absorbed dose) measures the amount of energy actually absorbed by a material, such as human tissue (Gray = 100 rads).

- Roentgen is a measure of exposure; it describes the amount of radiation energy, in the form of gamma or x-rays, in the air.

- Rem (roentgen equivalent man) measures the biological damage of radiation. It takes into account both the amount, or dose, of radiation and the biological effect of the type of radiation in question. A millirem is one one-thousandth of a rem (Sievert = 100 rems).

- Curie is a unit of radioactivity. One curie refers to the amount of any radionuclide that undergoes 37 billion atomic transformations a second. A nanocurie is one one-billionth of a curie (37 Becquerel = 1 nanocurie).

What levels of radiation are people exposed to in everyday life?

To put an emergency situation in perspective, it helps to be aware of the radiation levels people encounter in everyday life. Individual exposures vary, but humans are exposed routinely to radiation from both natural sources, such as cosmic rays from the sun and indoor radon, and from manufactured sources, such as televisions and medical x-rays. Even the human body contains natural radioactive elements.

Because individual human exposures to radiation are usually small, the millirem (one one-thousandth of a rem) is generally used to express the doses humans receive.

Table 41.1. Average Radiation Doses from Common Sources of Human Exposure

Radiation Source	Dose (millirems)
Chest x-ray	10
Mammogram	30
Cosmic rays	31 (annually)
Human body	39 (annually)
Household radon	200 (annually)
Cross-country airplane flight	5

Are there any legal limits for radiation exposure?

Another way to help put a radiological emergency into perspective is to be aware of the radiation exposure limits for people who work with and around radioactive materials full time, as shown in the Table 41.2.

Table 41.2. Yearly Radiation Exposure Limits for Full Time Workers

Worker Category	Legal Limit
18-year old male	5 rem/year
Pregnant woman	500 millirem (mrem) during pregnancy

What are radiation's effects on humans?

Radiation effects fall into two broad categories: deterministic and stochastic. At the cellular level, high doses of ionizing radiation can result in severe dysfunction, even death, of cells. At the organ level, if a sufficient number of cells are so affected, the function of the organ is impaired. Such effects are called deterministic. Deterministic effects have definite threshold doses, which mean that the effect is not seen until the absorbed dose is greater than a certain level. Once above that threshold level, the severity of the effect increases with dose. Also, deterministic effects are usually manifested soon after exposure. Examples of such effects include radiation skin burning, blood count effects, and cataracts.

In contrast, stochastic effects are caused by more subtle radiation-induced cellular changes (usually DNA mutations) that are random in nature and have no threshold dose. The probability of such effects increases with dose, but the severity does not. Cancer is the only observed clinical manifestation of radiation-induced stochastic effects. Not only is the severity independent of dose, but also, there is a substantial delay between the time of exposure and the appearance of the cancer, ranging from several years for leukemia to decades for solid tumors. Cancer can result from some DNA changes in the somatic cells of the body, but radiation can also damage the germ cells (ova and sperm) to produce hereditary effects. These are also classified as stochastic; however, clinical manifestations of such effects have not been observed in humans at a statistically significant level. (Source: Los Alamos Science, No. 23, 1995.)

The nature and extent of damage caused by ionizing radiation depend on a number of factors, including the amount of exposure, the frequency of exposure, and the penetrating power of the radiation to which an individual is exposed. Rapid exposure to very large doses of ionizing radiation is rare, but can cause death within a few days or months. The sensitivity of the exposed cells also influences the extent of damage. For example, rapidly growing tissues, such as developing embryos, are particularly vulnerable to harm from ionizing radiation.

National Cancer Institute Information about Screening for Thyroid Disease

What is exposure to iodine-131?

Between 1951 and 1963, the United States conducted about one hundred above-ground nuclear weapons tests at the Nevada Test Site. These tests released radioactive materials, including iodine-131 (I-131), mainly during 1952, 1953, and 1957. I-131 released from the tests was carried by the wind and deposited on soil and vegetation throughout the United States. The areas most affected were downwind of the test site, to the north and east of Nevada. The areas least affected were on the West Coast of the United States. Because I-131 breaks down quickly, most exposure occurred within three months after each test.

The most common way people came in contact with I-131 was through contaminated milk. This was because the I-131 fell onto pasture grasses eaten by cows and goats, and was absorbed into their milk. The I-131 concentrated in the thyroid glands of people who drank milk. Children usually drink larger amounts of milk, so young children absorbed more I-131 than adults did. Children's thyroid glands are smaller as well, so the larger amount of I-131 was concentrated in less tissue. Children may have received 10 times the I-131 doses that adults did as a result of the Nevada tests. People, particularly children, who were exposed to I-131 from the tests, probably have an increased risk for thyroid disease.

What is the thyroid gland?

The thyroid gland is located in the front of the neck, just above the top of the breastbone and overlying the windpipe. In most people it cannot be seen or felt. The gland normally takes up iodine from the diet and the blood, and makes thyroid hormone. The thyroid controls many body processes, including heart rate, blood pressure, and body temperature, as well as childhood growth and development.

What is thyroid disease?

There are two main types of thyroid diseases: noncancerous thyroid disease and thyroid cancer.

Some thyroid diseases are caused by changes in the amount of thyroid hormones that enter the body from the thyroid gland. Doctors can screen for these with a simple blood test.

Noncancerous thyroid disease also includes lumps, or nodules, in the thyroid gland that are benign and not cancerous.

Thyroid cancer occurs when a lump, or nodule, in the thyroid gland is cancerous.

Symptoms of Too Little Thyroid Hormone

- Depression or feeling blue
- Trouble concentrating
- Tiredness

- Dry skin and hair
- Weight gain
- Feeling cold all the time

Symptoms of Too Much Thyroid Hormone

- Nervousness
- Anxiety
- Tremor (shaking)
- Fast, irregular pulse

Symptoms of Thyroid Cancer

- A lump in the neck, sometimes growing noticeably
- Pain in the neck, sometimes going up to the ears
- Persistent hoarseness

These symptoms may not be the result of a thyroid condition. They are also associated with other medical conditions. If you have any symptoms, discuss them with your doctor.

What is thyroid cancer?

Thyroid cancer is a slow-growing cancer that is highly treatable and usually curable. About 95 out of 100 people who are diagnosed with thyroid cancer survive the disease for at least five years.

How common is thyroid cancer?

Thyroid cancer is not common and accounts for less than 2 percent of cancers diagnosed in the United States. In the United States, about 2 in every 1,000 men and about 4 in every 1,000 women who are currently cancer-free and aged 50 years will eventually develop thyroid cancer in their remaining lifetime.

How common are other cancers?

Of 1,000 women who are currently cancer-free and aged 50 years, about 120 will eventually develop breast cancer in their remaining lifetime. Of 1,000 men who are currently cancer-free and aged 50 years, about 170 will eventually develop prostate cancer in their remaining lifetime.

About 203,500 women are diagnosed with breast cancer each year in the United States, while about 15,800 women are diagnosed with thyroid cancer. About 189,000 men are diagnosed with prostate cancer each year in the United States, while about 4,900 men are diagnosed with thyroid cancer. Breast and prostate cancer are both much more common than thyroid cancer.

Section 41.2

Estimating Personal Thyroid Cancer Risks

Excerpted from "Making Choices: Screening for Thyroid Disease,"
National Cancer Institute (NCI), September 2002.

What was your I-131 dose from the Nevada tests?

The dose of I-131 people likely got from the Nevada tests depends on:

- How old they were at the time.
- How much milk they drank at the time and whether that milk was processed.
- Where they lived at the time.

I-131 doses are measured in radiation absorbed doses (called rad). The National Cancer Institute estimates that the average dose to the adult population living in the United States at the time (between 1951 and 1963) was about 2 rad. Because children likely absorb more I-131, people younger than 15 at the time of testing may have absorbed higher doses of radiation. Their thyroid glands were still developing during the testing period. And children were more likely to have consumed milk contaminated with I-131.

You can roughly estimate your I-131 dose using the following chart. Find the year in which you were born in the column on the left. Next, locate the column for the kind and amount of milk you drank during the nuclear tests (between 1951 and 1963). Then read your estimated dose in rad.

Table 41.3. What Is Your Estimated I-131 Dose?

Doses in rad by amount and type of milk

Year of birth	No milk 0 cups/day	Processed milk 1–3 cups/day	4+ cups/day	Farm cow any amount	Farm goat any amount
Before 1933	Less than 1	2	4	6	30
1933–1937	Less than 1	3	6	9	45
1938–1942	Less than 1	5	10	15	75
1943–1947	Less than 1	7	14	21	105
1948–1957	Less than 1	10	20	30	150
1958–1963	Less than 1	1	2	3	15
After 1963	Less than 1	Less than 1	Less than 1	Less than 1	Less than 1

Example: If you were born between 1948 and 1957, and drank 1-3 cups of milk a day of store-bought milk, your estimated dose of I-131 is about 10 rad.

Example: If you were born between 1958 and 1962, and drank 4 or more cups of milk a day of store-bought milk, your estimated dose of I-131 is about 2 rad.

Where did you live?

Depending on where you lived, your likely dose could be much higher or lower than the doses provided on the chart.

High-dose areas: Some counties in these states received higher doses: Montana, Idaho, Utah, Colorado, Wyoming, North Dakota, South Dakota, Nebraska, Kansas, Missouri, Nevada, and Arkansas.

If you lived in one of these states, your likely dose may be 2 to 3 times greater than the dose shown for you on the chart.

Low-dose areas: Some counties in these states received much lower doses: Oregon, California, Arizona, and New Mexico.

If you lived in one of these states, you may have received a dose 10 times smaller than that shown on the chart.

How accurate are these doses?

Given the amount of time that has passed since the tests were conducted, scientists cannot be certain about how much exposure each person received. Because few data were collected at the time of the tests, scientists have used available information to make their best estimates.

Table 41.4. Chance of Thyroid Cancer Per 1,000 Men

RAD	Number of men per 1,000
150–200	17–22 in 1,000
100–149	12–17 in 1,000
75–99	10–12 in 1,000
50–74	7–10 in 1,000
30–49	5–7 in 1,000
20–29	4–5 in 1,000
10–19	3–4 in 1,000
3–9	2–3 in 1,000
1–3	About 2 in 1,000
Less than 1	About 2 in 1,000

Example: A 50-year-old cancer-free man who was exposed to about 10 rad has about 3 to 4 chances in 1,000 of eventually developing thyroid cancer. He has about 996 to 997 chances in 1,000 of not developing thyroid cancer.

Table 41.5. Chance of Thyroid Cancer Per 1,000 Women

RAD	Number of women per 1,000
150–200	34–45 in 1,000
100–149	24–34 in 1,000
75–99	19–24 in 1,000
50–74	14–19 in 1,000
30–49	10–14 in 1,000
20–29	8–10 in 1,000
10–19	6–8 in 1,000
3–9	4–6 in 1,000
1–3	About 4 in 1,000
Less than 1	About 4 in 1,000

Example: A 50-year-old cancer-free woman who was exposed to about 10 rad has about 6 to 8 chances in 1,000 of eventually developing thyroid cancer. She has about 992 to 994 chances in 1,000 of not developing thyroid cancer.

As a result of this uncertainty, these dose figures are very rough esti-mates. The uncertainty in the dose estimate may be up to 5 times lower or 5 times higher. For example, if you estimate your dose was 5 rad, your real dose was likely in the range of 1 to 25 rad.

What is your risk of thyroid cancer?

Now, you can use your dose estimate to roughly work out whether exposure to I-131 has affected your chance of developing thyroid can-cer.

The figures in Tables 41.4 and 41.5 are for people who are 50 years old and cancer-free. Look to find your dose in rad and read your chance in 1,000 of eventually developing thyroid cancer in your remaining lifetime.

If you want to calculate your exposure more accurately based on your county of residence, use the dose calculator on the National Can-cer Institute website at http://www.cancer.gov (search keyword: I-131).

Section 41.3

Facts about Thyroid Cancer Screening

Excerpted from "Making Choices: Screening for Thyroid Disease,"
National Cancer Institute (NCI), September 2002.

What is screening for thyroid disease?

Screening aims to detect thyroid disease early, before there are any symptoms.

- Many people think screening is always a good thing. But there are good reasons why you might choose not to be screened for thyroid disease. Screening tests are never 100 percent accurate. Some people who are screened for thyroid disease will get an abnormal screening result even though they do not have thyroid disease. Others may receive a normal screening even though they have thyroid disease. These things happen with all screen-ing tests.

- Whether you think it is worthwhile to get screened is your decision. There is no right or wrong choice. Some people will choose to be screened. And others will choose not to be screened.

- The information that follows will focus on the pros and cons of thyroid cancer screening. Screening for noncancerous thyroid disease that increases or decreases the amount of thyroid hormones in the body involves a simple blood test. It is unlikely to cause you any harm, other than the inconvenience and cost of the blood test. About 14 in 1,000 women and about 9 in 1,000 men aged 60 years or older probably have undetected thyroid disease involving abnormal thyroid hormone levels. Through screening, these people may be identified and treated. Treatment is likely to be effective for those with clearly abnormal thyroid hormone levels. There is no good evidence on whether treatment is helpful in people with only mildly abnormal thyroid hormone levels.

What is involved in thyroid cancer screening?

Cancer screening is not just a matter of having a quick test. You need to consider what might happen after you get your screening test result.

Doctors screen for thyroid cancer by feeling the gland, to check for a lump or nodule. If a doctor feels a nodule, it does not mean cancer is present. Most thyroid nodules are not cancer.

There are two methods of investigating a thyroid lump or nodule:

1.   Ultrasound, to locate and describe the lump, and

2.   Biopsy, to determine if the lump may be cancerous.

Thyroid ultrasound creates pictures by bouncing sound waves off the gland. This technique is painless and quick. But it cannot determine whether a lump is cancerous. The ultrasound device uses sound waves that people cannot hear. A computer uses the echoes to create a picture called a sonogram. From the picture, the doctor can see how many nodules are present, how big they are, and whether they are solid or filled with fluid.

If you choose to be screened by ultrasound, your doctor will arrange for you to have a scan at an x-ray practice or clinic. The scan is quick and painless. Thyroid nodules may be seen on the scan. If so, follow-up tests will generally be advised. These may be a repeat ultrasound scan in the future to see if the nodules have grown, fine needle aspiration, or surgery.

Confirmation of cancer requires biopsy, usually using a fine needle. Cells removed from the nodule during biopsy are directly examined in the laboratory.

What is fine needle aspiration?

A needle is put into the thyroid and cells are taken out. The cells are examined under a microscope. You may feel minor pain or get a bruise. A needle aspiration can usually tell whether there is cancer in the nodule. But in about 20 percent of cases the result is unhelpful, and people need to have another biopsy or surgery.

What are the pros of thyroid cancer screening?

1. **Reassurance** for people who do not have cancer. Most people who are screened do not have cancer. These people benefit by being reassured that they do not have cancer.

2. **Early detection** for people who do have cancer. A few people will have cancer. These people will have their cancer found earlier than they would have otherwise, perhaps while it is very small. So, they may require less complicated treatment and have better chances of survival.

What are the cons of thyroid cancer screening?

1. **False alarms for people who do not have cancer.** Some people will be falsely alarmed because a nodule is found. They may need to have repeat scans, fine needle aspiration, or surgery to see whether they have cancer. Ultimately, these people learn they do not have cancer. But they will have experienced stress and anxiety in the process of reaching a diagnosis, as well as inconvenience and possibly complications of unnecessary surgery.

2. **Uncertainty about the benefit of early treatment.** Scientists know that most thyroid cancers can be cured. It is unclear if finding and treating those cancers early offers an added benefit. There are no reliable studies about the long-term benefit of thyroid cancer screening. No one knows for certain if thyroid cancers found early require less treatment than those found later.

3. **False reassurance for some people who do have cancer.** Screening does not find all the cancers. A few people will be

falsely reassured. They do have cancer but their screening test is normal. So, they do not benefit from screening.

How many people have cancer correctly detected and how many people get false alarms?

The numbers of cancers detected and false alarms are different for screening by neck exam than for screening by ultrasound.

Following are the pros and cons of screening by neck exam and by ultrasound. The numbers are based on scientists' best guesses at how many people are affected. The exact numbers will vary for different places and people.

Pros and Cons of Screening 1,000 People by Neck Exam for Thyroid Cancer

- 920–960 people will be correctly assured they do not have cancer.

- 1–3 people will have cancer found early. They may need less complex treatment and may have better chances of cure.

- 40–80 people will have false alarms and will be offered follow-up tests:
  - 40–80 people will be offered ultrasound scan
  - 20–40 people will be offered fine needle aspiration as well as ultrasound
  - 3–10 people will be offered surgery as well as ultrasound and fine needle aspiration

- The 1–3 people who will have cancer found early may not have better chances of cure. They might just know for a longer time that they have cancer.

Pros and Cons of Screening 1,000 People by Ultrasound Exam for Thyroid Cancer

- 800–850 people will be correctly assured they do not have cancer.

- 4–6 people will have cancer found early. They may need less complex treatment and may have better chances of cure.

- 150–200 people will have false alarms and will be offered follow-up tests:
  - 70–120 people will be offered repeat ultrasounds and 70–80 people will be offered fine needle aspiration

- 10–15 people will be offered both surgery and fine needle aspiration
- The 4–6 people who will have cancer found early may not have better chances of cure. They might just know for a longer time that they have cancer.

What is thyroid surgery?

Thyroid surgery may be needed to detect thyroid cancer that is not found by fine needle aspiration. Thyroid surgery is generally very successful. Most of the time only a part of the thyroid gland is removed. Nevertheless some people have adverse effects, which can include:

- Damage to the parathyroid gland (next to the thyroid gland). This causes temporary low blood calcium and muscle cramps in 10 to 15 of every 1,000 people. A few people (about 7 of 1,000) will need to take calcium supplements permanently.

- Needing to take thyroid pills. If the entire gland is removed, thyroid hormone replacement pills must be taken. If part of the gland is removed, between 1 and 10 people out of every 1,000 will need to take hormone replacement pills.

- Damage to the vocal cords and having a hoarse voice afterwards. Generally this is temporary, but in about 7 of 1,000 people, the hoarseness is permanent.

- Getting an infection in the wound and needing antibiotics (about 3 out of 1,000 people).

- Bleeding during the operation and needing a blood transfusion (less than 1 of 1,000 people).

- Dying from the anesthetic (less than 1 of 1,000 people).

*These are average rates and will vary with different people, places, and surgeries.

How can you decide whether to be screened for thyroid cancer?

1. Continue with your usual health care. If you develop a symptom, see your doctor and have this symptom checked.

2. Ask your doctor to screen you by neck exam.

3. Ask your doctor to arrange an ultrasound.

Steps in making your decision

1. What is your estimated dose of I-131 from the Nevada tests?

2. What is your likely risk of developing thyroid cancer?

3. How important is each of the pros and cons of thyroid cancer screening to you?

4. Which of the two methods of screening is best for you?

5. What questions do you have before deciding?

6. Discuss your decision-making with your doctor.

Additional Information

National Cancer Institute (NCI)
6116 Executive Blvd., MSC 8322
Bethesda, MD 20892-8322
Toll-Free: 800-4-CANCER (800-422-6237)
Toll-Free TTY: 800-332-8615
Website: http://www.cancer.gov
E-mail: cancergovstaff@mail.nih.gov

Chapter 42

Staging and Treatments by Type of Thyroid Cancer

What Is Thyroid Cancer?

Thyroid cancer is a disease in which cancer (malignant) cells are found in the tissues of the thyroid gland. The thyroid gland is at the base of the throat. It has two lobes, one on the right side and one on the left. The thyroid gland makes important hormones that help the body function normally.

Certain factors may increase the risk of developing thyroid cancer.

- Thyroid cancer occurs more often in people between the ages of 25 and 65 years.

- People who have been exposed to radiation or received radiation treatments to the head and neck during infancy or childhood have a greater chance of developing thyroid cancer. The cancer may occur as early as 5 years after exposure or may occur 20 or more years later.

- People who have had goiter (enlarged thyroid) or a family history of thyroid disease have an increased risk of developing thyroid cancer.

- Thyroid cancer is more common in women than in men.

- Asian people have an increased risk of developing thyroid cancer.

PDQ® Cancer Information Summary. National Cancer Institute, Bethesda, MD. *Thyroid Cancer (PDQ®): Treatment–Patient.* Updated 03/23/2004. Available at http://cancergov. Accessed December 18, 2004.

A doctor should be seen if there is a lump or swelling in the front of the neck or in other parts of the neck.

If there are symptoms, a doctor will feel the patient's thyroid and check for lumps in the neck. The doctor may order blood tests and special scans to see whether a lump in the thyroid is making too many hormones. The doctor may want to take a small amount of tissue from the thyroid. This is called a biopsy. To do this, a small needle is inserted into the thyroid at the base of the throat and some tissue is drawn out. The tissue is then looked at under a microscope to see whether it contains cancer.

There are four main types of thyroid cancer (based on how the cancer cells look under a microscope):

- papillary   - follicular   - medullary   - anaplastic

Some types of thyroid cancer grow faster than others. The chance of recovery (prognosis) depends on the type of thyroid cancer, whether it is in the thyroid only or has spread to other parts of the body (stage), and the patient's age and overall health. The prognosis is better for patients younger than 40 years who have cancer that has not spread beyond the thyroid.

The genes in our cells carry the hereditary information from our parents. An abnormal gene has been found in patients with some forms of thyroid cancer. If medullary thyroid cancer is found, the patient may have been born with a certain abnormal gene which may have led to the cancer. Family members may have also inherited this abnormal gene. Tests have been developed to determine who has the genetic defect long before any cancer appears. It is important that the patient and his or her family members (children, grandchildren, parents, brothers, sisters, nieces, and nephews) see a doctor about tests that will show if the abnormal gene is present. These tests are confidential and can help the doctor help patients. Family members, including young children, who do not have cancer, but do have this abnormal gene, may reduce the chance of developing medullary thyroid cancer by having surgery to safely remove the thyroid gland (thyroidectomy).

Explanation of Thyroid Cancer Stages

Once thyroid cancer is found (diagnosed), more tests will be done to find out if cancer cells have spread to other parts of the body. This is called staging. A doctor needs to know the stage of the disease to plan treatment.

Papillary and Follicular Thyroid Cancer

Stage I:

- In patients younger than 45 years, cancer may have spread within the neck or upper chest and/or to nearby lymph nodes, but not to other parts of the body.
- In patients aged 45 years and older, the tumor is 2 centimeters (about ¾ inch) or smaller and in the thyroid only.

Stage II:

- In patients younger than 45 years, the cancer has spread to distant parts of the body, such as the lung or bone, and may have spread to nearby lymph nodes.
- In patients aged 45 years and older, the tumor is larger than 2 centimeters, but not larger than 4 centimeters (between ¾ and 1½ inches) in the thyroid only.

Stage III: The cancer is found in patients aged 45 years or older. The tumor either:

- is larger than 4 centimeters; or
- may be any size and has spread just outside the thyroid and/or to lymph nodes in the neck.

Stage IVA: The cancer is found in patients aged 45 years or older. The tumor may be any size and has spread within the neck and/or to lymph nodes in the neck or upper chest.

Stage IVB: The cancer is found in patients aged 45 years or older. The tumor may be any size and has spread to neck tissues near the backbone or around blood vessels in the neck or upper chest. Cancer may have spread to lymph nodes.

Stage IVC: The cancer has spread to other parts of the body, such as the lung or bone, and may have spread to nearby lymph nodes.

Medullary Thyroid Cancer

Stage 0: No tumor is found in the thyroid but the cancer is detected by screening tests. Stage 0 is also called carcinoma in situ.

Stage I: The tumor is 2 centimeters or smaller and in the thyroid only.

Stage II: The tumor is larger than 2 centimeters but not larger than 4 centimeters and is in the thyroid only.

Stage III: The tumor either:

- is larger than 4 centimeters; or
- may be any size and has spread just outside the thyroid and/or to lymph nodes in the neck.

Stage IVA: The tumor may be any size and has spread within the neck and/or to lymph nodes in the neck or upper chest.

Stage IVB: The tumor may be any size and has spread to neck tissues near the backbone or around blood vessels in the neck or upper chest. Cancer may have spread to lymph nodes.

Stage IVC: Cancer has spread to other parts of the body, such as the lung or bone, and may have spread to nearby lymph nodes.

Anaplastic Thyroid Cancer

Anaplastic thyroid cancer is considered to be stage IV thyroid cancer. It grows quickly and has usually spread within the neck when it is found. Anaplastic thyroid cancer develops most often in older people.

Recurrent Thyroid Cancer

Recurrent disease means that the cancer has come back (recurred) after it has been treated. It may come back in the thyroid or in other parts of the body.

Treatment Option Overview

How Thyroid Cancer Is Treated

There are treatments for all patients with thyroid cancer. Four types of treatment are used:

- Surgery (taking out the cancer).
- Radiation therapy (using high-dose x-rays or other high-energy rays to kill cancer cells).

- Hormone therapy (using hormones to stop cancer cells from growing).
- Chemotherapy (using drugs to kill cancer cells).

Surgery is the most common treatment of thyroid cancer. A doctor may remove the cancer using one of the following operations:

- Lobectomy removes only the side of the thyroid where the cancer is found. Lymph nodes in the area may be taken out (biopsied) to see if they contain cancer.
- Near-total thyroidectomy removes all of the thyroid except for a small part.
- Total thyroidectomy removes the entire thyroid.
- Lymph node dissection removes lymph nodes in the neck that contain cancer.

Radiation therapy uses high-energy x-rays to kill cancer cells and shrink tumors. Radiation for thyroid cancer may come from a machine outside the body (external radiation therapy) or from drinking a liquid that contains radioactive iodine. Because the thyroid takes up iodine, the radioactive iodine collects in any thyroid tissue remaining in the body and kills the cancer cells.

Hormone therapy uses hormones to stop cancer cells from growing. In treating thyroid cancer, hormones can be used to stop the body from making other hormones that might make cancer cells grow. Hormones are usually given as pills.

Chemotherapy uses drugs to kill cancer cells. Chemotherapy may be taken by pill, or it may be put into the body by a needle in the vein or muscle. Chemotherapy is called a systemic treatment because the drug enters the bloodstream, travels through the body, and can kill cancer cells outside the thyroid.

Treatment by Stage

Treatment of thyroid cancer depends on the type and stage of the disease, and the patient's age and overall health. Standard treatment may be considered because of its effectiveness in patients in past studies, or participation in a clinical trial may be considered. Not all patients are cured with standard therapy, and some standard treatments may have more side effects than are desired. For these reasons, clinical trials are designed to find better ways to treat cancer patients and are based on the most up-to-date information. Clinical trials are ongoing in many parts of the country for some patients with thyroid cancer.

Stage I and II Papillary and Follicular Thyroid Cancer

Treatment may be one of the following:

1. Surgery to remove the thyroid (total thyroidectomy). This may be followed by hormone therapy and radioactive iodine.

2. Surgery to remove one lobe of the thyroid (lobectomy), followed by hormone therapy. Radioactive iodine also may be given following surgery.

Stage III Papillary and Follicular Thyroid Cancer

Treatment may be one of the following:

1. Surgery to remove the entire thyroid (total thyroidectomy) and lymph nodes where cancer has spread.

2. Total thyroidectomy followed by radiation therapy with radioactive iodine or external-beam radiation therapy.

Stage IV Papillary and Follicular Thyroid Cancer

Treatment may be one of the following:

1. Radioactive iodine.

2. External-beam radiation therapy.

3. Surgery to remove the cancer from places where it has spread.

4. Hormone therapy.

5. A clinical trial of new treatments, including chemotherapy.

Medullary Thyroid Cancer

Treatment may be one of the following:

1. Total thyroidectomy for tumors in the thyroid only. Lymph nodes in the neck may also be removed.

2. Radiation therapy for tumors that come back in the thyroid as palliative treatment to relieve symptoms and improve the patient's quality of life.

3. Chemotherapy for cancer that has spread to other parts of the body, as palliative treatment to relieve symptoms and improve the patient's quality of life.

Anaplastic Thyroid Cancer

Treatment may be one of the following:

1. Surgery to create an opening in the windpipe, for tumors that block the airway. This is called a tracheostomy.

2. Total thyroidectomy to reduce symptoms if the tumor is in the area of the thyroid only.

3. External-beam radiation therapy.

4. Chemotherapy.

5. Clinical trials of chemotherapy and radiation therapy following thyroidectomy.

6. Clinical trials studying new methods of treatment of thyroid cancer.

Recurrent Thyroid Cancer

The choice of treatment depends on the type of thyroid cancer the patient has, the kind of treatment the patient had before, and where the cancer comes back. Treatment may be one of the following:

1. Surgery with or without radioactive iodine. A second surgery may be done to remove tumor that remains.

2. Radioactive iodine.

3. External-beam radiation therapy or radiation therapy given during surgery to relieve symptoms caused by the cancer.

4. Chemotherapy.

5. Clinical trials of new treatments.

Additional Information

National Cancer Institute (NCI)
6116 Executive Boulevard, MSC8322
Bethesda, MD 20892-8322
Toll-Free: 800-422-6237

TTY Toll-Free: 800-332-8615
Website: http://www.cancer.gov
E-mail: cancergovstaff@mail.nih.gov

The NCI has booklets and other materials for patients, health professionals, and the public. These publications discuss types of cancer, methods of cancer treatment, coping with cancer, and clinical trials. Some publications provide information on tests for cancer, cancer causes and prevention, cancer statistics, and NCI research activities.

Chapter 43

Medullary Thyroid Cancer

Medullary Thyroid Cancer Overview

Medullary tumors are the third most common of all thyroid cancers (about 5 to 8 percent). Unlike papillary and follicular thyroid cancers which arise from thyroid hormone producing cells, medullary cancer of the thyroid originates from the parafollicular cells (also called C cells) of the thyroid. These C cells make a different hormone called calcitonin (thus their name) which has nothing to do with the control of metabolism the way thyroid hormone does. As you will see, the production of this hormone can be measured after an operation to determine if the cancer is still present, and if it is growing. This cancer has a much lower cure rate than does the well differentiated thyroid cancers (papillary and follicular), but cure rates are higher than they are for anaplastic thyroid cancer. Overall 10 year survival rates are 90% when all the disease is confined to the thyroid gland, 70% with spread to cervical lymph nodes, and 20 when spread to distant sites is present.

This chapter begins with "Medullary Thyroid Cancer Overview," by James Norman, M.D., Norman Endocrine Surgery Clinic, Tampa, FL. © 2003 Norman Endocrine Surgery Clinic. Reprinted with permission. Text under the heading "Genetics of Medullary Thyroid Cancer" is from PDQ® Cancer Information Summary. National Cancer Institute; Bethesda, MD. *Genetics of Medullary Thyroid Cancer (PDQ®): Genetics–Health Professional*. Updated 11/22/2004. Available at http://cancer.gov. Accessed 12/18/2004.

Characteristics of Medullary Thyroid Cancer

- Occurs in 4 clinical settings and can be associated with other endocrine tumors.

- Females more common than males (except for inherited cancers).

- Regional metastases (spread to neck lymph nodes) occur early in the course of the disease.

- Spread to distant organs (metastasis) occurs late and can be to the liver, bone, brain, and adrenal medulla.

- Not associated with radiation exposure.

- Usually originates in the upper central lobe of the thyroid.

- Poor prognostic factors include age over 50, male, distant spread (metastases), and MEN II-B.

- Residual disease (following surgery) or recurrence can be detected by measuring calcitonin.

Medullary Thyroid Cancer Occurs in Four Clinical Settings

1. *Sporadic:* Accounts for 80% of all cases of medullary thyroid cancer. They are typically unilateral and there are no associated endocrinopathies (not associated with disease in other endocrine glands. Peak onset 40–60 years of age. Females outnumber males by a ratio of 3:2. One-third will present with intractable diarrhea. Diarrhea is caused by increased gastrointestinal secretion and hypermotility due to the hormones secreted by the tumor (calcitonin, prostaglandins, serotonin, or VIP).

2. *MEN II-A (Sipple Syndrome):* Multiple Endocrine Neoplasia Syndromes (abbreviated as MEN and pronounced M, E, N) are a group of endocrine disorders which occur together in the same patient and typically are found in families because they are inherited. Syndromes are medical conditions which occur in groups of three. Sipple syndrome has 1) bilateral medullary carcinoma or C cell hyperplasia, 2) pheochromocytoma, and 3) hyperparathyroidism. This syndrome is inherited, and is due to a defect of a gene (DNA) which helps control the normal growth of endocrine tissues. This inherited syndrome is passed on to all children who get the gene (inherited in an autosomal dominant fashion), which theoretically, would be

50% of all offspring of a person with this defective gene. Because of this, males and females are equally affected. Peak incidence of medullary carcinoma in these patients is in their 30s.

3. *MEN II-B:* This syndrome also has 1) medullary carcinoma and 2) pheochromocytoma, but only rarely will have hyperparathyroidism. Instead these patients have 3) an unusual appearance which is characterized by mucosal ganglioneuromas (tumors in the mouth) and a Marfanoid habitus. Inheritance is autosomal dominant as in MEN II-A, or it can occur sporadically (without being inherited). MEN II-B patients usually get medullary carcinoma in their 30s, and males and females are equally effected. As with MEN II-A, pheochromocytomas must be detected prior to any operation. The idea here is to remove the pheochromocytoma first to remove the risk of severe hypertensive episodes while the thyroid or parathyroid is being operated on.

4. *Inherited medullary carcinoma* without associated endocrinopathies. This form of medullary carcinoma is the least aggressive. Like other types of thyroid cancers, the peak incidence is between the ages of 40 and 50.

Management of Medullary Thyroid Cancer

In contrast to papillary and follicular cancers, little controversy exits when discussing the management of medullary thyroid cancer. After assessment and treatment of associated endocrine conditions (such as pheochromocytomas if present) by an endocrinologist, all patients should receive total thyroidectomy—a complete central neck dissection (removal of all lymph nodes and fatty tissues in the central area of the neck), and removal of all lymph nodes and surrounding fatty tissues within the side of the neck which harbored the tumor.

The Use of Radioactive Iodine Post-Operatively

Although thyroid cells have the cellular mechanism to absorb iodine, medullary thyroid cancer does not arise from this type of thyroid cell. Therefore, radioactive iodine therapy is not useful for the treatment of medullary thyroid cancer. Similarly, if medullary cancer spreads to distant sites, it cannot be found by iodine scanning the way that distant spread from papillary or follicular cancer can.

What Kind of Long-Term Follow-Up Is Necessary?

In addition to the usual cancer follow-up, patients should receive a yearly chest x-ray as well as calcitonin levels. Serum calcitonin is very useful in follow-up of medullary thyroid cancer because no other cells of the body make this hormone. A high serum calcitonin level that had previously been low following total thyroidectomy is indicative of recurrence. Under the best circumstances, surgery will remove all of the thyroid and all lymph nodes in the neck which harbor metastatic spread. In this case, post-operative calcitonin levels will go to zero. This is often not the case, and calcitonin levels remain elevated, but less than pre-operatively. These levels should still be checked every 6 months, and when they begin to rise, a more diligent examination is in order to find the source.

Genetics of Medullary Thyroid Cancer

Medullary Thyroid Cancer

Thyroid cancer represents approximately 1% of malignancies occurring in the United States, accounting for an estimated 23,600 cancer diagnoses and 1,460[1] cancer deaths per year. Of these cancers, 2% to 3% are medullary thyroid cancer (MTC).[2] Average survival for MTC is lower than that for more common thyroid cancers, e.g., 83% 5-year survival for MTC compared with 90% to 94% 5-year survival for papillary and follicular thyroid cancer.[3, 4] Survival is correlated with stage at diagnosis, and decreased survival in MTC can be accounted for in part by a high proportion of late-stage diagnoses.[3-5] A Surveillance, Epidemiology, and End Results (SEER) population-based study of papillary, follicular, and medullary thyroid cancers found that survival varied by extent of local disease. For example, among men, 5-year survival rates ranged from 84% for disease confined to the thyroid gland to 35% for extensive, locally advanced disease.[4]

MTC arises from the parafollicular calcitonin-secreting cells of the thyroid gland. MTC occurs in sporadic and familial forms, and may be preceded by C-cell hyperplasia (CCH), although CCH is a relatively common abnormality in middle-aged adults. In a population-based study in Sweden, 26% of patients with MTC were familial.[6] A French national registry and a U.S. clinical series both reported a higher proportion of familial cases (43% and 44%, respectively).[5, 7] Familial cases often indicate the presence of multiple endocrine neoplasia type 2 (MEN 2), a group of autosomal dominant genetic disorders caused by inherited mutations in the *RET* oncogene.

In addition to early stage at diagnosis, other factors associated with improved survival in MTC include smaller tumor size, younger age at diagnosis, familial versus sporadic, and diagnosis by biochemical screening (that is, screening for calcitonin elevation) versus symptoms.[5-7]

References

1. *American Cancer Society: Cancer Facts and Figures 2004.* Atlanta, GA: American Cancer Society, 2004. Also available online. Last accessed November 15, 2004.

2. *Incidence: Thyroid Cancer.* Bethesda, MD: National Cancer Institute, SEER, 2004. Available online. Last accessed October 19, 2004.

3. Hundahl SA, Fleming ID, Fremgen AM, et al.: A National Cancer Data Base report on 53,856 cases of thyroid carcinoma treated in the U.S., 1985-1995 *Cancer* 83 (12): 2638-48, 1998.

4. Bhattacharyya N: A population-based analysis of survival factors in differentiated and medullary thyroid carcinoma. *Otolaryngol Head Neck Surg* 128 (1): 115-23, 2003.

5. Modigliani E, Vasen HM, Raue K, et al.: Pheochromocytoma in multiple endocrine neoplasia type 2: European study. The Euromen Study Group. *J Intern Med* 238 (4): 363-7, 1995.

6. Bergholm U, Bergström R, Ekbom A: Long-term follow-up of patients with medullary carcinoma of the thyroid. *Cancer* 79 (1): 132-8, 1997.

7. Kebebew E, Ituarte PH, Siperstein AE, et al.: Medullary thyroid carcinoma: clinical characteristics, treatment, prognostic factors, and a comparison of staging systems. *Cancer* 88 (5): 1139-48, 2000.

Multiple Endocrine Neoplasia Type 2

Multiple endocrine neoplasia type 2 (MEN 2) is a genetic disorder associated with a high lifetime risk of medullary thyroid cancer (MTC). It is caused by germline mutations in the *RET* proto-oncogene.

The disorder is classified into 3 subtypes based on the presence of other clinical complications: MEN 2A, familial medullary thyroid carcinoma (FMTC), and MEN 2B. All 3 subtypes have a high risk of developing MTC; MEN 2A has an increased risk of pheochromocytoma and parathyroid adenoma and/or hyperplasia. MEN 2B has an increased risk of pheochromocytoma, and includes additional clinical features such as mucosal neuromas of the lips and tongue, distinctive facies with enlarged lips, ganglioneuromatosis of the gastrointestinal tract, and an asthenic Marfanoid body habitus.

The age of onset of MTC varies in different subtypes of MEN 2. MTC typically occurs in early childhood for MEN 2B, early adulthood for MEN 2A, and middle age for FMTC.

All MEN 2 subtypes are inherited in an autosomal dominant manner. Offspring of affected individuals have a 50% chance of inheriting the gene mutation.

DNA-based testing of the *RET* gene (chromosomal region 10q11) identifies disease-causing mutations in about 95% of individuals with MEN 2A and MEN 2B and in about 85% of individuals with FMTC.

Prevalence: The prevalence of MEN 2 has been estimated to be 1 in 30,000. A study in the United Kingdom estimated the incidence of MTC at 20 to 25 new cases per year among a population of 55 million.[6]

Medullary Thyroid Cancer and C-Cell Hyperplasia

Medullary thyroid cancer (MTC) originates in calcitonin-producing cells (C-cells) of the thyroid gland. MTC is diagnosed when nests of C-cells appear to extend beyond the basement membrane and to infiltrate and destroy thyroid follicles. C-cell hyperplasia (CCH) is diagnosed histologically by the presence of an increased number of diffusely scattered or clustered C-cells. Not all CCH proceeds to MTC in individuals with disease-associated *RET* mutations.[7, 8] MTC and CCH are suspected in the presence of an elevated plasma calcitonin concentration. In provocative testing, plasma calcitonin concentration is measured before (basal level) and at 2 and 5 minutes after intravenous administration of calcium (stimulated level). A positive test is one in which the peak stimulated level is more than 3 times the basal level, or exceeds 300 picograms per milliliter.[8] CCH associated with a positive calcitonin stimulation test occurs in about 5% of the general population; therefore, the plasma calcitonin responses to stimulation do not always distinguish CCH from small MTC.[7, 8]

MTC accounts for 2% to 3% of new cases of thyroid cancer diagnosed annually in the United States,[9] although this figure may be an under representation of true incidence due to changes in diagnostic techniques. A study of 10,864 patients with nodular thyroid disease found 44 (1/250) cases of MTC after stimulation with calcitonin, none of which were clinically suspected. Consequently, half of these patients had no evidence of MTC on fine-needle biopsy and thus might not have undergone surgery without the positive calcitonin stimulation test.[10] The total number of new cases of MTC diagnosed annually is between 1,000 and 1,200, about 75% of which are sporadic; that is, they occur in the absence of a family history of either MTC or other endocrine abnormalities seen in MEN 2. The peak incidence of the sporadic form is in the fifth and sixth decades of life.[2, 11] In the absence of a positive family history, MEN 2 may be suspected when MTC occurs at an early age or is multifocal. While small series of apparently sporadic MTC cases have suggested a higher prevalence of germline *RET* mutations,[12, 13] the two largest series indicate a prevalence range of 1.5% to 12.5%.[14, 15] It is widely recommended that *RET* gene mutation testing be performed for all cases of MTC.[1, 16, 17]

Pheochromocytoma

Pheochromocytoma is suspected among patients with refractory hypertension or when biochemical screening reveals elevated excretion of catecholamines and catecholamine metabolites (i.e., norepinephrine, epinephrine, metanephrine, and vanillylmandelic acid) in 24-hour urine collections. Abdominal MRI is usually performed when a pheochromocytoma is suspected clinically or when urinary catecholamine values are increased. It is unusual for an individual with pheochromocytoma and no family history of endocrine tumors to have MEN 2A or a disease-causing mutation in the *RET* gene.[18-20] When pheochromocytoma is diagnosed in a person suspected of having MEN 2, I-131-metaiodobenzylguanidine (MIBG) scintigraphy or positron emission tomography (PET) imaging may be used for further evaluation because of the high frequency of multiple tumors.[8, 21, 22]

MEN 2 is not the only genetic disorder that includes a predisposition to pheochromocytoma. Other disorders include neurofibromatosis 1 (NF1), von Hippel-Lindau disease (VHL),[23] and the hereditary paraganglioma syndromes.[24] A recent report detailed molecular genetic analyses of a consecutive series of 271 patients with apparently sporadic pheochromocytoma and documented 13 patients (5%) who had a germline mutation in the *RET* gene.[25] An additional 20% of patients had a germline mutation in one of the other pheochromocytoma susceptibility genes (i.e., *VHL*, *SDHD*, and *SDHB*). During subsequent follow-up, 6 of 13 patients with *RET* mutations and 12 of 30 patients with *VHL* mutations developed a personal or family history of other tumors related to their genetic disorders. Possible explanations for the detection of germline mutations in persons with apparently sporadic pheochromocytoma include the following:

- The presence of new germline mutations.
- Reduced penetrance of the relevant gene, resulting in less-dramatically affected families.
- Parental imprinting (e.g., *SDHD*—hereditary paraganglioma).
- Incomplete family history information.

These data indicate that almost one fourth of apparently sporadic pheochromocytoma patients may be carriers of germline genetic mutations, a substantial proportion of which are attributable to *RET*. These findings raise the possibility that routine analysis for mutations in a panel of these genes, including *RET*, might be considered in sporadic pheochromocytoma patients, in order to identify important cancer susceptibility syndromes that might otherwise be missed.

Diagnosis of MEN 2 Subtypes

The diagnosis of the 3 MEN 2 clinical subtypes relies on a combination of clinical findings, family history, and molecular genetic testing of the *RET* gene (chromosomal region 10q11).

MEN 2A

MEN 2A is diagnosed clinically by the occurrence of 2 or more specific endocrine tumors (MTC, pheochromocytoma, or parathyroid adenoma/hyperplasia) in a single individual or in close relatives.

The MEN 2A subtype makes up about 60% to 90% of MEN 2 cases. The MEN 2A subtype was initially called Sipple syndrome.[26] Since genetic testing for *RET* mutations has become available, it has become apparent that about 95% of individuals with MEN 2A will develop MTC, about 50% will develop pheochromocytoma, and about 20% to 30% will develop hyperparathyroidism.[27]

MTC is generally the first manifestation of MEN 2A. In asymptomatic, young, at-risk individuals, provocative testing may reveal elevated plasma calcitonin levels and the presence of CCH or MTC. In families with MEN 2A, the biochemical manifestations of MTC generally appear between the ages of 5 and 25 years (mean, 15 years).[8] If presymptomatic screening is not done, MTC typically presents as a neck mass or neck pain at about age 5 to 20 years. More than 50%

of such patients have cervical lymph node metastases.[2] Diarrhea, the most frequent systemic symptom, occurs in patients with a plasma calcitonin level of more than 10 nanograms per milliliter and implies a poor prognosis.[2] Up to 30% of patients with MTC present with diarrhea and advanced disease.[28]

Pheochromocytomas usually present after MTC, typically with intractable hypertension, and are often bilateral.[5] Sudden death from anesthesia-induced hypertensive crisis has been described in patients with MEN 2A and unsuspected pheochromocytoma.[2] Malignant transformation is uncommon and is estimated to occur in about 4% of familial cases.[29]

A series of 56 patients with MEN 2-related hyperparathyroidism has been reported by the French Calcitonin Tumors Study Group.[30] The median age at diagnosis was 38 years, documenting that this disorder is rarely the first manifestation of MEN 2. Parathyroid abnormalities were found concomitantly with surgery for medullary thyroid carcinoma in 43 patients (77%). Two-thirds of the patients were asymptomatic. Among the 53 parathyroid glands removed surgically, there were 24 single adenomas, 4 double adenomas, and 25 hyperplastic glands. Notably, other genetic causes of familial hyperparathyroidism have been identified, including the hyperparathyroidism–jaw tumor syndrome, MEN 1, and NF1.[31, 32] Germline mutations in the *HRPT2* tumor suppressor gene have been described in several families with familial isolated hyperparathyroidism.[31]

A small number of families with MEN 2A have pruritic skin lesions known as cutaneous lichen amyloidosis. This lichenoid skin lesion is located over the upper portion of the back and may appear before the onset of MTC.[33, 34]

Familial Medullary Thyroid Carcinoma

Familial medullary thyroid carcinoma (FMTC) subtype makes up about 5% to 35% of MEN 2 cases and is diagnosed in families with 4 or more cases of MTC in the absence of pheochromocytoma or parathyroid adenoma/hyperplasia.[27] Families in which there are 2 or 3 cases of MTC and incompletely documented screening for pheochromocytoma and parathyroid disease may represent MEN 2A; it has been suggested that these families should be considered unclassified.[6] Misclassification of families with MEN 2A as having FMTC (due to small family size or later onset of other manifestations of MEN 2A) may result in overlooking the risk of pheochromocytoma, a disease with significant morbidity and mortality.

MEN 2B

MEN 2B is diagnosed clinically by the presence of mucosal neuromas of the lips and tongue, as well as medullated corneal nerve fibers, distinctive facies with enlarged lips, an asthenic Marfanoid body habitus, and MTC.[35-37]

The MEN 2B subtype makes up about 5% of MEN 2 cases. MEN 2B is characterized by the early development of an aggressive form of MTC in all patients.[38, 39] Patients with MEN 2B who do not undergo thyroidectomy at an early age (approximately 1 year) are likely to develop metastatic MTC at an early age. Before intervention with early prophylactic thyroidectomy, the average age of death in patients with MEN 2B was 21 years. Pheochromocytomas occur in about 50% of MEN 2B cases; about half are multiple and often bilateral. Patients with undiagnosed pheochromocytoma may die from a cardiovascular crisis perioperatively. Clinically apparent parathyroid disease is very uncommon.[4, 27, 40]

Patients with MEN 2B may be identified in infancy or early childhood by a distinctive facial appearance and the presence of mucosal neuromas on the anterior dorsal surface of the tongue, palate, or pharynx. The lips become prominent over time, and submucosal nodules may be present on the vermilion border of the lips. Neuromas of the eyelids may cause thickening and eversion of the upper eyelid margins. Prominent thickened corneal nerves may be seen by slit lamp examination.

About 40% of patients have diffuse ganglioneuromatosis of the gastrointestinal tract. Associated symptoms include abdominal distension, megacolon, constipation, and diarrhea. About 75% of patients have a Marfanoid habitus, often with kyphoscoliosis or lordosis, joint laxity, and decreased subcutaneous fat. Proximal muscle wasting and weakness can also be seen.[36, 37]

Other Subtypes

The International *RET* Mutation Consortium classified MEN 2 into 6 separate phenotypes for the purpose of correlating specific mutations with clinical expression.[12, 27] They specified 3 forms of MEN 2A: MEN 2A(1), MEN 2A(2), MEN 2A(3), and single forms of MEN 2B, FMTC, and other, which included families that did not conform to the other phenotypes or were not objectively documented. The clinical usefulness of these additional subtypes for MEN 2A has not been demonstrated, although these classifications were created as a tool for evaluation of genotype-phenotype correlations.

Genetically Related Disorders

Hirschsprung Disease: Hirschsprung disease (HSCR), a disorder of the enteric plexus of the colon that typically results in enlargement of the bowel and constipation or obstipation in neonates, is observed in a small number of individuals with MEN 2A, FMTC, or very rarely, MEN 2B.[41] Up to 40% of familial cases of HSCR, and 3% to 7% of sporadic cases are associated with germline mutations in the *RET* proto-oncogene and are designated HSCR1.[42, 43] Some of these *RET* mutations are located in codons that lead to the development of MEN 2A or FMTC (i.e., codons Cys609, Cys618, and Cys620).[41, 44]

Multiple Endocrine Neoplasia Type 1: Multiple endocrine neoplasia type 1 (MEN 1) is an autosomal dominant endocrinopathy that is genetically and clinically distinct from MEN 2; however, the similar nomenclature for MEN 1 and MEN 2 may cause confusion. MEN 1 is caused by mutations in the *MEN1* gene (chromosomal region 11q13). MEN 1 is characterized by a triad of pituitary adenomas, pancreatic islet cell tumors, and parathyroid disease consisting of hyperplasia or adenoma. Patients can also have adrenal cortical tumors, carcinoid tumors, and lipomas.[45] Rarely, patients with MEN 1 have pituitary adenomas and pheochromocytomas, which has led to the hypothesis of an overlap syndrome with MEN 2.[46]

Molecular Genetics of MEN 2

MEN 2 syndromes are due to inherited mutations in the *RET* gene, located on chromosome region 10q11.[47-49] The *RET* gene is a proto-oncogene composed of 21 exons over 55 kilobase of genomic material.[50, 51] A partial sequence was cloned in 1988.[52] Renumbering of the full-length sequence added 254 codons to the original assignments.[53] Early publications that described allelic variants utilized the codon numbering for the partial sequence. Neutral sequence variants that do not alter the risk of the disease have been described.[54, 55]

Mutation Analysis

At least 95% of families with MEN 2A have a *RET* mutation in exon 10 or 11.[14, 53, 61] Mutations of codon Cys634 in exon 11 occur in about 85% of families; mutation of cysteine codons at amino acid positions 609, 611, 618, and 620 in exon 10 together account for the remainder of identifiable mutations.[14] Other rare mutations have been reported in single families.[62-64]

409

Approximately 85% of families with FMTC have an identifiable *RET* mutation.[53, 61] These mutations typically affect 1 of the 5 cysteine residues (codons 618, 620, 634, 609, and 611), with mutations of the first three each accounting for 25% to 35% of all mutations.

Approximately 95% of individuals with the MEN 2B phenotype have a single point mutation in the tyrosine kinase domain of the *RET* gene at codon Met918 in exon 16, which substitutes a threonine for methionine (Met918Thr).[70, 71] A second mutation at codon Ala883 in exon 15 has now been identified in at least 4 MEN 2B patients without a Met918Thr mutation.[72, 73]

Functional Effects of RET *Mutations and Genotype-Phenotype Correlations*

The following genotype-phenotype correlations have been suggested for *RET* mutations:

- *RET* germline Met918Thr and A883F mutations are associated only with MEN 2B. Somatic mutations in these codons are frequently observed in sporadic MTC.[71, 78, 79]

- Mutations at codons 768 or 804 may be FMTC-specific[27] and might represent important contributors to apparently sporadic MTC.[80]

- Mutations involving the cysteine codons 609, 618, and 620 are associated with either MEN 2A, FMTC, or HSCR1. Mutations in these codons are detected in about 10% of families with MEN 2A and 65% of families with FMTC.[27]

- Mutations in codons Glu768 in exon 13 and Val804 in exon 14 may only be associated with the development of MTC, since these mutations have been identified primarily in the FMTC subtype.[14, 27, 66, 81]

- Any *RET* mutation at codon Cys634 in exon 11 results in higher incidence of pheochromocytomas and hyperparathyroidism.[27, 53]

- Among the mutations at codon Cys634, it has been reported that Cys634Arg significantly correlates with the presence of hyperparathyroidism,[27, 53] but other studies do not confirm this correlation.[82, 83] This discrepancy may be explained by differences in study methodology.

- Some mutations, such as those involving cysteine codons 609, 618, and 620 in exon 10 and Val804 in exon 14, may be associated with milder forms of the disease.[27, 61, 84, 85]

- Possible correlation between the presence of mutations in codon Cys634 in the *RET* gene and the skin lesion cutaneous lichen amyloidosis has been noted.[27, 86, 87]

Genetic Testing

MEN 2 is a well-defined hereditary cancer syndrome for which genetic testing is considered an important part of the management for at-risk family members; it meets the criteria related to indications for genetic testing for cancer susceptibility outlined by the American Society of Clinical Oncology (ASCO) in its most recent genetic testing policy statement.[90] At-risk individuals are defined as first-degree relatives (parents, siblings, and children) of a person known to have MEN 2. Testing allows the identification of people with asymptomatic MEN 2 who can be offered prophylactic thyroidectomy and biochemical screening as preventive measures. A negative mutation analysis in at-risk relatives, however, is informative only after a disease-causing mutation has been identified in an affected relative. Because early detection of at-risk individuals affects medical management, testing of children who have no symptoms is considered beneficial.[91, 92]

Table 43.1. Testing Used in the Molecular Diagnosis of MEN 2

Disease Name	Mutation Detection Rate	Test Type
MEN 2A	~95%	DNA-based
FMTC	~85%	DNA-based
MEN 2B	~95%	DNA-based

Testing for the common mutations in exons 10, 11, 13, 14, and 16 is available at a number of clinical laboratories; some laboratories also include analysis of some of the rarer mutations. Methods used to detect mutations in *RET* include polymerase chain reaction (PCR) followed by restriction enzyme digestion of PCR products, heteroduplex analysis, single-strand conformation polymorphism analysis, and DNA sequencing.[54, 93-95]

A small number of families with MEN 2 have been described without detectable abnormalities in the *RET* coding sequence. There is considerable diversity in the approach to *RET* mutation testing among the various laboratories that perform this procedure. These range from

411

selective testing of those exons most likely to harbor MEN 2 mutations, to full sequencing of the entire gene. These differences represent important considerations for selecting a laboratory to perform a test and in interpreting the test result. There is no evidence, however, for involvement of other genetic loci, and all mutation-negative families analyzed to date have demonstrated linkage to the *RET* gene.

Linkage Analysis: When a disease-causing mutation in the *RET* gene cannot be identified, linkage analysis can be considered in families with more than 1 affected family member in 2 or more generations. Linkage studies are based on accurate clinical diagnosis of MTC and/or pheochromocytoma in the affected family members and accurate understanding of the genetic relationships in the family. Linkage analysis is dependent on the availability and willingness of all family members to be tested. The markers used for linkage are highly informative and very tightly linked to the *RET* gene; thus, they can be used in more than 95% of informative families with MEN 2 with greater than 95% accuracy.[96]

Linkage testing is not possible in families in which there is a single affected individual.

Interventions

Prophylactic Thyroidectomy

Prophylactic thyroidectomy with reimplantation of 1 or more parathyroid glands into the neck or nondominant forearm is a preventive option for all subtypes of MEN 2. In order to implement this management strategy, biochemical screening to identify CCH or genetic testing to identify persons who carry causative *RET* mutations is needed to identify candidates for prophylactic surgery. The optimal timing of surgery, however, is controversial.[3] Current recommendations are based on clinical experience and vary for different MEN 2 subtypes.

In a study of biochemical screening in a large family with MEN 2A done before mutation analysis became available, 22 family members without evidence of clinical disease had elevated calcitonin and underwent thyroidectomy. During a mean follow-up period of 11 years, all remained free of clinical disease, and 3 out of 22 had transient elevation of postoperative calcitonin levels.[97]

In the most comprehensive literature review published to date, 260 MEN 2A subjects aged 0 to 20 years were identified as having undergone either "early total thyroidectomy" (ages 1-5) [n=42], or late thyroidectomy (ages 6-20) [n=218].[100] There was a significantly lower rate of invasive or metastatic MTC among those operated on at an early age (57%) compared with those operated on late (76%). Follow-up information was available on only 28% of the cohort, due to the limitations of study design, with a median follow-up of only 2 years for this non-systematically selected subgroup. Persistent or recurrent disease was reported among 0 of 9 early-surgery subjects, versus 21 of 65 late-surgery subjects. Both findings are consistent with the hypothesis that patients undergoing surgery prior to age 6 have a more favorable outcome, but the nature of the data prevent this being a definitive conclusion. Finally, there was evidence to suggest that subjects carrying the Cys634 mutation were much more likely to present with invasive or metastatic MTC, and more likely to develop persistent or recurrent disease, than were those with the Cys804, Cys618, or Cys620 mutations.

In these and other studies, thyroid glands removed from individuals with a disease-causing mutation who had normal plasma calcitonin levels have been found to contain MTC.[8, 38] Therefore, although thyroidectomy prior to biochemical evidence of disease may reduce the risk of recurrent disease, continued monitoring for residual or recurrent MTC is still recommended.[3] All individuals who have undergone thyroidectomy and autotransplantation of the parathyroids need thyroid hormone replacement therapy and monitoring for possible hypoparathyroidism.

Questions remain concerning the natural history of MEN 2. As more information is acquired, recommendations regarding the optimal age for thyroidectomy and the potential role for genetics and biochemical screening may change. For example, a case report documents MTC before age 5 in 2 siblings with MEN 2A.[101] Conversely, another case report documents onset of cancer in midlife or later in some families with FMTC, as well as in elderly relatives who carry the FMTC genotype, but have not developed cancer.[102] The possibility that certain specific mutations (e.g., Cys634) might convey a significantly worse prognosis, if confirmed, may permit tailoring intervention based on knowing the specific *RET* mutation.[100] These clinical observations suggest that the natural history of the MEN 2 syndromes is variable and could be subject to modifying effects related to specific *RET* mutations, other genes, behavioral factors, or environmental exposures.

There is controversy about the age at which to perform prophylactic thyroidectomy, in part because outcome data are limited to uncontrolled studies or relatively small populations. Observational studies of the genotype-phenotype correlations suggest significant differences in biological aggressiveness of the medullary thyroid cancers that occur in MEN 2A, MEN 2B, and FMTC.[16, 87]

A summary of current practice in referral centers suggests the following:[104]

- *MEN 2A:* In most centers, thyroidectomy is performed in patients by the age of 5 years or when a mutation is identified.[16, 17]

- *FMTC:* Some centers recommend management similar to that for MEN 2A.

- *MEN 2B:* In most centers, surgery is performed within the first 6 months of life, preferably within the first month, because of the very early age of MTC onset and the particularly aggressive biologic behavior of MTC in the patients.[16]

Screening of At-Risk Individuals for Pheochromocytoma

The presence of a functioning pheochromocytoma should be excluded by appropriate biochemical screening before thyroidectomy in any patient with MEN 2A or MEN 2B. In addition, annual biochemical screening is recommended, followed by MRI only if the biochemical results are abnormal.[29, 104] Other screening studies, such as abdominal ultrasound examination or CT scan, may be warranted in some patients. In addition to surgery, there are other clinical situations in which patients with catecholamine excess face special risk. An example is the healthy at-risk female patient who becomes pregnant. Pregnancy, labor, or delivery may precipitate a hypertensive crisis in persons who carry an unrecognized pheochromocytoma. Pregnant patients who are found to have catecholamine excess require appropriate pharmacotherapy before delivery. Typical surveillance recommendations are as follows:

- *MEN 2A:* Annual biochemical screening.

- *FMTC:* Screening as for MEN 2A because not all families classified as FMTC are MTC-only.[84]

- *MEN 2B:* Same as MEN 2A.[104]

- *Unclassified:* Same as MEN 2A.

Screening of At-Risk Individuals for Parathyroid Hyperplasia or Adenoma

MEN 2-related hyperparathyroidism is generally associated with mild, often asymptomatic hypercalcemia early in the natural history of the disease—which, if left untreated, may become symptomatic.[30]

Annual biochemical screening is recommended for those patients who have not had parathyroidectomy and autotransplantation, as follows:

- *MEN 2A:* Starting at the time of diagnosis.[104]

- *FMTC:* Screening as for MEN 2A because not all families classified as FMTC are MTC-only.[84]

- *MEN 2B:* Same as MEN 2A although clinically apparent hyperparathyroidism is seldom observed in MEN 2B.[104]

- *Unclassified:* Same as MEN 2A.

Screening of At-Risk Individuals in Groups of Genetically-Related People without an Identifiable RET Mutation

- *MEN 2A:* Prophylactic thyroidectomy is not offered routinely to at-risk individuals in whom the disorder has not been confirmed. The screening protocol for MTC is an annual calcitonin stimulation test; however, caution needs to be used in interpreting test results because CCH that is not a precursor to MTC occurs in about 5% of the population.[7, 8, 105] In addition, there is significant risk of false-negative test results in patients younger than 15 years.[8] Screening for pheochromocytoma and parathyroid disease is the same as described earlier.

- *FMTC:* Annual screening for MTC, as for MEN 2A.

Treatment for Those with MTC

Standard treatment for MTC is surgical removal of the entire thyroid gland, including the posterior capsule, and central lymph node dissection. Chemotherapy and radiation are not effective against this type of cancer.[3, 106, 107]

Treatment for Those with Pheochromocytoma

Pheochromocytoma may be either unilateral or bilateral in patients with MEN 2. Laparoscopic adrenalectomy is recommended by some authorities for the treatment of unilateral pheochromocytoma.[16] It is unclear whether bilateral adrenalectomy should be performed routinely in patients with MEN 2-related pheochromocytoma, in the absence of bilateral pheochromocytomas.

Unilateral adrenalectomy appears to represent a reasonable management strategy for unilateral pheochromocytoma in patients with

MEN 2,[109, 110] when coupled with periodic surveillance (serum or urinary catecholamine measurements) for the development of disease in the contralateral adrenal gland.

Cortical-sparing adrenalectomy represents an additional approach to disease management in patients with bilateral pheochromocytomas.[111] Fourteen (93%) of 15 patients undergoing laparotomy for bilateral pheochromocytomas were treated with a procedure that spared as much normal-appearing adrenal cortex as possible. Thirteen patients did not require postoperative steroid hormone supplementation, and none experienced acute adrenal insufficiency. Three patients developed recurrent pheochromocytomas at 10 to 27 years after surgery. Similar results were obtained in a series of 26 patients undergoing cortex-sparing surgery for hereditary pheochromocytoma (including MEN 2).[112] Adrenal cortex-sparing surgery may also be accomplished laparoscopically, with intraoperative ultrasound guidance.[113] These approaches require long-term patient follow-up, as recurrence may develop many years after the initial operation.

Treatment for Those with Parathyroid Hyperplasia or Adenoma

Most patients with MEN 2-related parathyroid disease are either asymptomatic or diagnosed incidentally at the time of thyroidectomy. Typically, the hypercalcemia (when present) is mild, although it may be associated with increased urinary excretion of calcium and nephrolithiasis. As a consequence, the indications for surgical intervention are generally similar to those recommended for patients with sporadic, primary hyperparathyroidism.[16] In general, fewer than 4 of the parathyroid glands are involved at the time of detected abnormalities in calcium metabolism. Uncertainty exists regarding the criteria that would indicate parathyroidectomy and the role of parathyroid autotransplantation in the management of these patients.

Cure of hyperparathyroidism was achieved surgically in 89% of 1 large series of patients;[30] however, 22% of resected patients in this study developed postoperative hypoparathyroidism. Five patients (9%) had recurrent hyperparathyroidism. This series employed various surgical techniques, including total parathyroidectomy with autotransplantation to the nondominant forearm, subtotal thyroidectomy, and resection only of glands that were macroscopically enlarged. Postoperative hypoparathyroidism developed in 4 (36%) of 11 patients, 6 (50%) of 12 patients, and 3 (10%) of 29 patients, respectively. These data indicate that excision of only those parathyroid glands that are enlarged appears to be sufficient in most cases.

Some investigators have suggested using the MEN 2 subtype to decide where to place the parathyroid glands that are identified at the time of thyroid surgery. For patients with MEN 2B, in whom the risk of parathyroid disease is quite low, the parathyroid glands may be left in the neck. For patients with MEN 2A and FMTC, it is suggested that the glands be implanted in the nondominant forearm to minimize the need for further surgery on the neck after prophylactic thyroidectomy and a central lymph node dissection.[114]

Genetic Counseling

Mode of Inheritance

All of the MEN 2 subtypes are inherited in an autosomal dominant manner. For the child of someone with MEN 2, the risk of inheriting the MEN 2 mutation is 50%. Some individuals with MEN 2, however, carry a de novo mutation; that is, they carry a new mutation that was not present in previous generations of their family, and thus do not have an affected parent. The proportion of individuals with MEN 2 who have an affected parent varies by subtype.

- *MEN 2A:* About 95% of affected individuals have an affected parent. It is appropriate to evaluate the parents of an individual with MEN 2A for manifestations of the disorder. In the 5% of cases that are not familial, either de novo gene mutations or incomplete penetrance of the mutant allele is possible.[115]

- *FMTC:* Multiple family members are affected, and thus all affected individuals have inherited the mutant gene from a parent.

- *MEN 2B:* About 50% of affected individuals have de novo *RET* gene mutations, and 50% have inherited the mutation from a parent.[116, 117] The majority of de novo mutations are paternal in origin, but cases of maternal origin have been reported.[118]

- *Siblings of a proband:* The risk to siblings depends on the genetic status of the parent, which can be clarified by pedigree analysis and/or DNA-based testing. In situations of apparent de novo gene mutations, germline mosaicism in an apparently unaffected parent needs to be considered, even though such an occurrence has not yet been reported.

Psychosocial Issues

The psychosocial impact of genetic testing for MEN 2 has not been extensively studied. Published studies have had limitations such as small sample size and heterogenous populations; thus, the clinical relevance of these findings should be interpreted with caution. Identification as the carrier of a deleterious mutation may affect self-esteem, family relationships, and quality of life. In addition, misconceptions about genetic disease may result in familial blame and guilt.[119, 120] Several review articles outline both the medical and psychological issues, especially those related to the testing of children.[121-124] The medical value of early screening and prophylactic treatment are contrasted with the loss of decision-making autonomy for the individual. Lack of agreement between parents about the value and timing of genetic testing and surgery may spur the development of emotional problems within the family.

One study examined levels of psychological distress in the interval between submitting a blood sample and receiving genetic test results. Those individuals who experienced the highest level of distress were young (<25 years of age), single, and had a history of responding to distressful situations with anxiety.[125] Mutation-positive parents whose children received negative test results did not seem to be reassured, questioned the reliability of the DNA test, and were eager to continue screening of their non-carrier children.[126]

A small qualitative study (N=21) evaluated how patients with MEN 2A and family members conceptualized participation in lifelong high-risk surveillance.[127] Ongoing surveillance was viewed as a reminder of a health threat. Acceptance and incorporation of lifelong surveillance into routine health care was essential for coping with the implications of this condition. Concern about genetic predisposition to cancer was peripheral to concerns about surveillance. Supportive interventions, such as internet discussion forums, can serve as an ongoing means of addressing informational and support needs of patients with medullary thyroid carcinoma undergoing lifelong surveillance.[128]

References

1. Lips CJ: Clinical management of the multiple endocrine neoplasia syndromes: results of a computerized opinion poll at the Sixth International Workshop on Multiple Endocrine Neoplasia and von Hippel-Lindau disease. *J Intern Med* 243 (6): 589-94, 1998.

2. Robbins J, Merino MJ, Boice JD Jr, et al.: Thyroid cancer: a lethal endocrine neoplasm. *Ann Intern Med* 115 (2): 133-47, 1991.

3. Moley JF, Debenedetti MK, Dilley WG, et al.: Surgical management of patients with persistent or recurrent medullary thyroid cancer. *J Intern Med* 243 (6): 521-6, 1998.

4. Eng C: Seminars in medicine of the Beth Israel Hospital, Boston. The *RET* proto-oncogene in multiple endocrine neoplasia type 2 and Hirschsprung's disease. *N Engl J Med* 335 (13): 943-51, 1996.

5. Conte-Devolx B, Schuffenecker I, Niccoli P, et al.: Multiple endocrine neoplasia type 2: management of patients and subjects at risk. French Study Group on Calcitonin-Secreting Tumors (GETC). *Horm Res* 47 (4-6): 221-6, 1997.

6. Ponder BA: Multiple endocrine neoplasia type 2. In: Vogelstein B, Kinzler KW, eds.: *The Genetic Basis of Human Cancer*. New York, NY: McGraw-Hill, 2002, pp 501-513.

7. Landsvater RM, Rombouts AG, te Meerman GJ, et al.: The clinical implications of a positive calcitonin test for C-cell hyperplasia in genetically unaffected members of an MEN2A kindred. *Am J Hum Genet* 52 (2): 335-42, 1993.

8. Lips CJ, Landsvater RM, Höppener JW, et al.: Clinical screening as compared with DNA analysis in families with multiple endocrine neoplasia type 2A. *N Engl J Med* 331 (13): 828-35, 1994.

9. *Incidence: Thyroid Cancer.* Bethesda, Md: National Cancer Institute, SEER, 2004. Available online. Last accessed October 19, 2004.

10. Elisei R, Bottici V, Luchetti F, et al.: Impact of routine measurement of serum calcitonin on the diagnosis and outcome of medullary thyroid cancer: experience in 10,864 patients with nodular thyroid disorders. *J Clin Endocrinol Metab* 89 (1): 163-8, 2004.

11. Gharib H, McConahey WM, Tiegs RD, et al.: Medullary thyroid carcinoma: clinicopathologic features and long-term follow-up of 65 patients treated during 1946 through 1970. *Mayo Clin Proc* 67 (10): 934-40, 1992.

12. Decker RA, Peacock ML, Borst MJ, et al.: Progress in genetic screening of multiple endocrine neoplasia type 2A: is calcitonin

testing obsolete? *Surgery* 118 (2): 257-63; discussion 263-4, 1995.

13. Kitamura Y, Goodfellow PJ, Shimizu K, et al.: Novel germline *RET* proto-oncogene mutations associated with medullary thyroid carcinoma (MTC): mutation analysis in Japanese patients with MTC. *Oncogene* 14 (25): 3103-6, 1997.

14. Eng C, Mulligan LM, Smith DP, et al.: Low frequency of germline mutations in the *RET* proto-oncogene in patients with apparently sporadic medullary thyroid carcinoma. *Clin Endocrinol* (Oxf) 43 (1): 123-7, 1995.

15. Wohllk N, Cote GJ, Bugalho MM, et al.: Relevance of *RET* proto-oncogene mutations in sporadic medullary thyroid carcinoma. *J Clin Endocrinol Metab* 81 (10): 3740-5, 1996.

16. Brandi ML, Gagel RF, Angeli A, et al.: Guidelines for diagnosis and therapy of MEN type 1 and type 2. *J Clin Endocrinol Metab* 86 (12): 5658-71, 2001.

17. National Comprehensive Cancer Network.: *NCCN Clinical Practice Guidelines in Oncology*. Rockledge, Pa : National Comprehensive Cancer Network, 2003. Available online. Last accessed September 30, 2004.

18. Crossey PA, Eng C, Ginalska-Malinowska M, et al.: Molecular genetic diagnosis of von Hippel-Lindau disease in familial phaeochromocytoma. *J Med Genet* 32 (11): 885-6, 1995.

19. Bar M, Friedman E, Jakobovitz O, et al.: Sporadic phaeochromocytomas are rarely associated with germline mutations in the von Hippel-Lindau and *RET* genes. *Clin Endocrinol* (Oxf) 47 (6): 707-12, 1997.

20. Woodward ER, Eng C, McMahon R, et al.: Genetic predisposition to phaeochromocytoma: analysis of candidate genes *GDNF, RET* and *VHL*. *Hum Mol Genet* 6 (7): 1051-6, 1997.

21. van der Harst E, de Herder WW, Bruining HA, et al.: [(123)I]metaiodobenzylguanidine and [(111)In]octreotide uptake in benign and malignant pheochromocytomas. *J Clin Endocrinol Metab* 86 (2): 685-93, 2001.

22. Pacak K, Linehan WM, Eisenhofer G, et al.: Recent advances in genetics, diagnosis, localization, and treatment of pheochromocytoma. *Ann Intern Med* 134 (4): 315-29, 2001.

23. Kaelin WG Jr: Molecular basis of the VHL hereditary cancer syndrome. *Nat Rev Cancer* 2 (9): 673-82, 2002.

24. Maher ER, Eng C: The pressure rises: update on the genetics of phaeochromocytoma. *Hum Mol Genet* 11 (20): 2347-54, 2002.

25. Neumann HP, Bausch B, McWhinney SR, et al.: Germ-line mutations in nonsyndromic pheochromocytoma. *N Engl J Med* 346 (19): 1459-66, 2002.

26. Sipple JH: The association of pheochromocytoma with carcinoma of the thyroid gland. *Am J Med* 31: 163-166, 1961.

27. Eng C, Clayton D, Schuffenecker I, et al.: The relationship between specific *RET* proto-oncogene mutations and disease phenotype in multiple endocrine neoplasia type 2. International *RET* mutation consortium analysis. *JAMA* 276 (19): 1575-9, 1996.

28. Raue F, Frank-Raue K, Grauer A: Multiple endocrine neoplasia type 2. Clinical features and screening. *Endocrinol Metab Clin North Am* 23 (1): 137-56, 1994.

29. Modigliani E, Vasen HM, Raue K, et al.: Pheochromocytoma in multiple endocrine neoplasia type 2: European study. The Euromen Study Group. *J Intern Med* 238 (4): 363-7, 1995.

30. Kraimps JL, Denizot A, Carnaille B, et al.: Primary hyperparathyroidism in multiple endocrine neoplasia type IIa: retrospective French multicentric study. Groupe d'Etude des Tumeurs á Calcitonine (GETC, French Calcitonin Tumors Study Group), French Association of Endocrine Surgeons. *World J Surg* 20 (7): 808-12; discussion 812-3, 1996.

31. Villablanca A, Calender A, Forsberg L, et al.: Germline and de novo mutations in the *HRPT2* tumour suppressor gene in familial isolated hyperparathyroidism (FIHP). *J Med Genet* 41 (3): e32, 2004.

32. Marx SJ, Simonds WF, Agarwal SK, et al.: Hyperparathyroidism in hereditary syndromes: special expressions and special managements. *J Bone Miner Res* 17 (Suppl 2): N37-43, 2002.

33. Bugalho MJ, Limbert E, Sobrinho LG, et al.: A kindred with multiple endocrine neoplasia type 2A associated with pruritic skin lesions. *Cancer* 70 (11): 2664-7, 1992.

34. Robinson MF, Furst EJ, Nunziata V, et al.: Characterization of the clinical features of five families with hereditary primary cutaneous lichen amyloidosis and multiple endocrine neoplasia type 2. *Henry Ford Hosp Med J* 40 (3-4): 249-52, 1992.

35. Morrison PJ, Nevin NC: Multiple endocrine neoplasia type 2B (mucosal neuroma syndrome, Wagenmann-Froboese syndrome). *J Med Genet* 33 (9): 779-82, 1996.

36. Gorlin RJ, Sedano HO, Vickers RA, et al.: Multiple mucosal neuromas, pheochromocytoma and medullary carcinoma of the thyroid—a syndrome. *Cancer* 22 (2): 293-9 passim, 1968.

37. Gorlin RJ, Vickers RA: Multiple mucosal neuromas, pheochromocytoma, medullary carcinoma of the thyroid and marfanoid body build with muscle wasting. *Birth Defects Orig Artic Ser* 7 (6): 69-72, 1971.

38. Skinner MA, DeBenedetti MK, Moley JF, et al.: Medullary thyroid carcinoma in children with multiple endocrine neoplasia types 2A and 2B. *J Pediatr Surg* 31 (1): 177-81; discussion 181-2, 1996.

39. O'Riordain DS, O'Brien T, Weaver AL, et al.: Medullary thyroid carcinoma in multiple endocrine neoplasia types 2A and 2B. *Surgery* 116 (6): 1017-23, 1994.

40. Vasen HF, van der Feltz M, Raue F, et al.: The natural course of multiple endocrine neoplasia type IIb. A study of 18 cases. *Arch Intern Med* 152 (6): 1250-2, 1992.

41. Romeo G, Ceccherini I, Celli J, et al.: Association of multiple endocrine neoplasia type 2 and Hirschsprung disease. *J Intern Med* 243 (6): 515-20, 1998.

42. Decker RA, Peacock ML, Watson P: Hirschsprung disease in MEN 2A: increased spectrum of *RET* exon 10 genotypes and strong genotype-phenotype correlation. *Hum Mol Genet* 7 (1): 129-34, 1998.

43. Carrasquillo MM, McCallion AS, Puffenberger EG, et al.: Genome-wide association study and mouse model identify interaction between *RET* and EDNRB pathways in Hirschsprung disease. *Nat Genet* 32 (2): 237-44, 2002.

44. Mulligan LM, Eng C, Attié T, et al.: Diverse phenotypes associated with exon 10 mutations of the *RET* proto-oncogene. *Hum Mol Genet* 3 (12): 2163-7, 1994.

45. Giraud S, Zhang CX, Serova-Sinilnikova O, et al.: Germ-line mutation analysis in patients with multiple endocrine neoplasia type 1 and related disorders. *Am J Hum Genet* 63 (2): 455-67, 1998.

46. Schimke RN: Multiple endocrine neoplasia: how many syndromes? *Am J Med Genet* 37 (3): 375-83, 1990.

47. Gardner E, Papi L, Easton DF, et al.: Genetic linkage studies map the multiple endocrine neoplasia type 2 loci to a small interval on chromosome 10q11.2. *Hum Mol Genet* 2 (3): 241-6, 1993.

48. Mole SE, Mulligan LM, Healey CS, et al.: Localization of the gene for multiple endocrine neoplasia type 2A to a 480 kb region in chromosome band 10q11.2. *Hum Mol Genet* 2 (3): 247-52, 1993.

49. Takahashi M, Ritz J, Cooper GM: Activation of a novel human transforming gene, *RET*, by DNA rearrangement. *Cell* 42 (2): 581-8, 1985.

50. Kwok JB, Gardner E, Warner JP, et al.: Structural analysis of the human *RET* proto-oncogene using exon trapping. *Oncogene* 8 (9): 2575-82, 1993.

51. Myers SM, Eng C, Ponder BA, et al.: Characterization of *RET* proto-oncogene 3' splicing variants and polyadenylation sites: a novel C-terminus for *RET*. *Oncogene* 11 (10): 2039-45, 1995.

52. Takahashi M, Buma Y, Iwamoto T, et al.: Cloning and expression of the *RET* proto-oncogene encoding a tyrosine kinase with two potential transmembrane domains. *Oncogene* 3 (5): 571-8, 1988.

53. Mulligan LM, Eng C, Healey CS, et al.: Specific mutations of the *RET* proto-oncogene are related to disease phenotype in MEN 2A and FMTC. *Nat Genet* 6 (1): 70-4, 1994.

54. Ceccherini I, Hofstra RM, Luo Y, et al.: DNA polymorphisms and conditions for SSCP analysis of the 20 exons of the *RET* proto-oncogene. *Oncogene* 9 (10): 3025-9, 1994.

55. Ceccherini I, Hofstra RM, Luo Y, et al.: DNA polymorphisms and conditions for SSCP analysis of the 20 exons of the *RET* proto-oncogene. *Oncogene* 10 (6): 1257, 1995.

56. Airaksinen MS, Saarma M: The *GDNF* family: signaling, biological functions and therapeutic value. *Nat Rev Neurosci* 3 (5): 383-94, 2002.

57. Takaya K, Yoshimasa T, Arai H, et al.: Expression of the *RET* proto-oncogene in normal human tissues, pheochromocytomas, and other tumors of neural crest origin. *J Mol Med* 74 (10): 617-21, 1996.

58. Kurokawa K, Kawai K, Hashimoto M, et al.: Cell signaling and gene expression mediated by *RET* tyrosine kinase. *J Intern Med* 253 (6): 627-33, 2003.

59. Manié S, Santoro M, Fusco A, et al.: The *RET* receptor: function in development and dysfunction in congenital malformation. *Trends Genet* 17 (10): 580-9, 2001.

60. Bounacer A, Du Villard JA, Wicker R, et al.: Association of *RET* codon 691 polymorphism in radiation-induced human thyroid tumours with C-cell hyperplasia in peritumoural tissue. *Br J Cancer* 86 (12): 1929-36, 2002.

61. Mulligan LM, Marsh DJ, Robinson BG, et al.: Genotype-phenotype correlation in multiple endocrine neoplasia type 2: report of the International *RET* Mutation Consortium. *J Intern Med* 238 (4): 343-6, 1995.

62. Höppner W, Ritter MM: A duplication of 12 bp in the critical cysteine rich domain of the *RET* proto-oncogene results in a distinct phenotype of multiple endocrine neoplasia type 2A. *Hum Mol Genet* 6 (4): 587-90, 1997.

63. Höppner W, Dralle H, Brabant G: Duplication of 9 base pairs in the critical cysteine-rich domain of the *RET* proto-oncogene causes multiple endocrine neoplasia type 2A. *Hum Mutat Suppl* (1): S128-30, 1998.

64. Pigny P, Bauters C, Wemeau JL, et al.: A novel 9-base pair duplication in *RET* exon 8 in familial medullary thyroid carcinoma. *J Clin Endocrinol Metab* 84 (5): 1700-4, 1999.

65. Berndt I, Reuter M, Saller B, et al.: A new hot spot for mutations in the *RET* protooncogene causing familial medullary thyroid carcinoma and multiple endocrine neoplasia type 2A. *J Clin Endocrinol Metab* 83 (3): 770-4, 1998.

66. Bolino A, Schuffenecker I, Luo Y, et al.: *RET* mutations in exons 13 and 14 of FMTC patients. *Oncogene* 10 (12): 2415-9, 1995.

67. Eng C, Smith DP, Mulligan LM, et al.: A novel point mutation in the tyrosine kinase domain of the *RET* proto-oncogene in

sporadic medullary thyroid carcinoma and in a family with FMTC. *Oncogene* 10 (3): 509-13, 1995.

68. Hofstra RM, Fattoruso O, Quadro L, et al.: A novel point mutation in the intracellular domain of the *RET* protooncogene in a family with medullary thyroid carcinoma. *J Clin Endocrinol Metab* 82 (12): 4176-8, 1997.

69. Komminoth P, Kunz EK, Matias-Guiu X, et al.: Analysis of *RET* protooncogene point mutations distinguishes heritable from nonheritable medullary thyroid carcinomas. *Cancer* 76 (3): 479-89, 1995.

70. Carlson KM, Dou S, Chi D, et al.: Single missense mutation in the tyrosine kinase catalytic domain of the *RET* protooncogene is associated with multiple endocrine neoplasia type 2B. *Proc Natl Acad Sci U S A* 91 (4): 1579-83, 1994.

71. Eng C, Smith DP, Mulligan LM, et al.: Point mutation within the tyrosine kinase domain of the *RET* proto-oncogene in multiple endocrine neoplasia type 2B and related sporadic tumours. *Hum Mol Genet* 3 (2): 237-41, 1994.

72. Gimm O, Marsh DJ, Andrew SD, et al.: Germline dinucleotide mutation in codon 883 of the *RET* proto-oncogene in multiple endocrine neoplasia type 2B without codon 918 mutation. *J Clin Endocrinol Metab* 82 (11): 3902-4, 1997.

73. Smith DP, Houghton C, Ponder BA: Germline mutation of *RET* codon 883 in two cases of de novo MEN 2B. *Oncogene* 15 (10): 1213-7, 1997.

74. Santoro M, Carlomagno F, Romano A, et al.: Activation of *RET* as a dominant transforming gene by germline mutations of MEN2A and MEN2B. *Science* 267 (5196): 381-3, 1995.

75. Takahashi M, Asai N, Iwashita T, et al.: Molecular mechanisms of development of multiple endocrine neoplasia 2 by *RET* mutations. *J Intern Med* 243 (6): 509-13, 1998.

76. Songyang Z, Carraway KL 3rd, Eck MJ, et al.: Catalytic specificity of protein-tyrosine kinases is critical for selective signaling. *Nature* 373 (6514): 536-9, 1995.

77. Iwashita T, Murakami H, Asai N, et al.: Mechanism of *RET* dysfunction by Hirschsprung mutations affecting its extracellular domain. *Hum Mol Genet* 5 (10): 1577-80, 1996.

78. Zedenius J, Wallin G, Hamberger B, et al.: Somatic and MEN 2A de novo mutations identified in the *RET* proto-oncogene by screening of sporadic MTCs. *Hum Mol Genet* 3 (8): 1259-62, 1994.

79. Eng C, Mulligan LM, Healey CS, et al.: Heterogeneous mutation of the *RET* proto-oncogene in subpopulations of medullary thyroid carcinoma. *Cancer Res* 56 (9): 2167-70, 1996.

80. Shannon KE, Gimm O, Hinze R: Germline V804M mutation in the *RET* protooncogene in 2 apparently sporadic cases of MTC presenting in the 7th decade of life. *The Journal of Endocrine Genetics* 1 (1): 39-46, 1999.

81. Boccia LM, Green JS, Joyce C, et al.: Mutation of *RET* codon 768 is associated with the FMTC phenotype. *Clin Genet* 51 (2): 81-5, 1997.

82. Schuffenecker I, Billaud M, Calender A, et al.: *RET* proto-oncogene mutations in French MEN 2A and FMTC families. *Hum Mol Genet* 3 (11): 1939-43, 1994.

83. Frank-Raue K, Höppner W, Frilling A, et al.: Mutations of the *RET* protooncogene in German multiple endocrine neoplasia families: relation between genotype and phenotype. German Medullary Thyroid Carcinoma Study Group. *J Clin Endocrinol Metab* 81 (5): 1780-3, 1996.

84. Moers AM, Landsvater RM, Schaap C, et al.: Familial medullary thyroid carcinoma: not a distinct entity? Genotype-phenotype correlation in a large family. *Am J Med* 101 (6): 635-41, 1996.

85. Niccoli-Sire P, Murat A, Rohmer V, et al.: Familial medullary thyroid carcinoma with non-cysteine *RET* mutations: phenotype-genotype relationship in a large series of patients. *J Clin Endocrinol Metab* 86 (8): 3746-53, 2001.

86. Seri M, Celli I, Betsos N, et al.: A Cys634Gly substitution of the *RET* proto-oncogene in a family with recurrence of multiple endocrine neoplasia type 2A and cutaneous lichen amyloidosis. *Clin Genet* 51 (2): 86-90, 1997.

87. Yip L, Cote GJ, Shapiro SE, et al.: Multiple endocrine neoplasia type 2: evaluation of the genotype-phenotype relationship. *Arch Surg* 138 (4): 409-16; discussion 416, 2003.

88. Borrego S, Wright FA, Fernández RM, et al.: A founding locus within the *RET* proto-oncogene may account for a large proportion of apparently sporadic Hirschsprung disease and a subset of cases of sporadic medullary thyroid carcinoma. *Am J Hum Genet* 72 (1): 88-100, 2003.

89. Griseri P, Pesce B, Patrone G, et al.: A rare haplotype of the *RET* proto-oncogene is a risk-modifying allele in Hirschsprung disease. *Am J Hum Genet* 71 (4): 969-74, 2002.

90. American Society of Clinical Oncology.: American Society of Clinical Oncology policy statement update: genetic testing for cancer susceptibility. *J Clin Oncol* 21 (12): 2397-406, 2003.

91. Statement of the American Society of Clinical Oncology: genetic testing for cancer susceptibility, Adopted on February 20, 1996. *J Clin Oncol* 14 (5): 1730-6; discussion 1737-40, 1996.

92. Points to consider: ethical, legal, and psychosocial implications of genetic testing in children and adolescents. American Society of Human Genetics Board of Directors, American College of Medical Genetics Board of Directors. *Am J Hum Genet* 57 (5): 1233-41, 1995.

93. Xue F, Yu H, Maurer LH, et al.: Germline *RET* mutations in MEN 2A and FMTC and their detection by simple DNA diagnostic tests. *Hum Mol Genet* 3 (4): 635-8, 1994.

94. McMahon R, Mulligan LM, Healey CS, et al.: Direct, non-radioactive detection of mutations in multiple endocrine neoplasia type 2A families. *Hum Mol Genet* 3 (4): 643-6, 1994.

95. Kambouris M, Jackson CE, Feldman GL: Diagnosis of multiple endocrine neoplasia [MEN] 2A, 2B and familial medullary thyroid cancer [FMTC] by multiplex PCR and heteroduplex analyses of *RET* proto-oncogene mutations. *Hum Mutat* 8 (1): 64-70, 1996.

96. Howe JR, Lairmore TC, Mishra SK, et al.: Improved predictive test for MEN2, using flanking dinucleotide repeats and RFLPs. *Am J Hum Genet* 51 (6): 1430-42, 1992.

97. Gagel RF, Tashjian AH Jr, Cummings T, et al.: The clinical outcome of prospective screening for multiple endocrine neoplasia type 2a. An 18-year experience. *N Engl J Med* 318 (8): 478-84, 1988.

98. Niccoli-Sire P, Murat A, Baudin E, et al.: Early or prophylactic thyroidectomy in MEN 2/FMTC gene carriers: results in 71 thyroidectomized patients. The French Calcitonin Tumours Study Group (GETC). *Eur J Endocrinol* 141 (5): 468-74, 1999.

99. Wells SA Jr, Skinner MA: Prophylactic thyroidectomy, based on direct genetic testing, in patients at risk for the multiple endocrine neoplasia type 2 syndromes. *Exp Clin Endocrinol Diabetes* 106 (1): 29-34, 1998.

100. Szinnai G, Meier C, Komminoth P, et al.: Review of multiple endocrine neoplasia type 2A in children: therapeutic results of early thyroidectomy and prognostic value of codon analysis. *Pediatrics* 111 (2): E132-9, 2003.

101. van Heurn LW, Schaap C, Sie G, et al.: Predictive DNA testing for multiple endocrine neoplasia 2: a therapeutic challenge of prophylactic thyroidectomy in very young children. *J Pediatr Surg* 34 (4): 568-71, 1999.

102. Hansen HS, Torring H, Godballe C, et al.: Is thyroidectomy necessary in *RET* mutations carriers of the familial medullary thyroid carcinoma syndrome? *Cancer* 89 (4): 863-7, 2000.

103. Machens A, Niccoli-Sire P, Hoegel J, et al.: Early malignant progression of hereditary medullary thyroid cancer. *N Engl J Med* 349 (16): 1517-25, 2003.

104. Wells SA Jr, Donis-Keller H: Current perspectives on the diagnosis and management of patients with multiple endocrine neoplasia type 2 syndromes. *Endocrinol Metab Clin North Am* 23 (1): 215-28, 1994.

105. Marsh DJ, McDowall D, Hyland VJ, et al.: The identification of false positive responses to the pentagastrin stimulation test in *RET* mutation negative members of MEN 2A families. *Clin Endocrinol* (Oxf) 44 (2): 213-20, 1996.

106. Samaan NA, Schultz PN, Hickey RC: Medullary thyroid carcinoma: prognosis of familial versus nonfamilial disease and the role of radiotherapy. *Horm Metab Res Suppl* 21: 21-5, 1989.

107. Scherübl H, Raue F, Ziegler R: Combination chemotherapy of advanced medullary and differentiated thyroid cancer. Phase II study. *J Cancer Res Clin Oncol* 116 (1): 21-3, 1990.

108. Lairmore TC, Ball DW, Baylin SB, et al.: Management of pheochromocytomas in patients with multiple endocrine neoplasia

type 2 syndromes. *Ann Surg* 217 (6): 595-601; discussion 601-3, 1993.

109. Okamoto T, Obara T, Ito Y, et al.: Bilateral adrenalectomy with autotransplantation of adrenocortical tissue or unilateral adrenalectomy: treatment options for pheochromocytomas in multiple endocrine neoplasia type 2A. *Endocr J* 43 (2): 169-75, 1996.

110. Inabnet WB, Caragliano P, Pertsemlidis D: Pheochromocytoma: inherited associations, bilaterality, and cortex preservation. *Surgery* 128 (6): 1007-11; discussion 1011-2, 2000.

111. Lee JE, Curley SA, Gagel RF, et al.: Cortical-sparing adrenalectomy for patients with bilateral pheochromocytoma. *Surgery* 120 (6): 1064-70; discussion 1070-1, 1996.

112. Yip L, Lee JE, Shapiro SE, et al.: Surgical management of hereditary pheochromocytoma. *J Am Coll Surg* 198 (4): 525-34; discussion 534-5, 2004.

113. Pautler SE, Choyke PL, Pavlovich CP, et al.: Intraoperative ultrasound aids in dissection during laparoscopic partial adrenalectomy. *J Urol* 168 (4 Pt 1): 1352-5, 2002.

114. Norton JA, Brennan MF, Wells SA Jr: Surgical Management of Hyperparathyroidism. In: Bilezikian JP, Marcus R, Levine MA: *The Parathyroids: Basic and Clinical Concepts*. New York: Raven Press, 1994, pp 531-551.

115. Schuffenecker I, Ginet N, Goldgar D, et al.: Prevalence and parental origin of de novo *RET* mutations in multiple endocrine neoplasia type 2A and familial medullary thyroid carcinoma. Le Groupe d'Etude des Tumeurs a Calcitonine. *Am J Hum Genet* 60 (1): 233-7, 1997.

116. Norum RA, Lafreniere RG, O'Neal LW, et al.: Linkage of the multiple endocrine neoplasia type 2B gene (MEN2B) to chromosome 10 markers linked to MEN2A. *Genomics* 8 (2): 313-7, 1990.

117. Carlson KM, Bracamontes J, Jackson CE, et al.: Parent-of-origin effects in multiple endocrine neoplasia type 2B. *Am J Hum Genet* 55 (6): 1076-82, 1994.

118. Kitamura Y, Scavarda N, Wells SA Jr, et al.: Two maternally derived missense mutations in the tyrosine kinase domain of the *RET* protooncogene in a patient with de novo MEN 2B. *Hum Mol Genet* 4 (10): 1987-8, 1995.

119. Freyer G, Dazord A, Schlumberger M, et al.: Psychosocial impact of genetic testing in familial medullary-thyroid carcinoma: a multicentric pilot-evaluation. *Ann Oncol* 10 (1): 87-95, 1999.

120. Grosfeld FJ, Lips CJ, Ten Kroode HF, et al.: Psychosocial consequences of DNA analysis for MEN type 2. *Oncology* (Huntingt) 10 (2): 141-6; discussion 146, 152, 157, 1996.

121. Johnston LB, Chew SL, Trainer PJ, et al.: Screening children at risk of developing inherited endocrine neoplasia syndromes. *Clin Endocrinol* (Oxf) 52 (2): 127-36, 2000.

122. MacDonald DJ, Lessick M: Hereditary cancers in children and ethical and psychosocial implications. *J Pediatr Nurs* 15 (4): 217-25, 2000.

123. Grosfeld FJ, Lips CJ, Beemer FA, et al.: Psychological risks of genetically testing children for a hereditary cancer syndrome. *Patient Educ Couns* 32 (1-2): 63-7, 1997 Sept.-Oct.

124. Giarelli E: Multiple endocrine neoplasia type 2a (MEN2a): a call for psycho-social research. *Psychooncology* 11 (1): 59-73, 2002 Jan-Feb.

125. Grosfeld FJ, Lips CJ, Beemer FA, et al.: Distress in MEN 2 family members and partners prior to DNA test disclosure. Multiple endocrine neoplasia type 2. *Am J Med Genet* 91 (1): 1-7, 2000.

126. Grosfeld FJ, Beemer FA, Lips CJ, et al.: Parents' responses to disclosure of genetic test results of their children. *Am J Med Genet* 94 (4): 316-23, 2000.

127. Giarelli E: Bringing threat to the fore: participating in lifelong surveillance for genetic risk of cancer. *Oncol Nurs Forum* 30 (6): 945-55, 2003 Nov-Dec.

128. Schultz PN: Providing information to patients with a rare cancer: using Internet discussion forums to address the needs of patients with medullary thyroid carcinoma. *Clin J Oncol Nurs* 6 (4): 219-22, 2002 July-Aug.

Chapter 44

Parathyroid Cancer

Parathyroid cancer, a very rare cancer, is a disease in which cancer (malignant) cells are found in the tissues of the parathyroid gland. The parathyroid gland is at the base of the neck, near the thyroid gland. The parathyroid gland makes a hormone called parathyroid hormone (PTH), or parathormone, which helps the body store and use calcium.

Problems with the parathyroid gland are common and are usually not caused by cancer. If parathyroid cancer is found, the parathyroid gland may be making too much PTH. This causes too much calcium to be found in the blood. The extra PTH also takes calcium from the bones, which causes pain in the bones, kidney problems, and other types of problems. There are other conditions that can cause the parathyroid gland to make too much PTH. It is important for a doctor to determine what is causing the extra PTH. Hyperparathyroidism is a condition which can cause the body to make extra PTH. If hyperparathyroidism runs in the family, there is a greater chance of getting this type of cancer.

A doctor should be seen if there are the following symptoms: bone pain, a lump in the neck, pain in the upper part of the back, weak muscles, difficulty speaking, or vomiting. If there are symptoms, the doctor will conduct a physical examination and feel for lumps in the throat. The doctor may also order blood tests and other tests to check for cancer or other types of tumors that may not be cancer (benign tumors).

PDQ® Cancer Information summary. National Cancer Institute; Bethesda, MD. *Parathyroid Cancer (PDQ®): Treatment–Patient.* Updated 06/062003. Available at http://cancer.gov. Accessed 12/18/2004.

The chance of recovery (prognosis) depends on whether the cancer is just in the parathyroid gland or has spread to other parts of the body (stage) and the patient's general health.

Explanation of Parathyroid Cancer Stages

Once parathyroid cancer is found, more tests will be done to find out if cancer cells have spread to other parts of the body. This is called staging. A doctor needs to know the stage of the disease to plan treatment. The following stages are used for parathyroid cancer.

Localized

The cancer is only on the parathyroid gland and has not spread to tissues next to the parathyroid.

Metastatic

The cancer has spread to lymph nodes in the area or to other parts of the body, such as the lungs (lymph nodes are small bean-shaped structures that are found throughout the body; they produce and store infection-fighting cells).

Recurrent

Recurrent disease means that the cancer has come back (recurred) after it has been treated. It may come back in the original place or in another part of the body.

Treatment Option Overview

How Parathyroid Cancer Is Treated

There are treatments for all patients with parathyroid cancer. Two kinds of treatment are used:

1. Surgery (taking out the cancer).
2. Radiation therapy (using high-dose x-rays or other high-energy rays to kill cancer cells).

Surgery is the most common treatment of parathyroid cancer. A doctor may remove the parathyroid gland (parathyroidectomy) and the half of the thyroid on the same side as the cancer (ipsilateral thyroidectomy).

Radiation therapy uses high-energy x-rays to kill cancer cells and shrink tumors. Radiation may come from a machine outside the body (external radiation therapy) or from putting materials that produce radiation (radioisotopes) through thin plastic tubes in the area where the cancer cells are found (internal radiation therapy).

Chemotherapy (using drugs to kill cancer cells) is being studied in clinical trials. Chemotherapy uses drugs to kill cancer cells. Chemotherapy may be taken by pill, or it may be put into the body by a needle in the vein or muscle. Chemotherapy is called a systemic treatment because the drug enters the bloodstream, travels through the body, and can kill cancer cells outside the parathyroid gland.

Treatment by Stage

Treatment for parathyroid cancer depends on the type and stage of the disease and the patient's age and overall health.

Standard treatment may be considered because of its effectiveness in patients in past studies, or participation in a clinical trial may be considered. Not all patients are cured with standard therapy and some standard treatments may have more side effects than are desired. For these reasons, clinical trials are designed to find better ways to treat cancer patients and are based on the most up-to-date information. Clinical trials are ongoing in some parts of the country for patients with parathyroid cancer.

Localized Parathyroid Cancer

Treatment may be one of the following:

1. Surgery to remove the parathyroid gland (parathyroidectomy) and the half of the thyroid on the same side as the cancer (ipsilateral thyroidectomy).

2. A clinical trial of surgery followed by radiation therapy.

3. A clinical trial of radiation therapy.

Metastatic Parathyroid Cancer

Treatment may be one of the following:

1. Surgery to remove the parathyroid gland (parathyroidectomy) and other tissues around the thyroid if they contain cancer.

2. Surgery to remove as much of the parathyroid gland as possible in order to reduce production of PTH.

3. Medical treatment to reduce the amount of calcium in the blood.

4. A clinical trial of surgery followed by radiation therapy.

5. A clinical trial of radiation therapy.

6. A clinical trial of chemotherapy.

Recurrent Parathyroid Cancer

Recurrent disease can occur as late as 34 years after the first tumor. Treatment may be one of the following:

1. Surgery to remove the parathyroid gland (parathyroidectomy) and other tissues around the thyroid if they contain cancer.

2. Surgery to remove as much of the parathyroid gland as possible in order to reduce production of PTH.

3. Medical treatment to reduce the amount of calcium in the blood.

4. A clinical trial of surgery followed by radiation therapy.

5. A clinical trial of radiation therapy.

5. A clinical trial of chemotherapy.

Additional Information

National Cancer Institute
6116 Executive Boulevard, MSC8322
Bethesda, MD 20892-8322
Toll-Free: 800-422-6237
Toll-Free TTY: 800-332-8615
Website: http://www.cancer.gov
E-mail: cancergovstaff@mail.nih.gov

The NCI has booklets and other materials for patients, health professionals, and the public. These publications discuss types of cancer, methods of cancer treatment, coping with cancer, and clinical trials. Some publications provide information on tests for cancer, cancer causes and prevention, cancer statistics, and NCI research activities.

Part Eight

Thyroid and Parathyroid Disorder Treatments

Chapter 45

Thyroid Hormones: Drug Information for Hypothyroidism

Drug Information: Thyroid

Brand name(s): Armour Thyroid; S-P-T; Thyrar; Thyroid Strong; Westhroid

Other name(s): Desiccated thyroid; thyroid extract; thyroid gland

Important Warning

Thyroid hormone should not be used to treat obesity in patients with normal thyroid function. Thyroid medication is ineffective for weight reduction in normal thyroid patients and may cause serious or life-threatening toxicity, especially when taken with amphetamines. Talk to your doctor about the potential risks associated with this medication.

Why is this medication prescribed?

Thyroid is a hormone produced by the body. When taken correctly, thyroid reverses the symptoms of hypothyroidism, a condition where

---

This chapter begins with "Drug Information: Thyroid," Medmaster, American Society of Health-System Pharmacists, Bethesda, MD, 1998, Revised 2003. Reprinted with permission. Additional text is from "Thyroid Hormones (Systemic)," USP DI® System: Klasco RK (ed). USP DI® Vol. II Advice for the Patient®. © 2004 Thomson MICROMEDEX, Greenwood Village, Colorado (Volume 122, Expires 1/2005). Reprinted with permission.

the thyroid gland does not produce enough thyroid hormone. Without thyroid hormone, the body cannot function properly, resulting in poor growth, slow speech, lack of energy, weight gain, hair loss, dry thick skin, and increased sensitivity to cold. Thyroid also is used to treat goiter (enlarged thyroid gland).

This medication is sometimes prescribed for other uses; ask your doctor or pharmacist for more information.

How should this medicine be used?

Thyroid comes as a tablet and a capsule to take by mouth. It usually is taken as a single dose every day before breakfast. To control the symptoms of hypothyroidism, you probably will need to take thyroid for the rest of your life. It may take about 2 weeks before you notice any change in your symptoms. Follow the directions on your prescription label carefully, and ask your doctor or pharmacist to explain any part you do not understand. Take thyroid exactly as directed. Do not take more or less of it or take it more often than prescribed by your doctor.

Continue to take thyroid even if you feel well. Do not stop taking thyroid without talking to your doctor.

What special precautions should I follow?

Before taking thyroid:

- Tell your doctor and pharmacist if you are allergic to thyroid; foods such as pork, beef, soybean oil, or corn; or any other drugs.
- Tell your doctor and pharmacist what prescription and nonprescription medications you are taking, especially amphetamines, anticoagulants (blood thinners) such as warfarin (Coumadin), arthritis medications, aspirin, cholesterol-lowering resins such as cholestyramine (Questran) or colestipol (Colestid), diabetes medications (insulin and tablets), digoxin (Lanoxin), estrogens, oral contraceptives, steroids, and vitamins.
- If you take cholestyramine (Questran) or colestipol (Colestid), take it at least 4 hours before or 1 hour after taking your thyroid medication.
- Tell your doctor if you have or have ever had diabetes; hardening of the arteries (atherosclerosis); kidney disease; hepatitis; cardiovascular disease such as high blood pressure, chest pain (angina), arrhythmias, or heart attack; or an underactive adrenal or pituitary gland.

- Tell your doctor if you are pregnant, plan to become pregnant, or are breastfeeding. If you become pregnant while taking thyroid, call your doctor.

- If you are having surgery, including dental surgery, tell the doctor or dentist that you are taking thyroid.

- Tell your doctor if you drink alcoholic beverages. It is important not to drink alcohol while taking thyroid.

What should I do if I forget a dose?

Take the missed dose as soon as you remember it. However, if it is almost time for the next dose, skip the missed dose and continue your regular dosing schedule. Do not take a double dose to make up for a missed one.

What side effects can this medication cause?

Although side effects from thyroid are not common, they can occur. Tell your doctor if any of these symptoms are severe or do not go away:

- weight loss
- tremor
- headache
- upset stomach
- vomiting
- diarrhea
- stomach cramps
- nervousness
- irritability
- insomnia
- excessive sweating
- increased appetite
- fever
- changes in menstrual cycle
- sensitivity to heat
- temporary hair loss, particularly in children during the first month of therapy

If you experience any of the following symptoms, call your doctor immediately:

- severe skin rash
- difficulty breathing or swallowing
- chest pain (angina)
- rapid or irregular heartbeat or pulse

What storage conditions are needed for this medicine?

Keep this medication in the container it came in, tightly closed, and out of reach of children. Store it at room temperature and away from excess heat and moisture (not in the bathroom). Throw away any medication that is outdated or no longer needed. Talk to your pharmacist about the proper disposal of your medication.

What should be done in case of emergency or overdose?

In case of overdose, call your local poison control center at 800-222-1222. If the victim has collapsed or is not breathing, call local emergency services at 911.

What other information should I know?

- Keep all appointments with your doctor and the laboratory. Your doctor will order certain lab tests to check your response to thyroid.

- Learn the brand name and generic name of your medication. Do not switch brands without talking to your doctor or pharmacist, as each brand of thyroid contains a slightly different amount of medication.

- Do not let anyone else take your medication. Ask your pharmacist any questions you have about refilling your prescription.

Drug Information: Thyroid Hormones (Systemic)

Brand Names

Common U.S. Brand Names

- Armour Thyroid [5]
- Cytomel [2]

- Levo-T [1]
- Levothroid [1]
- Levoxyl [1]
- Synthroid [1]
- Thyrar [5]
- Thyroid Strong [5]
- Thyrolar [3]
- Triostat [2]
- Westhroid [5]

Common Canadian Brand Names

- Cytomel [2]
- Eltroxin [1]
- PMS-Levothyroxine Sodium [1]
- Synthroid [1]

Note: For quick reference, the following thyroid hormones are numbered to match the corresponding brand names.

1. Levothyroxine (lee-voe-thye-ROX-een) [t]
2 Liothyronine (lye-oh-THYE-roe-neen) [t]
3. Liotrix (LYE-oh-trix) [**]
4. Thyroglobulin (thye-roe-GLOB-yoo-lin) [*]
5. Thyroid (THYE-roid) [t]

[t] Generic name product may be available in the U.S.

[a] Generic name product may be available in Canada

[*] Not commercially available in the U.S.

[**] Not commercially available in Canada

Category

- **Antineoplastic:** Levothyroxine; Liothyronine; Liotrix; Thyroglobulin; Thyroid

- **Diagnostic aid, thyroid function:** Levothyroxine; Liothyronine

441

- **Thyroid hormone:** Levothyroxine; Liothyronine; Liotrix; Thyroglobulin; Thyroid

Description

Thyroid medicines belong to the general group of medicines called hormones. They are used when the thyroid gland does not produce enough hormone. They are also used to help decrease the size of enlarged thyroid glands (known as goiter) and to treat thyroid cancer.

These medicines are available only with your doctor's prescription, in the following dosage forms:

Oral

- Levothyroxine—Tablets (U.S. and Canada)
- Liothyronine—Tablets (U.S. and Canada)
- Liotrix—Tablets (U.S.)
- Thyroglobulin—Tablets (not commercially available in the U.S.)
- Thyroid—Tablets (U.S. and Canada)

Parenteral

- Levothyroxine—Injection (U.S. and Canada)
- Liothyronine—Injection (U.S.)

Before Using This Medicine

In deciding to use a medicine, the risks of taking the medicine must be weighed against the good it will do. This is a decision you and your doctor will make. For thyroid hormones, the following should be considered:

Allergies: Tell your doctor if you have ever had any unusual or allergic reaction to thyroid hormones. Also tell your health care professional if you are allergic to any other substances, such as foods, preservatives, or dyes.

Pregnancy: Use of proper amounts of thyroid hormone during pregnancy has not been shown to cause birth defects or other problems. However, your doctor may want you to change your dose while you are pregnant. This will make regular visits to your doctor important.

Breastfeeding: Use of proper amounts of thyroid hormones by mothers has not been shown to cause problems in nursing babies.

Children: Thyroid hormones have been tested in children and have not been shown to cause different side effects or problems in children than they do in adults.

Older adults: This medicine has been tested and has not been shown to cause different side effects or problems in older people than it does in younger adults. However, a different dose may be needed in the elderly. Therefore, it is important to take the medicine only as directed by the doctor.

Other medicines: Although certain medicines should not be used together at all, in other cases two different medicines may be used together even if an interaction might occur. In these cases, your doctor may want to change the dose, or other precautions may be necessary. When you are taking thyroid hormones, it is especially important that your health care professional know if you are taking any of the following:

- Amphetamines
- Anticoagulants (blood thinners)
- Appetite suppressants (diet pills)
- Cholestyramine (e.g., Questran)
- Colestipol (e.g., Colestid)
- Medicine for asthma or other breathing problems
- Medicine for colds, sinus problems, or hay fever or other allergies (including nose drops or sprays)

Other medical problems: The presence of other medical problems may affect the use of thyroid hormones. Make sure you tell your doctor if you have any other medical problems especially:

- Diabetes mellitus (sugar diabetes)
- Hardening of the arteries
- Heart disease
- High blood pressure
- Overactive thyroid (history of)
- Underactive adrenal gland
- Underactive pituitary gland

Proper Use of This Medicine

Use this medicine only as directed by your doctor. Do not use more or less of it, and do not use it more often than your doctor ordered. Your doctor has prescribed the exact amount your body needs and if you take different amounts, you may experience symptoms of an overactive or underactive thyroid. Take it at the same time each day to make sure it always has the same effect.

If your condition is due to a lack of thyroid hormone, you may have to take this medicine for the rest of your life. It is very important that you do not stop taking this medicine without first checking with your doctor.

Dosing: The dose of these medicines will be different for different patients. Follow your doctor's orders or the directions on the label. The following information includes only the average doses of these medicines. If your dose is different, do not change it unless your doctor tells you to do so.

The number of tablets that you take depends on the strength of the medicine. The amount of thyroid hormone that you need to take every day depends on the results of your thyroid tests. However, treatment is usually started with lower doses that are increased a little at a time until you are taking the full amount. This helps prevent side effects.

Levothyroxine

For oral dosage form (tablets): For replacing the thyroid hormone:

- Adults and teenagers: At first, 0.0125 to 0.05 milligrams (mg) once a day. Then, your doctor may increase your dose a little at a time to 0.075 to 0.125 mg a day. The dose is usually no higher than 0.15 mg once a day.

- Children less than 6 months of age: The dose is based on body weight and must be determined by your doctor. The usual dose is 0.025 to 0.05 mg once a day.

- Children 6 months to 12 months of age: The dose is based on body weight and must be determined by your doctor. The usual dose is 0.05 to 0.075 mg once a day.

- Children 1 to 5 years of age: The dose is based on body weight and must be determined by your doctor. The usual dose is 0.075 to 0.1 mg once a day.

- Children 6 to 10 years of age: The dose is based on body weight and must be determined by your doctor. The usual dose is 0.1 to 0.15 mg once a day.

- Children over 10 years of age: The dose is based on body weight and must be determined by your doctor. The usual dose is 0.15 to 0.2 mg once a day.

For injection dosage form: For replacing the thyroid hormone:

- Adults and teenagers: 50 to 100 micrograms (mcg) injected into a muscle or into a vein once a day. People with very serious conditions caused by too little thyroid hormone may need higher doses.

- Children less than 6 months of age: The dose is based on body weight and must be determined by your doctor. The usual dose is 0.019 to 0.038 mg once a day.

- Children 6 months to 12 months of age: The dose is based on body weight and must be determined by your doctor. The usual dose is 0.038 to 0.056 mg once a day.

- Children 1 to 5 years of age: The dose is based on body weight and must be determined by your doctor. The usual dose is 0.056 to 0.075 mg once a day.

- Children 6 to 10 years of age: The dose is based on body weight and must be determined by your doctor. The usual dose is 0.075 to 0.113 mg once a day.

- Children over 10 years of age: The dose is based on body weight and must be determined by your doctor. The usual dose is 0.113 to 0.15 mg once a day.

Liothyronine Sodium

For oral dosage form (tablets):

- For replacing the thyroid hormone:
  - Adults and teenagers: At first, 25 micrograms (mcg) a day. Some patients with very serious conditions caused by too little thyroid hormone may need to take only 2.5 to 5 mcg a day at first. Also, some patients with heart disease or the elderly may need lower doses at first. Then, your doctor may increase your dose a little at a time to up to 50 mcg a day if

needed. Your doctor may want you to divide your dose into smaller amounts that are taken two or more times a day.

- For treating a large thyroid gland (goiter):
  - Adults: At first, 5 mcg a day. Some patients with heart disease or the elderly may need lower doses at first. Then, your doctor may increase your dose a little at a time to 50 to 100 mcg a day.

For injection dosage form:

- For replacing the thyroid hormone in very serious conditions (myxedema coma):
  - Adults: At first, 10 to 50 mcg injected into a vein every four to twelve hours. Then, your doctor may want to adjust your dose depending on your condition.
  - Children: Use and dose must be determined by your doctor.

Liotrix (Levothyroxine and Liothyronine Combination)

For oral dosage form (tablets): For replacing the thyroid hormone:

- Adults, teenagers, and children: At first, 50 micrograms (mcg) of levothyroxine and 12.5 mcg of liothyronine once a day. Some people with very serious conditions caused by too little thyroid hormone may need only 12.5 mcg of levothyroxine and 3.1 mcg of liothyronine once a day. Also, some elderly patients may need lower doses at first. Then, your doctor may want to increase your dose a little at a time to up to 100 mcg of levothyroxine and 25 mcg of liothyronine.

Thyroglobulin

For oral dosage form (tablets): For replacing the thyroid hormone:

- Adults, teenagers, and children: At first, 32 milligrams (mg) a day. Some people with very serious conditions caused by too little thyroid hormone may need to take only 16 to 32 mg a day at first. Then, the doctor may want you to increase your dose a little at a time to 65 to 160 mg a day.

Thyroid

For oral dosage form (tablets): For replacing thyroid hormone:

- Adults, teenagers, and children: 60 milligrams (mg) a day. Some people with very serious conditions caused by too little thyroid hormone may need to take only 15 mg a day at first. Also, some elderly patients may need lower doses at first. Then, your doctor may want you to increase your dose a little at a time to 60 to 120 mg a day.

Missed dose: If you miss a dose of this medicine, take it as soon as possible. However, if it is almost time for your next dose, skip the missed dose and go back to your regular dosing schedule. Do not double doses. If you miss 2 or more doses in a row or if you have any questions about this, check with your doctor.

Storage: To store this medicine:

- Keep out of the reach of children.
- Store away from heat and direct light.
- Do not store in the bathroom, near the kitchen sink, or in other damp places. Heat or moisture may cause the medicine to break down.
- Do not keep outdated medicine or medicine no longer needed. Be sure that any discarded medicine is out of the reach of children.

Precautions while Using This Medicine

- It is very important that your doctor check your progress at regular visits, to make sure that this medicine is working properly.
- If you have certain kinds of heart disease, this medicine may cause chest pain or shortness of breath when you exert yourself. If these occur, do not overdo exercise or physical work. If you have any questions about this, check with your doctor.
- Before having any kind of surgery (including dental surgery) or emergency treatment, tell the medical doctor or dentist in charge that you are taking this medicine.
- Do not take any other medicine unless prescribed by your doctor. Some medicines may increase or decrease the effects of thyroid on your body and cause problems in controlling your condition. Also, thyroid hormones may change the effects of other medicines.

Side Effects of This Medicine

Along with its needed effects, a medicine may cause some unwanted effects. Although not all of these side effects may occur, if they do occur they may need medical attention. Check with your doctor as soon as possible if any of the following side effects occur since they may indicate an overdose or an allergic reaction:

- **Less common or rare:** Headache (severe) in children; skin rash or hives

- **Signs and symptoms of overdose:** Chest pain; confusion; fast or irregular heartbeat; mood swings; muscle weakness; psychosis; restlessness (extreme); yellow eyes or skin; shortness of breath

For patients taking this medicine for underactive thyroid: This medicine usually takes several weeks to have a noticeable effect on your condition. Until it begins to work, you may experience no change in your symptoms. Check with your doctor if the following symptoms continue:

- Clumsiness; coldness; constipation; dry, puffy skin; listlessness; muscle aches; sleepiness; tiredness; weakness; weight gain.

Other effects may occur if the dose of the medicine is not exactly right. These side effects will go away when the dose is corrected. Check with your doctor if any of the following symptoms occur:

- Changes in appetite; changes in menstrual periods; diarrhea; fever; hand tremors; headache; increased sensitivity to heat; irritability; leg cramps; nervousness; sweating; trouble in sleeping; vomiting; weight loss.

Other side effects not listed may also occur in some patients. If you notice any other effects, check with your doctor.

Chapter 46

Antithyroid Drugs for Hyperthyroidism

Antithyroid drugs are used to treat an overactive thyroid (hyperthyroidism) caused by Graves disease, an autoimmune condition. These drugs block the synthesis of thyroid hormone by the thyroid gland. They may also help control the disease by indirectly affecting the immune system.

Antithyroid drugs may be used as a short-term treatment to prepare people with Graves hyperthyroidism for thyroid surgery or radioiodine; alternatively, they may be used alone for long-term treatment. Long-term treatment is associated with a remission of Graves disease in 30 percent of patients. Antithyroid drugs may also be used to treat hyperthyroidism associated with toxic multinodular goiter or a toxic adenoma (hot nodule).

The use of antithyroid drugs has several benefits but some risks. It is therefore important to learn as much as you can about the treatment of Graves disease and to discuss all of the possible effects of antithyroid drugs with your doctor before selecting this treatment option.

Effects of Antithyroid Drugs

- Antithyroid drugs decrease the production and blood levels of thyroxine (T4) and triiodothyronine (T3).

Adapted with permission from: Douglas S. Ross, M.D., Patient Information: Antithyroid Drugs. In: UpToDate, Rose, BD (Ed), UpToDate, Wellesley, MA, 2004. Copyright 2004 UpToDate, Inc. For more information visit www .uptodate.com.

- Antithyroid drugs require at least three weeks (usually six to eight weeks or longer) to lower thyroid hormone levels because they only block synthesis of new T4 and T3; they do not alter the effects of the T3 and T4 that are already present in the thyroid and the bloodstream.

- Approximately 30 percent of people with Graves disease will have a remission after prolonged treatment with antithyroid drugs.

Types of Antithyroid Drugs

Two antithyroid drugs are currently available in the United States: propylthiouracil (PTU) and methimazole (MMI, brand name Tapazole). A third drug, carbimazole, is available in Europe, but not in the United States; the body converts carbimazole to MMI. Doctors usually first recommend MMI for the medical treatment of Graves disease, but PTU is recommended during pregnancy or nursing.

Methimazole (MMI)—MMI is usually preferred over PTU because MMI reverses hyperthyroidism more quickly and has fewer side effects. MMI requires an average of 5.8 weeks to lower T4 levels to normal.

MMI can be administered once per day. When used before radioiodine treatment, MMI is less likely than PTU to be associated with failure of the radioiodine treatment.

Propylthiouracil (PTU)—PTU has an added effect on thyroid hormones: PTU blocks the conversion of T4 to T3 in non-thyroid tissue. Nonetheless, PTU does not reverse hyperthyroidism as rapidly as does MMI. PTU requires an average of 16.8 weeks to effectively lower T4 levels.

PTU must be taken in several doses throughout the day, and many tablets are often needed to achieve an effective dose.

Despite these drawbacks, PTU is an alternative for people who have intolerable side effects when taking MMI. PTU is also the preferred antithyroid drug for pregnant and nursing women. In fact, MMI has been associated with scalp problems in the baby. PTU is less likely to cross the placenta and to be transferred into breast milk. Both MMI and PTU can cause goiter and hypothyroidism in the baby. Women taking antithyroid drugs should not get pregnant until they have discussed these possibilities with their doctor if they are considering pregnancy.

Dose

The optimal dose of antithyroid drug for each person will depend on many factors, including the medication selected, the stage of treatment, the size of any goiter, and the degree of hyperthyroidism.

Higher doses of antithyroid drug are often prescribed early in treatment and for people with large goiters and severe hyperthyroidism. Spreading these higher total daily doses out over the course of the day can help minimize gastrointestinal side effects.

Methimazole (MMI)—MMI may be initially prescribed at doses ranging from 10 to 40 milligrams per day. Once the hyperthyroidism is under control, doses of 5 to 15 milligrams per day are sufficient to control hyperthyroidism in most people.

Propylthiouracil (PTU)—PTU may be initially prescribed at doses ranging from 300 to 600 milligrams per day. Once the hyperthyroidism is under control, doses of 100 to 200 milligrams per day are sufficient to control hyperthyroidism in most people.

Monitoring—Doctors usually monitor the effectiveness of antithyroid drug treatment by checking blood thyroid hormone levels periodically. This monitoring includes measurement of T4, T3, and thyroid-stimulating hormone (TSH) levels. Antithyroid drugs typically reduce levels of both T3 and T4, but levels of T3 may take longer to return to normal in some people. TSH levels usually take the longest to return to normal.

Prolonged Remission

About 30 percent of people who take an antithyroid drug for one to two years will have prolonged remission of Graves disease. It is not known for sure if the antithyroid drug plays an active role in this remission, or if it simply controls hyperthyroidism until spontaneous remission occurs.

Factors Associated with Prolonged Remission

It is not possible to tell for certain which people with Graves disease will achieve prolonged remission with antithyroid drug treatment. However, several factors seem to play a role in prolonged remission.

Antibodies to TSH receptors

People who do not have antibodies to their TSH receptors are more likely to have remission, and disappearance of these antibodies during antithyroid drug treatment is associated with a 70 percent chance of remission.

Other Individual Factors

Remission is more likely in women; in people with mild (versus moderate or severe) hyperthyroidism; in people with a small goiter or with goiters that shrink during treatment; in people over the age of 40 years, and in people with high levels of antibodies to thyroid peroxidase.

Dose of Antithyroid Drug

Studies disagree about the role of the dose of antithyroid drug in promoting prolonged remission. Most studies suggest that small doses are just as effective as large doses in achieving prolonged remission.

Duration of Treatment with an Antithyroid Drug

The likelihood of remission may increase with the duration of treatment. In the United States, doctors currently recommend one to two years of antithyroid drug treatment followed by re-evaluation of the activity of Graves disease, but in some countries remission rates are doubled by prolonged treatment, e.g., 10 years.

Checking for Remission and Recurrence

None of the currently available tests reliably predict remission of Graves disease. Therefore, it is not easy to identify people who no longer need to take antithyroid drug.

Usually, after one to two years of treatment, doctors simply recommend discontinuation of the antithyroid drug, combined with blood tests to monitor for remission or the recurrence of hyperthyroidism. T4, T3, and TSH levels are usually measured two to three weeks after stopping the antithyroid drug and are repeated periodically over six months.

Recurrence is signaled by low levels of TSH; this recurrence can occur within 10 days of stopping antithyroid drug treatment, or it can occur several years later. If levels of T3, T4, and TSH remain normal for six months, the prognosis is good; relapse after this time occurs in only 8 to 10 percent of people.

Side Effects

Most of the side effects of antithyroid drugs are minor, but major side effects can occur. Because there is no way to predict who will experience side effects, it is important to discuss all possible side effects with your doctor before starting treatment.

Minor Side Effects

Up to 15 percent of people who take an antithyroid drug have minor side effects. Both MMI and PTU can cause itching, rash, hives, joint pain and swelling, fever, altered taste sensation, nausea, and vomiting. If one medication causes side effects, your doctor may recommend switching to the other drug. However, half of the people who have side effects with one drug will also have side effects with the other drug. The nausea and vomiting may depend on the amount of drug taken in each dose; therefore, spreading large total daily doses out over the day might reduce these side effects.

Major Side Effects

Fortunately, the major side effects of antithyroid drugs are rare.

Agranulocytosis is characterized by a decrease in the production of white blood cells. This condition is serious, but affects only 0.2 to 0.5 percent of all people who take an antithyroid drug. Elderly people taking PTU and very high doses of MMI may be more susceptible to this side effect.

Agranulocytosis is more likely to occur within the first three months of starting treatment with an antithyroid drug. Doctors recommend that a white blood cell count be done immediately if you have a sore throat, fever, or evidence of any infection.

Once the antithyroid drug is stopped, agranulocytosis usually resolves in a few days, although serious illness and death are possible.

Liver damage: Some people taking antithyroid drugs may develop liver damage. MMI and PTU are about equally likely to cause this side effect, but the type of liver damage seen with PTU can be more serious. Most people recover fully when the drug is stopped.

Aplastic anemia: A rare, but very serious complication associated with the use of an antithyroid drug is aplastic anemia (failure of the bone marrow to produce blood cells).

Vasculitis: Another rare complication, associated primarily with the use of PTU, is vasculitis (inflammation of blood vessels).

References

1. Franklyn, JA. Drug therapy: The management of hyperthyroidism. *N Engl J Med* 1994; 330:1731.

2. Torring, O, Tallstedt, L, Wallin, G, et al. Graves hyperthyroidism: Treatment with antithyroid drugs, surgery, or radioiodine a prospective, randomized study. *J Clin Endocronol Metab* 1996; 81:2986.

3. Vitti, P, Rayo, T, Chiovato, L, et al. Clinical features of patients with Graves disease undergoing remission after antithyroid drug treatment. *Thyroid* 1997; 7:369.

4. Allahabadia, A, Daykin, J, Holder, RL, et al. Age and gender predict the outcome of treatment for Graves hyperthyroidism. *J Clin Endocrinol Me*tab 2000; 85:1038.

Your doctor is the best resource for finding out important information related to your particular case. Not all patients with hyperthyroidism are alike, and it is important that your situation is evaluated by someone who knows you as a whole person.

Additional Information

American Thyroid Association
6066 Leesburg Pike, Suite 550
Falls Church, VA 22041
Toll-Free: 800-THYROID (849-7643)
Phone: 703-998-8890
Fax: 703-998-8893
Website: http://www.thyroid.org
E-mail: admin@thyroid.org

Hormone Foundation
8401 Connecticut Ave., Suite 900
Chevy Chase, MD 20815-5817
Toll-Free: 800-HORMONE (467-6663)
Website: http://www.hormone.org

Thyroid Foundation of America
One Longfellow Place, Suite 1518
Boston, MA 02114
Toll-Free: 800-832-8321
Phone: 617-534-1500
Fax: 617-534-1515
Website: http://www.allthyroid.org
E-mail: info@allthyroid.org

Chapter 47

Thyroiditis: Diagnosis and Management

Thyroiditis refers to a group of inflammatory diseases affecting the thyroid gland (Table 47.1). With the help of historical information, a physical examination and diagnostic tests, physicians can classify the type of thyroiditis and initiate appropriate treatment.

Chronic Lymphocytic Thyroiditis

Chronic lymphocytic thyroiditis (Hashimoto thyroiditis) is the most common inflammatory condition of the thyroid gland and the most common cause of goiter in the United States.[1, 2] It is an autoimmune condition characterized by high titers of circulating antibodies to thyroid peroxidase and thyroglobulin.[3]

Epidemiology

Chronic lymphocytic thyroiditis is the most common cause of hypothyroidism in the United States, and euthyroid persons with Hashimoto disease develop hypothyroidism at a rate of approximately 5 percent per year.[4] Up to 95 percent of cases of chronic lymphocytic thyroiditis occur in women, usually between 30 and 50 years of age.[5] Chronic lymphocytic thyroiditis is also the most common cause of sporadic goiter in children.[5, 6] The incidence of Hashimoto disease has risen exponentially over the past 50 years, and this increase may be related to an increased iodine content in the North American diet.[6]

A genetic predisposition to thyroid autoimmunity exists; it is inherited as a dominant trait.[7] Hashimoto disease has been linked to other autoimmune diseases, including systemic lupus erythematosus, rheumatoid arthritis, pernicious anemia, diabetes mellitus, and Sjögren's syndrome.[5] A rare but serious complication of chronic autoimmune thyroiditis is thyroid lymphoma.[7] These lymphomas, generally the B-cell, non-Hodgkin's type, tend to occur in women 50 to 80 years of age and are usually limited to the thyroid gland.[7]

Clinical Manifestations

Chronic lymphocytic thyroiditis (Hashimoto thyroiditis) is the most common cause of goiter in the United States. Although Hashimoto thyroiditis is usually asymptomatic, some patients may complain of a feeling of tightness or fullness in the neck; however, neck pain and tenderness are rare [6,7] At the time of diagnosis, symptoms of hypothyroidism are present in 20 percent of patients.[6] Physical examination generally reveals a firm, irregular, nontender goiter.[7] The erythrocyte sedimentation rate (ESR) and white blood cell count are normal. The definitive indicator of chronic lymphocytic thyroiditis is the presence of thyroid-specific autoantibodies in the serum. The three main targets for thyroid antibodies are thyroglobulin (a protein carrier for thyroid hormones), thyroid microsomal antigen (also called thyroid peroxidase), and the thyroid-stimulating hormone (TSH) receptor.[7] Low

Table 47.1. Classification of Thyroiditis

Histologic classification	Synonyms
Chronic lymphocytic	Chronic lymphocytic thyroiditis, Hashimoto thyroiditis
Subacute lymphocytic	Subacute lymphocytic thyroiditis: (1) postpartum thyroiditis and (2) sporadic painless thyroiditis
Granulomatous	Subacute granulomatous thyroiditis, de Quervain's thyroiditis
Microbial inflammatory	Suppurative thyroiditis, acute thyroiditis
Invasive fibrous	Riedel's struma, Riedel's thyroiditis

levels of circulating antibodies are common in other thyroid diseases, such as multinodular goiter and thyroid malignancy. Antithyroid microsomal antibodies in titers greater than 1:6,400 or antithyroid peroxidase antibodies in excess of 200 IU per mL, however, are strongly suggestive of chronic autoimmune thyroiditis.[7] Testing of thyroid autoantibodies and measurement of serum thyroglobulin levels will confirm the diagnosis.[7] Radioactive iodine uptake (RAIU) is variable and can be depressed, normal, or increased, depending on the extent of follicular destruction. Patchy uptake is common, providing little diagnostically useful information.[7] Ultrasonography shows an enlarged gland with a diffusely hypoechogenic pattern in most patients.[7] RAIU and thyroid ultrasonography are not necessary parts of the work-up for this disease. A dominant nodule in a patient with Hashimoto disease should prompt a fine-needle aspiration biopsy to exclude malignancy.[7]

Clinical Management

Because thyroiditis is usually asymptomatic and the goiter is small, many patients do not require treatment.[6] When hypothyroidism is present, treatment with thyroxine (T4) is indicated.[7] Thyroid hormone replacement therapy is also indicated in patients with a TSH level in the normal range, to reduce goiter size and prevent progression to overt hypothyroidism in high-risk patients.[7] Lifetime replacement of levothyroxine is indicated in hypothyroid patients, at a starting dosage of 25 to 50 µg per day, with gradual titration to an average daily dosage of 75 to 150 µg. A lower starting dosage (12.5 to 25 µg per day) and a more gradual titration are recommended in elderly patients and in patients with cardiovascular disease. The dosage may be increased in these patients 25 to 50 µg every four to six weeks until the TSH level is normal.[6, 7]

In patients with an elevated TSH level and a normal thyroxine (T4) level (subclinical hypothyroidism), indications for treatment are less clear. If the TSH level is greater than 20 mU per mL (20 mU per L) with a normal T4 level, there is a high probability that the patient will develop hypothyroidism. If the TSH level is elevated but is less than 20 mU per mL and the antimicrosomal antibody titer is greater than 1:1,600, hypothyroidism will develop in 80 percent of patients.[5] Therefore, it is recommended that treatment be initiated in patients with symptoms of hypothyroidism, in patients with a serum TSH level greater than 10 mU per mL (10 mU per L), and in patients with a high risk of progression to hypothyroidism (e.g., those with high antibody titers).[7] Because of the risk of developing hypothyroidism, patients with a history of chronic lymphocytic thyroiditis require annual assessment of thyroid function.[6]

Subacute Lymphocytic Thyroiditis

Subacute lymphocytic thyroiditis occurs most often in the postpartum period, but may also occur sporadically.[7] Therefore, it is subdivided into two groups, postpartum thyroiditis and sporadic painless thyroiditis. Antimicrosomal antibodies are present in 50 to 80 percent of patients, while antithyroid peroxidase antibodies are present in nearly all patients.[3, 6, 7] Subacute lymphocytic thyroiditis starts with an initial hyperthyroid phase, followed by subsequent hypothyroidism, and finally, a return to the euthyroid state. In the postpartum patient, thyrotoxicosis usually develops in the first three months following delivery and lasts for one or two months. Then the patient returns to a euthyroid state or hyperthyroidism ensues for several months.[8] Patients with an initial episode of postpartum subacute lymphocytic thyroiditis have a notably high risk of recurrence in subsequent pregnancies.[1, 6, 9] Serum TSH testing is indicated in symptomatic patients.

Epidemiology

Subacute lymphocytic thyroiditis comprises 29 to 50 percent of all cases of thyroiditis[3] and occurs most often in women between 30 and 50 years of age.[6, 9] There is a higher incidence of antimicrosomal antibodies in the postpartum form (80 percent) of the disease than in the sporadic form (50 percent). A family history of autoimmune thyroid disease is found in 50 percent of patients with the postpartum form of thyroiditis. The severity of the hypothyroid phase correlates directly with the antimicrosomal antibody titer. A titer of 1:1,600 or greater early in pregnancy is associated with a high risk of postpartum hypothyroidism.[10] Approximately 6 percent of patients who have the postpartum form develop chronic hypothyroidism.[6]

Clinical Manifestations

Patients usually present with acute symptoms of hyperthyroidism, such as tachycardia, palpitations, heat intolerance, nervousness, and weight loss.[6, 9] A small painless goiter is present in 50 percent of patients.[6-9] The ESR and white blood cell count are normal. T4 and triiodothyronine (T3) levels are initially elevated, with a disproportionate increase in T4 compared with T3.[9] RAIU is decreased in the hyperthyroid phase of the disease and is almost always less than 3 percent. This situation contrasts markedly with the elevated RAIU found in patients with Graves disease.[3, 5, 8, 9]

Clinical Management

Acute symptoms of hyperthyroidism are managed primarily with beta blockers.[3, 6, 7, 9] Antithyroid drugs, which inhibit the production of new T4, are not indicated in the management of patients with hyperthyroidism because symptoms are caused by the release of pre-formed T3 and T4 from the damaged gland.[6, 9] Replacement of thyroid hormone in the hypothyroid phase is indicated if the patient's symptoms are severe or of long duration.[7] If the hypothyroid phase lasts longer than six months, permanent hypothyroidism is likely.[11]

Subacute Granulomatous Thyroiditis

Subacute granulomatous thyroiditis is the most common cause of a painful thyroid gland.[7] It is most likely caused by a viral infection and is generally preceded by an upper respiratory tract infection.[7] Numerous etiologic agents have been implicated, including mumps virus, echovirus, coxsackievirus, Epstein-Barr virus, influenza, and adenovirus.[3, 7]

Epidemiology

Women are three to five times more likely to be affected than men. The average age of onset is 30 to 50 years.[7] The disorder tends to be geographical and seasonal, occurring most often in the summer and fall.[6, 7] A painful thyroid following an upper respiratory tract infection is usually a sign of subacute granulomatous thyroiditis.

Clinical Manifestations

Subacute granulomatous thyroiditis presents clinically with acute onset of pain in the thyroid region. The pain may be exacerbated by turning the head or swallowing, and may radiate to the jaw, ear, or chest.[3, 5, 6] Symptoms of hypermetabolism may be present, and the ESR usually is markedly elevated.[6, 7] A normal ESR essentially rules out the diagnosis of subacute granulomatous thyroiditis.[7] The thyroid is firm, nodular and exquisitely tender to palpation. The leukocyte count is normal or slightly elevated.[7] Thyrotoxicosis is present in 50 percent of patients in the acute phase, and the serum T4 concentration is disproportionately elevated relative to the T3 level.[7] Serum TSH concentrations are low to undetectable.[7] Thyroglobulin is elevated. A normal thyroglobulin level essentially rules out the diagnosis of subacute granulomatous thyroiditis.[6] The RAIU is notably low, often less than 2 percent at 24 hours.[7] In summary, the physical examination, an elevated ESR, an elevated thyroglobulin level and a depressed RAIU confirm the diagnosis.

Clinical Management

The natural history of subacute granulomatous thyroiditis involves four phases that generally unfold over four to six months. The acute phase of thyroid pain and thyrotoxicosis may last three to six weeks or longer. Transient asymptomatic euthyroidism follows. Hypothyroidism often ensues and may last weeks to months or may be permanent (in up to 5 percent of patients).[5] The final phase is a recovery period, during which thyroid function tests normalize.

Therapy with antithyroid drugs is not indicated in patients with subacute granulomatous thyroiditis because this disorder is caused by the release of preformed thyroid hormone rather than synthesis of new T3 and T4.[6, 7] Therapy with beta blockers may be indicated for the symptomatic treatment of thyrotoxicosis. Nonsteroidal anti-inflammatory drugs are generally effective in reducing thyroid pain in patients with mild cases. Patients with more severe disease require a tapering dosage of prednisone (20 to 40 mg per day) given over two to four weeks.[3] Up to 20 percent of patients experience the recurrence of thyroid pain on discontinuation of prednisone.[7] RAIU can assist clinicians in determining patients at high risk for relapse. Low RAIU uptake implies ongoing inflammation, and steroid therapy should be continued.[3]

Microbial Inflammatory Thyroiditis

Microbial inflammatory thyroiditis, also known as acute suppurative thyroiditis, is a rare subtype most often caused by the presence of Gram-positive bacteria in the thyroid gland. Staphylococcus aureus is the most common infectious agent,[7] but other organisms have also been implicated. This disorder is rare because of the inherent resistance of the thyroid gland to infection. Microbial inflammatory thyroiditis occurs most often in women 20 to 40 years of age.[5, 9] Most patients have a preexisting thyroid disorder, usually nodular goiter.[3, 5, 9] Anterior neck pain and tenderness are common. Other clinical features include fever,

Table 47.2. Clinical Manifestations of Thyroiditis Subtypes

Subtype	Etiology	Neck pain	RAIU*	TSH*	T4*	Thyroid autoanti-bodies
Chronic lymphocytic (Hashimoto disease)	Autoimmune	No	Variable	Variable	Variable	Present
Subacute granulomatous	Viral	Yes	Decreased	Decreased	Increased	Absent
Subacute lymphocytic	Autoimmune	No	Decreased	Decreased	Increased	Present
Microbial inflammatory	Bacterial, fungal, parasitic	Yes	Variable	Normal	Normal	Absent
Hashitoxicosis	Autoimmune	No	Decreased	Decreased	Increased	Present
Invasive fibrous	Unknown	No	Variable	Normal	Normal	Variable

*RAIU = radioactive iodine uptake; TSH = thyroid-stimulating hormone; T4 = thyroxine.

pharyngitis, and dermal erythema.[5, 9] The pain is typically worse during swallowing and radiates locally.[5, 9, 12] Tachycardia is common, along with leukocytosis and an elevated ESR level.[3, 5, 9, 12] TSH, T4 and T3 levels are typically normal, while RAIU may be normal or show cold nodules in areas of abscess formation.[5, 9, 13] The cause of infection is first determined by culture and sensitivity of samples obtained through fine-needle aspiration.

When the cause of the infection is determined, appropriate parenteral antibiotics should be prescribed.[5, 9, 12] Patients with abscesses require surgical drainage, and possibly, a thyroid lobectomy.[5, 9, 12] Heat, rest, and aspirin provide symptomatic relief; steroids may offer additional benefit.[13] The disease is usually self-limited, lasting weeks to months.[13]

Invasive Fibrous Thyroiditis

First described by Riedel in 1898, this remains the rarest type of thyroiditis. In addition to the development of dense fibrosis of the thyroid gland itself, extra-cervical sites of fibrosis frequently occur as inflammatory fibrosclerotic processes, including sclerosing cholangitis, retroperitoneal fibrosis, and orbital pseudotumor.[9, 14, 15] Studies suggest that one-third of patients with fibrous thyroiditis develop multifocal fibrosclerosis.[14, 16] The mean age at presentation is 47.8 years, and 83 percent of all cases occur in females.[16] A stone-hard or woody mass that extends from the thyroid is common.[9, 14-16] Symptoms vary according to the structures involved and most commonly result from a thyroid mass that produces dyspnea, dysphagia, and occasionally, stridor.[9, 12, 14, 16] The thyroid mass may grow suddenly or slowly, and is usually unilateral.[14]

RAIU is decreased in affected areas of the gland.[12, 15] Most patients remain euthyroid, and the ESR is frequently elevated.[5, 9,14, 16] Thyroid autoantibodies are present in appreciable quantities in 45 percent of patients.[5, 9, 14, 16] Because of the similarity between fibrous thyroiditis and thyroid carcinoma, diagnosis must be made using open biopsy.[5, 9, 12, 14] The disease is usually self-limited, with surgical wedge resection of the thyroid isthmus being the mainstay of treatment in symptomatic patients.[5, 9, 12, 14]

Final Comment

Thyroiditis is a heterogeneous disease with several subtypes. These subtypes mimic other diseases as well as each other. Differentiation of the subtypes of thyroiditis requires an understanding of their unique clinical presentations, radiologic studies, laboratory data, and indications for pharmacotherapy.

References

1. Hamburger JI. The various presentations of thyroiditis. Diagnostic considerations. *Ann Intern Med* 1986;104:219-24.

2. Hay ID. Thyroiditis: a clinical update. *Mayo Clin Proc* 1985;60:836-43.

3. Farwell AP, Braverman LE. Inflammatory thyroid disorders. *Otolaryngol Clin North Am* 1996;29: 541-56.

4. Nagataki S. The concept of Hashimoto disease. In: Nagataki S, Mori T, Torizuka K, eds. Eighty years of Hashimoto disease. Amsterdam: *Elsevier Science*, 1993:539-45.

5. Sakiyama R. Thyroiditis: a clinical review. *Am Fam Physician* 1993;48:615-21.

6. Schubert MF, Kountz DS. Thyroiditis: a disease with many faces. *Postgrad Med* 1995;98:101-12.

7. Dayan CM, Daniels GH. Chronic autoimmune thyroiditis. *N Engl J Med* 1996;335:99-107.

8. Roti E, Emerson CH. Clinical review 29: postpartum thyroiditis. *J Clin Endocrinol Metab* 1992;74:3-5.

9. Singer PA: Thyroiditis: Acute, subacute, and chronic. *Med Clin North Am* 1991;75:61-77.

10. Jansson R, Bernander S, Karlsson A, Levin K, Nilsson G. Autoimmune thyroid dysfunction in the postpartum period. *J Clin Endocrinol Metab* 1984;58:681-7.

11. Braverman LE, Utiger RD, eds. Werner and Ingbar's *The thyroid: a fundamental and clinical text. 7ᵗʰ ed*. Philadelphia: Lippincott-Raven, 1997:583.

12. Levine SN. Current concepts of thyroiditis. *Arch Intern Med* 1983;143:1952-6.

13. Szabo SM, Allen DB. Thyroiditis: Differentiation of acute suppurative and subacute. *Clin Pediatr* [Phila] 1989;28:171-3.

14. Malotte MS, Chonkich GD, Zuppan CW. Riedel's thyroiditis. *Arch Otolaryngol Head Neck Surg* 1991;117:214-7.

15. Lange WE, Freling NJ, Molenaar WM, Doorenbos H. Invasive fibrous thyroiditis (Riedel's struma): a manifestation of multifocal fibrosclerosis? *Q J Med* 1989;72:709-717.

16. Schwaegerle SM, Bauer TW, Esselstyn CB Jr. Riedel's thyroiditis. *Am J Clin Pathol* 1988;90:715-22.

Chapter 48

Radiation Therapy

Radiation therapy may vary somewhat among different doctors, hospitals, and treatment centers. Therefore, your treatment or the advice of your doctor (the radiation oncologist) may be different from what you read here. Be sure to ask questions and discuss your concerns with your doctor, nurse, or radiation therapist. Ask whether they have any additional written information that might help you.

Facts about Radiation Therapy

- Radiation treatments are painless.
- External radiation treatment does not make you radioactive.
- Treatments are usually scheduled every day except Saturday and Sunday.
- You need to allow 30 minutes for each treatment session although the treatment itself takes only a few minutes.
- It is important to get plenty of rest and to eat a well-balanced diet during the course of your radiation therapy.
- Skin in the treated area may become sensitive and easily irritated.

Excerpted from "Radiation Therapy and You: A Guide to Self-Help during Cancer Treatment," National Cancer Institute (NCI), updated September 22, 1999. Reviewed in December 2004 by David A. Cooke, M.D., Diplomate, America Board of Internal Medicine.

- Side effects of radiation treatment are usually temporary, and they vary depending on the area of the body that is being treated.

What Is Radiation Therapy?

Radiation therapy (sometimes called radiotherapy, x-ray therapy, or irradiation) is the treatment of disease using penetrating beams of high energy waves or streams of particles called radiation.

Many years ago doctors learned how to use this energy to see inside the body and find disease. You have probably seen a chest x-ray or x-ray pictures of your teeth or your bones. At high doses (many times those used for x-ray exams), radiation is used to treat cancer and other illnesses.

The radiation used for cancer treatment comes from special machines or from radioactive substances. Radiation therapy equipment aims specific amounts of the radiation at tumors or areas of the body where there is disease.

How Does Radiation Therapy Work?

Radiation in high doses kills cells or keeps them from growing and dividing. Because cancer cells grow and divide more rapidly than most of the normal cells around them, radiation therapy can successfully treat many kinds of cancer. Normal cells are also affected by radiation, but unlike cancer cells, most of them recover from the effects of radiation.

To protect normal cells, doctors carefully limit the doses of radiation and spread the treatment out over time. They also shield as much normal tissue as possible while they aim the radiation at the site of the cancer.

What Are the Goals and Benefits of Radiation Therapy?

The goal of radiation therapy is to kill the cancer cells with as little risk as possible to normal cells. Radiation therapy can be used to treat many kinds of cancer in almost any part of the body. In fact, more than half of all people with cancer are treated with some form of radiation. For many cancer patients, radiation is the only kind of treatment they need. Thousands of people who have had radiation therapy alone or in combination with other types of cancer treatment are free of cancer.

Radiation treatment, like surgery, is a local treatment—it affects the cancer cells only in a specific area of the body. Sometimes doctors add radiation therapy to treatments that reach all parts of the body (systemic treatment), such as chemotherapy or biological therapy, to improve treatment results. You may hear your doctor use the term, adjuvant therapy, for a treatment that is added to, and given after, the primary therapy.

Radiation therapy is often used with surgery to treat cancer. Doctors may use radiation before surgery to shrink a tumor. This makes it easier to remove the cancerous tissue, and may allow the surgeon to perform less radical surgery.

Radiation therapy may be used after surgery to stop the growth of cancer cells that may remain. Your doctor may choose to use radiation therapy and surgery at the same time.

In some cases, instead of surgery, doctors use radiation along with anticancer drugs (chemotherapy) to destroy the cancer. Radiation may be given before, during, or after chemotherapy. Doctors carefully tailor this combination treatment to each patient's needs depending on the type of cancer, its location, and its size. The purpose of radiation treatment before or during chemotherapy is to make the tumor smaller and thus improve the effectiveness of the anticancer drugs. Doctors sometimes recommend that a patient complete chemotherapy, and then have radiation treatment to kill any cancer cells that might remain. When curing the cancer is not possible, radiation therapy can be used to shrink tumors and reduce pressure, pain, and other symptoms of cancer. This is called palliative care or palliation. Many cancer patients find that they have a better quality of life when radiation is used for this purpose.

What Are the Risks of Radiation Therapy?

The brief high doses of radiation that damage or destroy cancer cells can also injure or kill normal cells. These effects of radiation on normal cells cause treatment side effects. Most side effects of radiation treatment are well known, and with the help of your doctor and nurse, easily treated.

The risk of side effects is usually less than the benefit of killing cancer cells. Your doctor will not advise you to have any treatment unless the benefits—control of disease and relief from symptoms—are greater than the known risks.

How Is Radiation Therapy Given?

Radiation therapy can be given in one of two ways: external or internal. Some patients have both, one after the other.

Most people who receive radiation therapy for cancer have external radiation. It is usually given during outpatient visits to a hospital or treatment center. In external radiation therapy, a machine directs the high-energy rays at the cancer and a small margin of normal tissue surrounding it.

The various machines used for external radiation work in slightly different ways. Some are better for treating cancers near the skin surface; others work best on cancers deeper in the body. The most common type of machine used for radiation therapy is called a linear accelerator. Some radiation machines use a variety of radioactive substances (such as cobalt-60, for example) as the source of high-energy rays. Your doctor decides which type of radiation therapy machine is best for you..

When internal radiation therapy is used, the radiation source is placed inside the body. This method of radiation treatment is called brachytherapy or implant therapy. The source of the radiation (such as radioactive iodine, for example) sealed in a small holder is called an implant. Implants may be thin wires, plastic tubes (catheters), capsules, or seeds. An implant may be placed directly into a tumor or inserted into a body cavity. Sometimes, after a tumor has been removed by surgery, the implant is placed in the tumor bed—the area from which the tumor was removed—to kill any tumor cells that may remain.

Another type of internal radiation therapy uses unsealed radioactive materials which may be taken by mouth or injected into the body. If you have this type of treatment, you may need to stay in the hospital for several days.

Who Gives Radiation Treatments?

A doctor who specializes in using radiation to treat cancer—a radiation oncologist—will prescribe the type and amount of treatment that is right for you. The radiation oncologist is the person referred to as "your doctor" throughout this chapter. The radiation oncologist works closely with the other doctors and health care professionals involved in your care. This highly trained health care team may include:

- The radiation physicist, who makes sure that the equipment is working properly and that the machines deliver the right dose of radiation. The physicist also works closely with your doctor to plan your treatment.

- The dosimetrist, who works under the direction of your doctor and the radiation physicist, and helps carry out your treatment plan by calculating the amount of radiation to be delivered to the cancer and normal tissues that are nearby.

- The radiation therapist, who positions you for your treatments and runs the equipment that delivers the radiation.

- The radiation nurse, who will coordinate your care, help you learn about treatment, and tell you how to manage side effects. The nurse can also answer questions you or family members may have about your treatment.

Your health care team also may include a physician assistant, radiologist, dietitian, radiation oncologist, physical therapist, social worker, or other health care professional.

Is Radiation Treatment Expensive?

Treatment of cancer with radiation can be costly. It requires very complex equipment and the services of many health care professionals. The exact cost of your radiation therapy will depend on the type and number of treatments you need.

Most health insurance policies, including Part B of Medicare, cover charges for radiation therapy. It is a good idea to talk with your doctor's office staff or the hospital business office about your policy and how expected costs will be paid.

In some states, the Medicaid program may help you pay for treatments. You can find out from the office that handles social services in your city or county whether you are eligible for Medicaid and whether your radiation therapy is a covered expense.

If you need financial aid, contact the hospital social service office or the National Cancer Institute's (NCI) Cancer Information Service at 1-800-4-CANCER. They may be able to direct you to sources of help.

How Long Does the Treatment Take?

For most types of cancer, radiation therapy usually is given 5 days a week for 6 or 7 weeks. (When radiation is used for palliative care, the course of treatment is shorter, usually 2 to 3 weeks.) The total dose of radiation and the number of treatments you need will depend on the size, location, and kind of cancer you have, your general health, and other medical treatments you may be receiving.

471

Using many small doses of daily radiation rather than a few large doses helps protect normal body tissues in the treatment area. Weekend rest breaks allow normal cells to recover.

It is very important that you have all of your scheduled treatments to get the most benefit from your therapy. Missing or delaying treatments can lessen the effectiveness of your radiation treatment.

What Happens during the Treatment Visits?

Before each treatment, you may need to change into a hospital gown or robe. It is best to wear clothing that is easy to take off and put on again.

In the treatment room, the radiation therapist will use the marks on your skin to locate the treatment area and to position you correctly. You may sit in a special chair or lie down on a treatment table. For each external radiation therapy session, you will be in the treatment room about 15 to 30 minutes, but you will be getting radiation for only about 1 to 5 minutes of that time. Receiving external radiation treatments is painless, just like having an x-ray taken. You will not hear, see, or smell the radiation.

The radiation therapist may put special shields (or blocks) between the machine and certain parts of your body to help protect normal tissues and organs. There might also be plastic or plaster forms that help you stay in exactly the right place. You need to remain very still during the treatment so that the radiation reaches only the area where it is needed and the same area is treated each time. You do not have to hold your breath—just breathe normally.

The radiation therapist will leave the treatment room before your treatment begins. The radiation machine is controlled from a nearby area. You will be watched on a television screen or through a window in the control room. Although you may feel alone, keep in mind that the therapist can see and hear you and even talk with you using an intercom in the treatment room. If you should feel ill or very uncomfortable during the treatment, tell your therapist at once. The machine can be stopped at any time.

The machines used for radiation treatments are very large, and they make noises as they move around your body to aim at the treatment area from different angles. Their size and motion may be frightening at first. Remember that the machines are being moved and controlled by your radiation therapist. They are checked constantly to be sure they are working right. If you have concerns about anything that happens in the treatment room, discuss these concerns with the radiation therapist.

What Are the Side Effects of Treatment?

External radiation therapy does not cause your body to become radioactive. There is no need to avoid being with other people because you are undergoing treatment. Even hugging, kissing, or having sexual relations with others poses no risk of radiation exposure.

Most side effects of radiation therapy are related to the area that is being treated. Many patients have no side effects at all. Your doctor and nurse will tell you about the possible side effects you might expect, and how you should deal with them. You should contact your doctor or nurse if you have any unusual symptoms during your treatment, such as coughing, sweating, fever, or pain.

The side effects of radiation therapy, although unpleasant, are usually not serious and can be controlled with medication or diet. They usually go away within a few weeks after treatment ends, although some side effects can last longer. Always check with your doctor or nurse about how you should deal with side effects.

Throughout your treatment, your doctor will regularly check on the effects of the treatment. You may not be aware of changes in the cancer, but you probably will notice decreases in pain, bleeding, or other discomfort. You may continue to notice further improvement after your treatment is completed.

Your doctor may recommend periodic tests and physical exams to be sure that the radiation is causing as little damage to normal cells as possible. Depending on the area being treated, you may have routine blood tests to check the levels of red blood cells, white blood cells, platelets; radiation treatment can cause decreases in the levels of different blood cells.

What Can I Do To Take Care of Myself During Therapy?

Each patient's body responds to radiation therapy in its own way. That is why your doctor must plan, and sometimes adjust, your treatment. In addition, your doctor or nurse will give you suggestions for caring for yourself at home that are specific for your treatment and the possible side effects. Nearly all cancer patients receiving radiation therapy need to take special care to protect their health and to help the treatment succeed.

473

- Before starting treatment, be sure your doctor knows about any medicines you are taking and if you have any allergies. Do not start taking any medicine (whether prescription or over-the-counter) during your radiation therapy without first telling your doctor or nurse.

- Fatigue is common during radiation therapy. Your body will use a lot of extra energy over the course of your treatment, and you may feel very tired. Be sure to get plenty of rest and sleep as often as you feel the need. It is common for fatigue to last for 4 to 6 weeks after your treatment has been completed.

- Good nutrition is very important. Try to eat a balanced diet that will prevent weight loss.

- Check with your doctor before taking vitamin supplements or herbal preparations during treatment.

- Avoid wearing tight clothes such as girdles or close-fitting collars over the treatment area.

- Be extra kind to your skin in the treatment area:

  - Ask your doctor or nurse if you may use soaps, lotions, deodorants, sun blocks, medicines, perfumes, cosmetics, talcum powder, or other substances in the treated area.

  - Wear loose, soft cotton clothing over the treated area.

  - Do not wear starched or stiff clothing over the treated area.

  - Do not scratch, rub, or scrub treated skin.

  - Do not use adhesive tape on treated skin. If bandaging is necessary, use paper tape and apply it outside of the treatment area. Your nurse can help you place dressings so that you can avoid irritating the treated area.

  - Do not apply heat or cold (heating pad, ice pack, etc.) to the treated area. Use only lukewarm water for bathing the area.

  - Use an electric shaver if you must shave the treated area, but only after checking with your doctor or nurse. Do not use a pre-shave lotion or hair removal products on the treated area.

  - Protect the treatment area from the sun. Do not apply sunscreens just before a radiation treatment. If possible, cover treated skin (with light clothing) before going outside. Ask your doctor if you should use a sunscreen product. If so, select one with a protection factor of at least 15 and reapply it often. Ask your doctor or nurse how long after your treatments are completed you should continue to protect the treated skin from sunlight.

• If you have questions, ask your doctor or nurse. They are the only ones who can properly advise you about your treatment, its side effects, home care, and any other medical concerns you may have.

Managing Side Effects: Are Side Effects the Same for Everyone?

The side effects of radiation treatment vary from patient to patient. You may have no side effects or only a few mild ones through your course of treatment. Some people do experience serious side effects, however. The side effects that you have depend mostly on the radiation dose and the part of your body that is treated. Your general health also can affect how your body reacts to radiation therapy and whether you have side effects. Before beginning your treatment, your doctor and nurse will discuss the side effects you might experience, how long they might last, and how serious they might be.

Side effects may be acute or chronic. Acute side effects are sometimes referred to as early side effects. They occur soon after the treatment begins and usually are gone within a few weeks of finishing therapy. Chronic side effects, sometimes called late side effects, may take months or years to develop and usually are permanent.

The most common early side effects of radiation therapy are fatigue and skin changes. They can result from radiation to any treatment site. Other side effects are related to treatment of specific areas. For example, temporary or permanent hair loss may be a side effect of radiation treatment to the head. Appetite can be altered if treatment affects the mouth, stomach, or intestine.

Be sure to tell your doctor, nurse, or radiation therapist about any side effects that you notice. They can help you treat the problems and tell you how to lessen the chances that the side effects will come back.

What Side Effects Occur with Radiation Therapy to the Head and Neck?

Some people who receive radiation to the head and neck experience redness, irritation, and sores in the mouth; a dry mouth or thickened saliva; difficulty in swallowing; changes in taste; or nausea. Try not to let these symptoms keep you from eating.

Other problems that may occur during treatment to the head and neck are a loss of taste, which may diminish appetite and affect nutrition, and earaches (caused by hardening of ear wax). You may notice some swelling or drooping of the skin under your chin as well as changes in the skin texture. Your jaw may also feel stiff and you may be unable to open your mouth as wide as before treatment. Jaw exercises may help ease this problem. Report all side effects to your doctor or nurse, and ask what you should do about them.

If you are receiving radiation therapy to the head or neck, you need to take especially good care of your teeth, gums, mouth, and throat. Side effects from treatment to these areas commonly involve the mouth, which may be sore and dry. Here are a few tips that may help you manage mouth problems:

- Avoid spices and coarse foods such as raw vegetables, dry crackers, and nuts.

- Remember that acidic foods and liquids can cause mouth and throat irritation.

- Do not smoke, chew tobacco, or drink alcohol.

- Stay away from sugary snacks because they can promote tooth decay.

- Clean your mouth and teeth often, using the method your dentist or doctor recommends.

- Use only alcohol-free mouthwash; many commercial mouthwashes contain alcohol which has a drying effect on mouth tissues.

Mouth Care

Radiation treatment for head and neck cancer can increase your chances of getting cavities in your teeth. Mouth care designed to prevent problems will be a very important part of your treatment. Before starting radiation therapy, make an appointment for a complete dental/oral checkup. Ask your dentist and radiation oncologist to consult before your radiation treatments begin.

Your dentist probably will want to see you often during your radiation therapy to help you care for your mouth and teeth. This is a good way to reduce the risk of tooth decay and help you deal with possible problems such as soreness of the tissues in your mouth. It's important that you follow the dentist's advice while you're receiving radiation therapy. Most likely, your dentist will suggest that you:

- Clean your teeth and gums thoroughly with a soft brush at least 4 times a day (after meals and at bedtime).

- Use a fluoride toothpaste that contains no abrasives.

- Floss gently between teeth daily if you flossed regularly before your illness. Use waxed, non-shredding dental floss.

- Rinse your mouth gently and frequently with a salt and baking soda solution especially after you brush. Use ½ teaspoon of salt and ½ teaspoon of baking soda in a large glass of warm water. Follow with a plain water rinse.

- Apply fluoride regularly as prescribed by your dentist.

Your dentist can explain how to mix the salt and baking soda mouthwash and how to use the fluoride treatment method that best suits your needs. You can probably get printed instructions for proper dental care at the dentist's office. If dry mouth continues after your treatment is complete, you will need to continue the mouth care recommended during treatment. Always share your dentist's instructions with your radiation nurse.

Dealing with Mouth or Throat Problems

Soreness in your mouth or throat may appear in the second or third week of external radiation therapy, and it will most likely have disappeared within a month or so after your treatments have ended. You may have trouble swallowing during this time because your mouth feels dry. Your doctor or dentist can prescribe medicine for mouth discomfort, and tell you about methods to relieve other mouth problems during and following your radiation therapy. If you wear dentures, you may notice that they no longer fit well. This occurs if the radiation causes your gums to swell. You may need to stop wearing your dentures until your radiation therapy is over. It is important not to risk denture-induced gum sores because they may become infected and heal slowly.

Your salivary glands may produce less saliva than usual, making your mouth feel dry. Unfortunately dry mouth may continue to be a problem even after treatment is over. You may be given medication to help lessen this side effect. It is helpful to sip cool drinks throughout the day. Although many radiation therapy patients have said that drinking carbonated beverages helps relieve dry mouth, water probably is your best choice. In the morning, fill a large container with ice, add water, and carry it with you during the day so that you can take frequent sips. Keep a glass of cool water at your bedside at night, too. Sugar-free candy or gum also may help; be careful about overuse of these products as they can cause diarrhea in some people. Avoid tobacco and alcoholic drinks because they tend to dry and irritate your mouth tissues. Moisten food with gravies and sauces to make eating easier. If these measures are not enough, ask your dentist, radiation oncologist, or nurse about products that either replace or stimulate your own saliva. Artificial saliva and medication to increase saliva production are available.

Tips on Eating

You may find that it is difficult or painful to swallow. Some patients say that they feel as if something is stuck in their throat. Soreness or dryness in your mouth or throat can also make it hard to eat. The section on eating problems may be helpful. In addition, some of the following tips may help to make eating more comfortable:

- Choose foods that taste good to you and are easy to eat.
- Try changing the consistency of foods by adding fluids and using sauces and gravies to make them softer.
- Avoid highly spiced foods and textures that are dry and rough, such as crackers.
- Eat small meals, and eat more frequently than usual.
- Cut your food into small, bite-sized pieces.
- Ask your doctor for special liquid medicines to reduce the pain in your throat so that you can eat and swallow more easily.
- Ask your doctor about liquid food supplements that are easier to swallow than solids. They can help you get enough calories each day to avoid losing weight.
- If you are being treated for lung cancer, it's important to keep mucus and other secretions thin and manageable; drinking extra fluids can help.
- If familiar foods no longer taste good, try new foods and use different methods of food preparation. Additional helpful suggestions

can be found in the National Cancer Institute's booklet, "Eating Hints for Cancer Patients."

Follow-Up Care

Once you have completed your radiation treatments, it is important for your doctor to monitor the results of your therapy at regularly scheduled visits. These checkups are necessary to deal with radiation side effects and to detect any signs of recurrent disease. During these checkups your doctor will examine you and may order some lab tests and x-rays. The radiation oncologist also will want to see you for follow-up after your treatment ends and will coordinate follow-up care with your doctor. Follow-up care might include more cancer treatment, rehabilitation, and counseling. Taking good care of yourself is also an important part of following through after radiation treatments.

How Can I Help Myself after Radiation Therapy?

Patients who have had radiation therapy need to continue some of the special care they used during treatment, at least for a short while. For instance, you may have skin problems for several weeks after your treatments end. Continue to be gentle with skin in the treatment area until all signs of irritation are gone. Do not try to scrub off the marks in your treatment area. If tattoos were used to mark the treatment area, they are permanent and will not wash off. Your nurse can answer questions about skin care, and help you with other concerns you may have after your treatment has been completed.

You may find that you still need extra rest after your therapy is over while your healthy tissues are recovering and rebuilding. Keep taking naps as needed and try to get more sleep at night. It may take some time to get your strength back, so resume your normal schedule of activities gradually. If you feel that you need emotional or social support, ask your doctor, nurse, or a social worker for information about support groups or other ways to express your feelings and concerns.

When Should I Call the Doctor?

After treatment for cancer, you are likely to be more aware of your body and to notice even slight changes in how you feel from day to day. The doctor will want to know if you are having any unusual symptoms. Promptly tell your doctor about:

- A pain that does not go away, especially if it is always in the same place.
- New or unusual lumps, bumps, or swelling.
- Nausea, vomiting, diarrhea, or loss of appetite.
- Unexplained weight loss.
- A fever or cough that does not go away.
- Unusual rashes, bruises, or bleeding.
- Any symptoms that you are concerned about.
- Any other warning signs mentioned by your doctor or nurse.

Additional Information

National Cancer Institute
6116 Executive Blvd., MSC8322
Bethesda, MD 20892-8322
Toll-Free: 800-4-CANCER (800-422-6237)
Toll-Free TTY: 800-332-8615
Website: http://www.cancer.gov
E-mail: cancergovstaff@mail.nih.gov

Chapter 49

Radioiodine Therapy

What Is Radioiodine Therapy?

If you have an overactive thyroid gland or have been diagnosed with thyroid cancer, your endocrinologist may prescribe radioactive iodine (radioiodine) as part of your overall treatment. You, your family, and your coworkers may have some questions about this therapy.

Background

The thyroid gland produces hormones that regulate the body's metabolism. In order to produce these hormones, the thyroid gland requires large amounts of iodine, which is found in seafood, table salt, bread, and various other foods. Iodine is an essential ingredient in the creation of thyroid hormone. Each molecule of thyroid hormone contains either 4 (T4) or 3 (T3) molecules of iodine. Most overactive thyroid glands are quite hungry for iodine, and it was discovered in the 1940s that the diseased thyroid could be tricked into destroying itself by simply feeding it radioactive iodine. Your endocrinologist can also use radioiodine to treat some types of thyroid cancer. Fortunately, the radioiodine treatment itself will not cause you to feel bad, and very little radiation exposure occurs to the rest of the body.

Radioiodine has been used for more than 50 years in the treatment of thyroid diseases with remarkably few undesirable effects. However,

"Radioiodine Therapy: Information for Patients," © 2004 American Association of Clinical Endocrinologists. Reprinted with permission.

problems may rarely occur when very large doses are given, including decrease in taste sensation and irritation of the salivary glands, the gastrointestinal tract, or the urinary bladder. No increase has been seen in either the occurrence of malignant tumors in patients treated with radioiodine or the number of birth defects in children born later to women who have received this type of treatment.

Hyperthyroidism (Overactive Thyroid)

Before the development of current treatment options, the death rate from hyperthyroidism was as high as 50%. Now several effective treatments (antithyroid drugs, surgery, and radioiodine) are available, and death from hyperthyroidism is rare. Deciding which treatment is best depends on what caused the hyperthyroidism, its severity, and other conditions present. Endocrinologists are experienced in the management of thyroid diseases and can confidently diagnose the cause of hyperthyroidism, and prescribe and manage the best treatment program for each patient.

In the 50+ years, and hundreds of thousands of patients (including a former President of the United States and his wife), in which radioiodine has been used, no serious complications have been reported. Since the treatment appears to be extraordinarily safe, simple, and reliably effective, it is considered by most thyroid specialists in the United States to be the treatment of choice for those types of hyperthyroidism caused by overproduction of thyroid hormones.

Radioactive iodine is given by mouth, usually in capsule form, and is quickly absorbed from the bowel. It then enters the thyroid cells from the bloodstream and gradually destroys them. Although the radioactivity from this treatment is largely gone from the body within a few days, its effect on the thyroid gland usually takes between 1 and 3 months to develop, and maximal benefit is usually noted within 3 to 6 months.

It is not possible to reliably destroy part but not all of the diseased thyroid gland, since the effects of the radioiodine are slowly progressive on the thyroid cells. Therefore, most endocrinologists strive to completely destroy the diseased thyroid gland with a single dose of radioiodine. This results in the intentional development of an underactive thyroid state (hypothyroidism), which is easily, predictably, and inexpensively corrected by lifelong daily use of oral thyroid hormone replacement therapy. Although every effort is made to calculate the correct dose of radioiodine for each patient, not every treatment will successfully correct the hyperthyroidism, particularly if the goiter is quite large, in which case a second dose of radioiodine is occasionally needed.

Thyroid Cancer

The two most common types of thyroid cancer (papillary and follicular) can usually be treated with radioiodine because the cells are able to take up some iodine. Radioiodine is used in treating thyroid cancer in the following 2 general situations:

After Removal of the Thyroid

An experienced thyroid surgeon can remove most of the thyroid with a very low risk of surgical complications, and radioiodine can be used to destroy the remainder of the gland, since it might harbor additional microscopic clusters of cancer cells. In that case, you will be advised not to use thyroid hormone replacement for several weeks after the operation, in order to allow the thyroid levels to drop below normal. This will lead to maximal stimulation of the remaining thyroid cells to concentrate iodine and be destroyed when you receive a dose of radioiodine. This treatment significantly reduces the possibility of recurrent cancer in whatever thyroid tissue is left, and also improves the ability to detect and treat any future cancer recurrences that might develop.

During Follow-Up

All patients with thyroid cancer should have regular follow-up examinations by an endocrinologist. Additional doses of radioactive iodine may be recommended if thyroid cancer remains (which is called persistent) or reappears later (which is called recurrent). Your thyroid hormone replacement therapy will need to be stopped long enough to allow you to become hypothyroid, so that maximum response to the treatment will occur.

Patients with residual thyroid cancer in the neck or known distant metastatic (spreading) tumors can undergo a scan with a test amount of radioiodine. Scanning with radioiodine helps to determine the extent of persistent or recurrent thyroid cancer, whether it may respond to additional doses of radioactive iodine, and how much radioactive iodine to use for treatment. If any iodine is concentrated in the areas of the thyroid cancer, another dose of radioiodine can be given to try to destroy the tumor. This treatment is safe, well tolerated, and has successfully cured most cases of thyroid cancer even after the tumor has spread.

What happens to the radioiodine after a treatment?

Since surgery removes the vast majority of thyroid tissue, much of the radioiodine will not be absorbed and will leave the body primarily through the urine. Small amounts will also be excreted in saliva, sweat, tears, vaginal secretions, and feces. Nearly all the radioactive iodine will leave the body during the first 2 days after the dose has been given. Traces may still be present in the urine and blood for up to 1 week. Therefore, for the safety of laboratory workers, you may be advised not to have any blood or urine testing during this period.

What about breastfeeding during treatment?

Small amounts of radioactive iodine will also be excreted in breast milk. Therefore, since radioiodine could permanently damage the infants' thyroid, breastfeeding is not allowed.

- **Important:** Radioactive iodine treatment should never be given intentionally to a pregnant woman.

If radioiodine is inadvertently administered to a woman who is subsequently discovered to be pregnant, the advisability of terminating the pregnancy should be discussed with the patients' obstetrician and endocrinologist.

Are future pregnancies possible?

For safety's sake, male and female patients are advised to avoid fathering a child or becoming pregnant for several months after radioiodine treatment. This is because a theoretical risk to a developing fetus exists, even though the amount of radioactivity retained may be small, and there is no medical proof of an actual risk from radioiodine treatment. Such a precaution would essentially eliminate direct fetal exposure to radioactivity and markedly reduce the possibility of conception with sperm that might theoretically have been damaged by exposure to radioiodine. You may need to contact your physician for guidance about methods of contraception.

Regulations regarding the use of radioiodine therapy are made by the U.S. Nuclear Regulatory Commission (NRC). Physicians and hospitals that administer this therapy must have a license to administer radioiodine, and must adhere to stringent regulations regarding its use. If you have any questions before or after receiving your treatment, please do not hesitate to contact your physician or your hospital radiation safety officer for clarification.

Is hospitalization necessary for treatment with radioiodine?

Treatment for hyperthyroidism is almost always done on an outpatient basis because the dose required is relatively small in comparison with the doses typically used for treatment of thyroid cancer. If you have to take a larger dose of radioiodine for treatment of thyroid cancer, you may need to be admitted to the hospital for several days depending on your living environment, state of residence, and local practice patterns.

If you require hospitalization, your hospital room will have frequently handled items (such as the television control, table, phone, faucet handles, etc.), covered with protective material, and the floor will be partially covered. These precautions have nothing to do with you, but are merely designed to prevent the radioactive iodine from contaminating those items that will be reused by other patients after your dismissal from the hospital. To limit the contamination of your personal items, you should bring a minimal amount of belongings for your stay. All items will be monitored at your dismissal. Clothing should be limited to what you wear when you are admitted. You should use hospital gowns during your stay. Paperback books, magazines, and newspapers are preferred to hardback books, work papers, and craft items. Check with your endocrinologist about any other issues.

Recommendations for Reduction of Exposure to Others

For several days after treatment:

- Use private toilet facilities, if possible; flush twice after each use.
- Bathe daily and wash hands frequently.
- Drink normal amount of fluids.
- Use disposable eating utensils or wash your utensils separately from others.
- Sleep alone and avoid prolonged intimate contact.
- Launder your linens, towels, and clothes daily at home separately from others. No special cleaning of the washing machine is required between loads.
- Do not prepare food for others that requires prolonged handling with bare hands (such as mixing a meat loaf or kneading bread).

Brief periods of close contact, such as handshaking and hugging, are permitted. You may visit or shop in public places, attend concerts, or use public transportation at your convenience.

Your endocrinologist or radiation safety officer may recommend continued precautions for up to several weeks after treatment, depending on the amount of radioactivity administered. Patients receiving radioactive iodine should also carry information about their treatment with them in order to fully inform authorities who are in charge of screening for radioactive materials in public areas—an increasingly common occurrence.

After treatment, should contact with other people be limited?

The amount of radioactive exposure to other persons during your daily activities will depend on the duration of contact and the distance you are from them. As an example, a person 2 feet away receives only one-fourth the exposure of someone 1 foot away. Therefore, the general principle is to avoid prolonged, close contact with other people for several days.

If your work or daily activities involve prolonged contact with small children or pregnant women, you may want to wait for several days after your treatment to resume these activities. Those patients with infants at home should arrange for care to be provided by another person for the first several days after treatment. It will not be necessary for you personally to stay elsewhere after your treatment, although you will need to sleep alone for several days.

Additional Information

American Association of Clinical Endocrinologists
1000 Riverside Ave., Suite 205
Jacksonville, FL 32204
Phone: 904-353-7878
Fax: 904-353-8185
Website: http://www.aace.com
E-mail: info@aace.com

American Association of Clinical Endocrinologists (AACE) is a not-for-profit national organization of highly qualified specialists in hormonal and metabolic disorders whose primary professional activities focus on providing high-quality specialty care to patients with endocrine problems such as thyroid disease.

Chapter 50

Thyroid Surgery

Thyroid Surgery for Different Thyroid Diseases

There are several surgical options for the thyroid gland depending on the problem.

Which operation is performed on a thyroid gland depends upon two major factors. The first is the thyroid disease present which is necessitating the operation. The second is the anatomy of the thyroid gland itself as is illustrated in Figure 50.1.

1. If a dominant solitary nodule is present in a single lobe, then removal of that lobe is the preferred operation (if an operation is even warranted). If a massive goiter is compressing the trachea and esophagus, the goal of surgery will be to remove the mass and usually this means a near total or total thyroidectomy (occasionally a lobectomy will suffice). If a hot nodule is producing too much hormone resulting in hyperthyroidism, then removal of the lobe which harbors the hot nodule is all that is needed.

2. Most surgeons and endocrinologists recommend total or near total thyroidectomy in virtually all cases of thyroid carcinoma. In some patients with papillary carcinomas of small size, a less aggressive approach may be taken (lobectomy with removal

"Thyroid Operations," by James Norman, M.D., Norman Endocrine Surgery Clinic, Tampa, Florida. © 2003 Norman Endocrine Surgery Clinic. Reprinted with permission.

of the isthmus). A lymph node dissection within the anterior and lateral neck is indicated in patients with well differentiated (papillary or follicular) thyroid cancer if the lymph nodes can be palpated. This is a more extensive operation than is needed in the majority of thyroid cancer patients. All patients with medullary carcinoma of the thyroid require total thyroidectomy and aggressive lymph node dissection.

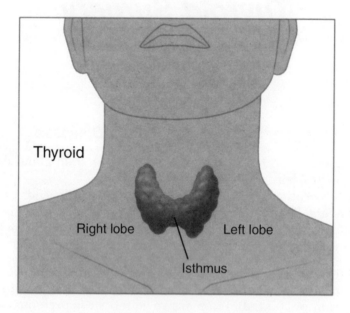

Figure 50.1. Thyroid Gland (Source: "What You Need to Know about Thyroid Cancer," National Cancer Institute, NIH Publication No. 01-4994, September 2001.

Surgical Options

Partial Thyroid Lobectomy

This operation is not performed very often because there are not many conditions which will allow this limited approach. Additionally, a benign lesion must be ideally located in the upper or lower portion of one lobe for this operation to be a choice.

Thyroid Lobectomy

This is typically the smallest operation performed on the thyroid gland. It is performed for solitary dominant nodules which are worrisome for cancer or those which are indeterminate following fine needle biopsy. Also appropriate for follicular adenomas, solitary hot or cold nodules, or goiters which are isolated to one lobe (not common).

Thyroid Lobectomy with Isthmusectomy

This simply means removal of a thyroid lobe and the isthmus (the part that connects the two lobes). This removes more thyroid tissue than a simple lobectomy, and is used when a larger margin of tissue is needed to assure that the problem has been removed. Appropriate for those indications listed under thyroid lobectomy as well as for Hürthle cell tumors, and some very small and non-aggressive thyroid cancers.

Subtotal Thyroidectomy

Just as the name implies, this operation removes all the problem side of the gland as well as the isthmus and the majority of the opposite lobe. This operation is typical for small, non-aggressive thyroid cancers. Also a common operation for goiters which are causing problems in the neck or even those which extend into the chest (substernal goiters).

Total Thyroidectomy

This operation is designed to remove all of the thyroid gland. It is the operation of choice for all thyroid cancers which are not small and non-aggressive in young patients. Many surgeons prefer this complete removal of thyroid tissue for all thyroid cancers regardless of the type.

Surgical Technique

The standard neck incision is made typically measuring about 4–5 inches in length although many endocrine surgeons are now performing this operation through an incision as small as 3 inches in thin patients. This incision is made in the lower part of the central neck and usually heals very well. It is almost unheard of to have an infection or other problem with this wound. The surgeon will then typically remove the part of the thyroid which contains the problem. As mentioned, for thyroid cancer, this will usually entail all of the thyroid lobe which harbors the malignancy, the isthmus, and a variable amount of the opposite lobe (ranging from 0 to 100% depending on the size and aggressive nature of the cancer, the cancer type, and the experience of the surgeon). The surgeon must be careful of the recurrent laryngeal nerves which are very close to the back side of the thyroid and are responsible for movement of the vocal cords. Damage to this nerve will cause hoarseness of the voice which is usually temporary but can be permanent. This is an uncommon complication (about 1 to 2 percent), but it gets lots of press because it is serious. The surgeon must also be careful to identify the parathyroid glands so their blood supply can be maintained. Another potential complication of thyroid surgery (although very rare) is hypoparathyroidism which is due to damage to all four parathyroid glands. Usually the only thyroid operations which have even a slight chance of this complication are the total or subtotal thyroidectomy. Although these complications can be serious, their risk should not be the sole determinant of whether or not to undergo surgery.

The thyroid gland and the voice box and parathyroid glands share the same blood supply, so the surgeon must take care to preserve the parathyroid artery and vein while ligating the vessels to the thyroid gland itself. This is usually not a problem, but sometimes it is not possible to save them all. In this case, the surgeon will usually implant the parathyroid gland into a muscle in the neck. The parathyroid will grow there and function normally—it is not a big deal, and you will never know the difference.

Often formal surgery is not needed to determine if a thyroid mass is cancerous. Because these masses can often be felt, a physician can stick a small needle into it to sample cells for malignancy. This is called fine needle aspiration biopsy (FNA)

Additional Information

Norman Endocrine Surgery Clinic
505 South Boulevard
Tampa, FL 33606
Phone: 813-991-6922
Fax: 813-991-6918
Website: http://www.endocrineweb.com

Chapter 51

Parathyroid Surgery

The Parathyroid Glands and Hyperparathyroidism

The parathyroid glands are 4 pea-sized glands which are usually located next to the thyroid gland in the neck (Figure 51.1).

Occasionally, a parathyroid gland can be found in other locations in the neck as well as in the upper chest. The parathyroid glands make parathyroid hormone (PTH), which controls the levels of calcium in the body. In patients with hyperparathyroidism, one or more parathyroid glands become enlarged and make too much parathyroid hormone. This causes the levels of calcium to rise in the blood. About 100,000 people in the U.S. develop hyperparathyroidism each year. Symptoms due to high calcium can include fatigue, loss of appetite, muscle aches, joint pain, and constipation. More severe symptoms include stomach ulcers, depression, loss of bone density, bone pain and/ or fractures, and kidney stones. The diagnosis of hyperparathyroidism is made based on a high blood calcium and a high blood PTH level.

A single enlarged parathyroid gland, or a parathyroid adenoma is the cause of the hyperparathyroidism in the majority (80%) of patients (Figure 51.2). In about 5% of patients, two parathyroid glands are

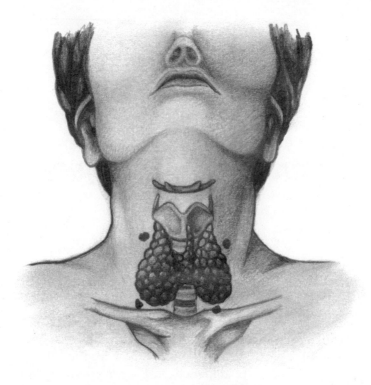

Figure 51.1. *Thyroid and Parathyroid Glands*

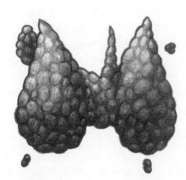

Figure 51.2. *Parathyroid Adenoma*

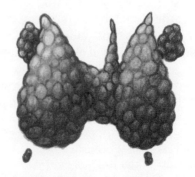

Figure 51.3. *Enlargement of Two Parathyroid Glands*

enlarged (abnormal) (Figure 51.3). In 15% of patients, all 4 glands are enlarged (Figure 51.4).

Parathyroid Scan

In most patients, it can be determined which parathyroid glands are abnormal before surgery using a parathyroid scan. Almost all patients will undergo a parathyroid scan prior to surgery. Some patients may have two scans. During a parathyroid scan, the patient receives a small injection of a radio-labeled compound which accumulates in the parathyroid glands. The patient lies on his/her back and rests while the scanner looks for the parathyroid glands. It is a painless, non-invasive procedure. If the scan detects one enlarged parathyroid gland, then the patient is a candidate for minimally invasive parathyroidectomy.

Radioguided Minimally Invasive or Targeted Parathyroidectomy (MIP)

On the day of surgery, the patient receives another injection of the radio-labeled compound about 1 hour before surgery. At the time of surgery, the surgeon will use a small probe to detect the exact location of the enlarged parathyroid gland. The surgeon will then make a small 0.5 inch to 2 inch incision directly over the parathyroid gland. The surgery can be performed under local or general anesthesia. After removal of the enlarged parathyroid gland, and while the patient is still under anesthesia, the surgeon will perform a blood test checking the patient's parathyroid hormone level in the operating room. This blood test will allow the surgeon to confirm that all enlarged parathyroid glands have been removed before the patient leaves the operating room.

Most patients go home the same day of surgery, but some may stay overnight in the hospital and go home the next morning.

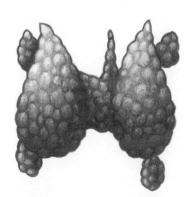

Figure 51.4. *Enlargement of All Four Parathyroid Glands*

Chapter 52

Clinical Trials: Researching New Treatments

Choosing to participate in a clinical trial is an important personal decision. The following frequently asked questions provide detailed information about clinical trials. In addition, it is often helpful to talk to a physician, family members, or friends about deciding to join a trial. After identifying some trial options, the next step is to contact the study research staff and ask questions about specific trials.

What is a clinical trial?

A clinical trial (also clinical research) is a research study in human volunteers to answer specific health questions. Carefully conducted clinical trials are the fastest and safest way to find treatments that work in people and ways to improve health. Interventional trials determine whether experimental treatments or new ways of using known therapies are safe and effective under controlled environments. Observational trials address health issues in large groups of people or populations in natural settings.

Why participate in a clinical trial?

Participants in clinical trials can play a more active role in their own health care, gain access to new research treatments before they are widely available, and help others by contributing to medical research

"Information on Clinical Trials and Human Research Studies," National Institutes of Health, (NIH), June 2003.

Who can participate in a clinical trial?

All clinical trials have guidelines about who can participate. Using inclusion/exclusion criteria is an important principle of medical research that helps to produce reliable results. The factors that allow someone to participate in a clinical trial are called inclusion criteria and those that disallow someone from participating are called exclusion criteria. These criteria are based on such factors as age, gender, the type and stage of a disease, previous treatment history, and other medical conditions. Before joining a clinical trial, a participant must qualify for the study. Some research studies seek participants with illnesses or conditions to be studied in the clinical trial, while others need healthy participants. It is important to note that inclusion and exclusion criteria are not used to reject people personally. Instead, the criteria are used to identify appropriate participants and keep them safe. The criteria help ensure that researchers will be able to answer the questions they plan to study.

What happens during a clinical trial?

The clinical trial process depends on the kind of trial being conducted The clinical trial team includes doctors and nurses as well as social workers and other health care professionals. They check the health of the participant at the beginning of the trial, give specific instructions for participating in the trial, monitor the participant carefully during the trial, and stay in touch after the trial is completed.

Some clinical trials involve more tests and doctor visits than the participant would normally have for an illness or condition. For all types of trials, the participant works with a research team. Clinical trial participation is most successful when the protocol is carefully followed, and there is frequent contact with the research staff.

What is informed consent?

Informed consent is the process of learning the key facts about a clinical trial before deciding whether or not to participate. It is also a continuing process throughout the study to provide information for participants. To help someone decide whether or not to participate, the doctors and nurses involved in the trial explain the details of the study. If the participant's native language is not English, translation assistance can be provided. Then the research team provides an informed consent document that includes details about the study, such as its purpose, duration, required procedures, and key contacts. Risks and potential benefits are explained in the informed consent document. The participant then decides whether or not to sign the document. Informed consent is not a contract, and the participant may withdraw from the trial at any time.

What are the benefits and risks of participating in a clinical trial?

Benefits: Clinical trials that are well-designed and well-executed are the best approach for eligible participants to:

- Play an active role in their own health care.
- Gain access to new research treatments before they are widely available.
- Obtain expert medical care at leading health care facilities during the trial.
- Help others by contributing to medical research.

Risks: There are risks to clinical trials.

- There may be unpleasant, serious, or even life-threatening side effects to treatment.
- The treatment may not be effective for the participant.
- The protocol may require more of their time and attention than would a non-protocol treatment, including trips to the study site, more treatments, hospital stays, or complex dosage requirements.

What are side effects and adverse reactions?

Side effects are any undesired actions or effects of drug or treatment. Negative or adverse effects may include headache, nausea, hair loss, skin irritation, or other physical problems. Experimental treatments must be evaluated for both immediate and long-term side effects.

How is the safety of the participant protected?

The ethical and legal codes that govern medical practice also apply to clinical trials. In addition, most clinical research is federally regulated with built-in safeguards to protect the participants. The trial follows a carefully controlled protocol, a study plan which details what researchers will do in the study. As a clinical trial progresses, researchers report the results of the trial at scientific meetings, to medical journals, and to various government agencies. Individual participants' names will remain secret and will not be mentioned in these reports.

What should people consider before participating in a trial?

People should know as much as possible about the clinical trial and feel comfortable asking the members of the health care team questions about it, the care expected while in a trial, and the cost of the trial. The following questions might be helpful for the participant to discuss with the health care team. Some of the answers to these questions are found in the informed consent document.

- What is the purpose of the study?
- Who is going to be in the study?
- Why do researchers believe the new treatment being tested may be effective? Has it been tested before?
- What kinds of tests and treatments are involved?
- How do the possible risks, side effects, and benefits in the study compare with my current treatment?
- How might this trial affect my daily life?
- How long will the trial last?
- Will hospitalization be required?
- Who will pay for the treatment?
- Will I be reimbursed for other expenses?
- What type of long-term follow-up care is part of this study?
- How will I know that the treatment is working? Will results of the trials be provided to me?
- Who will be in charge of my care?

What kind of preparation should a potential participant make for the meeting with the research coordinator or doctor?

- Plan ahead and write down possible questions to ask.
- Ask a friend or relative to come along for support and to hear the responses to the questions.
- Bring a tape recorder to record the discussion to replay later.

Every clinical trial in the U.S. must be approved and monitored by an Institutional Review Board (IRB) to make sure the risks are as low as possible and are worth any potential benefits. An IRB is an independent committee of physicians, statisticians, community advocates, and others that ensures that a clinical trial is ethical and the rights of study participants are protected. All institutions that conduct or support biomedical research involving people must, by federal regulation, have an IRB that initially approves and periodically reviews the research.

Does a participant continue to work with a primary health care provider while in a trial?

Yes. Most clinical trials provide short-term treatments related to a designated illness or condition, but do not provide extended or complete primary health care. In addition, by having the health care provider work with the research team, the participant can ensure that other medications or treatments will not conflict with the protocol.

Can a participant leave a clinical trial after it has begun?

Yes. A participant can leave a clinical trial, at any time. When withdrawing from the trial, the participant should let the research team know about it, and the reasons for leaving the study.

Where do the ideas for trials come from?

Ideas for clinical trials usually come from researchers. After researchers test new therapies or procedures in the laboratory and in animal studies, the treatments with the most promising laboratory results are moved into clinical trials. During a trial, more and more information is gained about a new treatment, its risks and how well it may or may not work.

Who sponsors clinical trials?

Clinical trials are sponsored or funded by a variety of organizations or individuals such as physicians, medical institutions, foundations, voluntary groups, and pharmaceutical companies, in addition to federal agencies such as the National Institutes of Health (NIH), the Department of Defense (DOD), and the Department of Veteran's Affairs (VA). Trials can take place in a variety of locations, such as hospitals, universities, doctors' offices, or community clinics.

What is a protocol?

A protocol is a study plan on which all clinical trials are based. The plan is carefully designed to safeguard the health of the participants as well as answer specific research questions. A protocol describes what types of people may participate in the trial; the schedule of tests, procedures, medications, and dosages; and the length of the study. While in a clinical trial, participants following a protocol are seen regularly by the research staff to monitor their health and to determine the safety and effectiveness of their treatment.

What is a placebo?

A placebo is an inactive pill, liquid, or powder that has no treatment value. In clinical trials, experimental treatments are often compared with placebos to assess the treatment's effectiveness. In some studies, the participants in the control group will receive a placebo instead of an active drug or treatment.

What is a control or control group?

A control is the standard by which experimental observations are evaluated. In many clinical trials, one group of patients will be given an experimental drug or treatment, while the control group is given either a standard treatment for the illness or a placebo.

What are the different types of clinical trials?

Treatment trials test new treatments, new combinations of drugs, or new approaches to surgery or radiation therapy.

Prevention trials look for better ways to prevent disease in people who have never had the disease or to prevent a disease from returning. These approaches may include medicines, vitamins, vaccines, minerals, or lifestyle changes.

Diagnostic trials are conducted to find better tests or procedures for diagnosing a particular disease or condition.

Screening trials test the best way to detect certain diseases or health conditions.

Quality of life trials (supportive care trials) explore ways to improve comfort and the quality of life for individuals with a chronic illness.

What are the phases of clinical trials?

Clinical trials are conducted in phases. The trials at each phase have a different purpose and help scientists answer different questions:

- **In Phase I trials**, researchers test a new drug or treatment in a small group of people (20–80) for the first time to evaluate its safety, determine a safe dosage range, and identify side effects.

- **In Phase II trials**, the study drug or treatment is given to a larger group of people (100–300) to see if it is effective and to further evaluate its safety.

- **In Phase III trials**, the study drug or treatment is given to large groups of people (1,000–3,000) to confirm its effectiveness, monitor side effects, compare it to commonly used treatments, and collect information that will allow the drug or treatment to be used safely.

- **In Phase IV trials**, post-marketing studies delineate additional information including the drug's risks, benefits, and optimal use.

What is an expanded access protocol?

Most human use of investigational new drugs takes place in controlled clinical trials conducted to assess safety and efficacy of new drugs. Data from the trials can serve as the basis for the drug marketing application. Sometimes, patients do not qualify for these carefully-controlled trials because of other health problems, age, or other factors. For patients who may benefit from the drug use but do not qualify for the trials, FDA regulations enable manufacturers of investigational new drugs to provide for expanded access use of the drug. For example, a treatment IND (Investigational New Drug application) or treatment protocol is a relatively unrestricted study. The primary intent of a treatment IND/protocol is to provide for access to the new drug for people with a life-threatening or serious disease for which there is no good alternative treatment. A secondary purpose for a treatment IND/protocol is to generate additional information about the drug, especially its safety. Expanded access protocols can be undertaken only if clinical investigators are actively studying the new treatment in well-controlled studies, or all studies have been completed. There must be evidence that the drug may be an effective treatment in patients like those to be treated under the protocol. The drug cannot expose patients to unreasonable risks given the severity of the disease to be treated.

Some investigational drugs are available from pharmaceutical manufacturers through expanded access programs listed in Clinical Trials available at http://clinicaltrials.gov on the Internet. Expanded access protocols are generally managed by the manufacturer, with the investigational treatment administered by researchers or doctors in office-based practice. If you, or a loved one, are interested in treatment with an investigational drug under an expanded access protocol listed in ClinicalTrials.gov, review the protocol eligibility criteria and location information and inquire at the contact information number.

Examples of Clinical Research Studies Recruiting New Patients as of January 2005

Evaluation of Patients with Thyroid Function Disorders

Number: 77-DK-0002

Summary: Participants in this study will be patients diagnosed with or suspected to have a thyroid function disorder. These conditions may include: hypothyroidism, hyperthyroidism, thyroid hormone resistance, Graves Dermopathy, and thyroid-stimulating hormone (TSH) secreting pituitary adenomas.

The main purpose of this study is to further understand the natural history, clinical presentation, and genetics of thyroid function disorders. Many of the tests performed are in the context of standard medical care that is offered to all patients with thyroid function disorders. In addition, blood and tissue samples may be taken for research and genetic studies.

Sponsoring Institute: National Institute of Diabetes and Digestive and Kidney Diseases (NIDDK)

Recruitment Detail:

- **Type:** Active accrual of new subjects
- **Gender:** Male and female

Referral Letter Required: Yes

Population Exclusion(s): None

Eligibility Criteria:

- **Inclusion Criteria:** Patients of any age with known or suspected thyroid abnormalities may be included in this study. These disorders can be broadly defined as hyper- or hypothyroid states and laboratory abnormalities.

  Special Instructions: Only a limited number of patients are being recruited at the present time. Current research aims are focusing on Graves Dermopathy, and TSH secreting pituitary tumors. If interested have your health care provider send a written referral letter summarizing your thyroid disorder plus all applicable laboratory, radiology, and/or nuclear medicine reports. This information will be reviewed by Principal Investigator to determine whether you are eligible for protocol enrollment.

Studies on Thyroid Nodules and Thyroid Cancer Protocol

Number: 77-DK-0096

Summary: Participants in this study will be patients diagnosed with or suspected to have a thyroid nodule or thyroid cancer.

The main purpose of this study is to further understand the methods for the diagnosis and treatment of thyroid nodules and thyroid cancer. Many of the tests performed are in the context of standard medical care that is offered to all patients with thyroid nodules or thyroid cancer. Other tests are performed for research purposes. In addition, blood and tissue samples will be taken for research and genetic studies.

Sponsoring Institute: National Institute of Diabetes and Digestive and Kidney Diseases (NIDDK)

Recruitment Detail:

- **Type:** Active accrual of new subjects
- **Gender:** Male and female

Referral Letter Required: Yes

Population Exclusion(s): None

Eligibility Criteria:

- **Inclusion Criteria:** Patients of any age at risk for thyroid carcinoma will be selected. The section of our study relevant to the detection and analysis of nRNA transcripts for specific genes in circulating thyrocytes in peripheral blood of patients with previously treated thyroid cancer will also include patients of all ages.

- **Exclusion Criteria:** All patients under age 18 (minors) will be excluded from the part of our study necessitating collection of specimens by fine needle aspiration of primary thyroid and metastatic lesions that are specifically and solely obtained for research purposes.

Special Instructions: Only a limited number of patients are being recruited at the present time. Our major research focus is the diagnosis and treatment of clinically aggressive thyroid cancer. Current research aims are focusing on patients requiring dosimetry measurements, patients with iodine non-avid disease, as well as patients with progressive disease despite optimal prior surgical and radioiodine therapies.

If interested, have your health care provider send a written referral letter summarizing your thyroid disorder plus all applicable laboratory, radiology, and nuclear medicine reports. All biopsy or surgery pathology reports and relevant slides must be included. This information will be reviewed by Principal Investigator to determine whether you are eligible for protocol enrollment.

Additional Information

Patient Recruitment and Public Liaison Office
10 Cloister Ct., Bldg. 61
Bethesda, MD 20892-4754
Toll Free: 800-411-1222
Toll-Free TTY: 866-411-1010
Fax: 301-480-9793
Website: http://clinicalstudies.info.nih.gov
E-mail: prpl@mail.cc.nih.gov

Part Nine

Thyroid Disorder Effects on Other Body Systems

Chapter 53

Thyroid Disease Can Increase the Risk of Heart Disease

Chapter Contents

Section 53.1

Understanding the
Thyroid/Cholesterol Connection

"Understanding the Thyroid-Cholesterol Connection," © 2000 American
Association of Clinical Endocrinologists. Reprinted with permission.

The Thyroid/Cholesterol Overlap

- An estimated 98 million American adults have high cholesterol
  or total blood cholesterol values of 200 milligram/deciliter (mg/
  dL) or higher.

- More than 13 million Americans have a thyroid disorder, yet
  nearly half remain undiagnosed.

- Hypothyroidism (underactive thyroid) is the most common secondary cause of high cholesterol after diet, according to the National Cholesterol Education Program (NCEP).

- Ninety percent of patients with overt hypothyroidism have increased cholesterol and/or triglycerides.

  - Average blood cholesterol levels of patients with underactive
    thyroid are often 30 to 50 percent higher than desirable
    (normal range is considered under 200 mg/dL).

  - People with unrecognized subclinical hypothyroidism gener-
    ally have elevated cholesterol levels as well.

- Thyroid disorders affect 20 percent of women over age 60.

- Coronary heart disease is the cause of death in more than 50
  percent of women over age 70.

Why Does Untreated Thyroid Disease Lead to Elevated Cholesterol Levels?

The thyroid gland produces hormones that regulate the body's metabolism. If the thyroid gland produces too little hormone, metabolism

can slow, having a direct impact on the body's ability to clear cholesterol from the bloodstream. As a result, the risk of cholesterol being
deposited in the arteries, and especially around the heart, is increased,
thereby increasing the risk for heart disease.

Implications of Untreated Thyroid and Cholesterol Conditions

Approximately 39 million American adults are at risk for heart
disease because they have cholesterol levels of 240 mg/dL or above.
Coronary heart disease costs the U.S. between $50 and $100 billion
each year, and NCEP reports suggest that prevention could greatly
reduce this.

Diagnosis and Treatment

- Since increased blood cholesterol is the most common cause of
  heart disease, the NCEP recommends that all adults age 20 and
  older have their blood cholesterol checked at least once every 5
  years.

  - The lipoprotein profile test measures LDL (low density lipo-
    proteins or bad cholesterol which is the main source of dam-
    aging build up in the arteries) and HDL (high density
    lipoproteins or good cholesterol which carries bad choles-
    terol to the liver to remove it from the body).

- The treatment of elevated cholesterol must be tailored to each
  individual patient after evaluating the patient's health history
  and determining other risk factors related to cardiac health.
  The treatment of choice for patients who require a medication is
  a statin, a type drug which is highly effective in lowering LDL-
  cholesterol.

- Because untreated hypothyroidism can increase LDL levels,
  the prescribing information on cholesterol-lowering statins recommends that all patients diagnosed with high LDL cholesterol
  be tested for thyroid disease prior to initiating a cholesterol-
  lowering therapy.

- The TSH (thyroid stimulating hormone) test is the most accurate and sensitive indicator of thyroid function.

- Treatment for thyroid disease is tailored to the type and severity of the disorder.

- Hypothyroidism: Treatment with levothyroxine sodium, a synthetic thyroid hormone tablet, corrects this by replacing the missing thyroid hormone in the body.

- Hyperthyroidism: Excess thyroid hormone production can be treated by ablative radioactive iodine treatment, anti-thyroid medication, or surgical removal. The patient often later develops hypothyroidism.

- Once hypothyroidism is treated with a thyroid hormone replacement, and the TSH level is restored to normal, the majority of patients show an estimated 20 to 30 percent reduction in cholesterol levels.

Additional Information

American Association of Clinical Endocrinologists
1000 Riverside Ave., Suite 205
Jacksonville, FL 32204
Phone: 904-353-7878
Fax: 904-353-8185
Website: http://www.aace.com
E-mail: info@aace.com

Section 53.2

Irregular Heartbeat and Over-Active Thyroid

"Irregular Heartbeat is Common Side Effect of Overactive Thyroid,"
September 20, 2003. Copyright The American Thyroid Association.
Reprinted with permission.

Irregular Heartbeat Is Common Side Effect of Over-Active Thyroid, Resists Treatment, and Leads to Death

An irregular heartbeat, called atrial fibrillation (AF), affects almost 10 percent of those with an over-active thyroid, known as hyperthyroidism. This problem often continues despite effective treatment of the thyroid condition, according to a study presented at the 75th Annual Meeting of the American Thyroid Association in September 2003. The study also found that hyperthyroid-induced AF is of particular concern for elderly males. Furthermore, this complication of the thyroid condition is associated with an increased risk of death.

"Physicians need to have a heightened awareness that this is a serious complication of hyperthyroidism," advised Jayne A. Franklyn, M.D., Ph.D., senior author and professor of medicine in the Division of Medical Sciences at the University of Birmingham and Queen Elizabeth Hospital in Edgbaston, Birmingham, United Kingdom. "In turn, this should prompt rapid treatment and specialist referral of patients with hyperthyroidism, preferably before development of atrial fibrillation."

Dr. Franklyn and colleagues had previously found that there is increased risk of death from cardiovascular diseases in patients with previous hyperthyroidism. Therefore, they wanted to investigate the issue further.

The researchers recruited 425 patients with overt hyperthyroidism, which can result in an increased metabolic rate, enlargement of the thyroid gland, rapid heart rate, and high blood pressure. Dr. Franklyn noted that the majority of all hyperthyroid patients have a rapid heart rate before thyroid treatment because excess thyroid hormones speed up the heart. Of the total group, 334 were female and 91 were male, with 35 of the group (8.2 percent) being diagnosed with AF.

511

Of those with AF, their average age was 71 years old, and men were over-represented in the group, at 11 percent. Ten of them had known AF, 20 newly onset AF, and five had sudden, temporary episodes of AF, known as paroxysmal AF, before and after thyroid treatment. All but two of the 35 patients were treated with anti-thyroid thionamides and radioactive iodine. Two returned to normal thyroid function immediately and four died during the follow-up period. Only 10 of the patients returned to a normal heart rhythm, either due to thyroid or heart-related treatment, the latter composed of drugs or electrical cardioversion.

"More effective means of managing those with this complication need to be developed," added Dr. Franklyn. "This might mean earlier intervention with drugs in an attempt to abolish the abnormal rhythm or development of new electrical methods to achieve a normal rhythm."

Additional Information

American Thyroid Association
6066 Leesburg Pike, Suite 550
Falls Church, VA 22041
Toll-Free: 800-THYROID (849-7643)
Phone: 703-998-8890
Fax: 703-998-8893
Website: http://www.thyroid.org
E-mail: admin@thyroid.org

Chapter 54

Thyroid-Related Eye Disease

Eye Enlargement and Inflammation

Any hyperthyroid patient, no matter what causes their hyperthyroidism, may experience elevation of the upper eyelid anytime the blood level of thyroid hormone is above normal. For example, patients who are hyperthyroid because of too much thyroid hormone medication may have raised upper eyelids causing their eyes to appear enlarged or staring. In this situation, however, the eyes do not actually protrude.

If you have Graves disease, you may develop protrusion and inflammation of your eyes without there being any evidence of infection. It is likely to begin about the time your thyroid becomes overactive, but it may precede your hyperthyroidism or occur years after your thyroid function has become normal. Very rarely, the eye disorder may occur without your having any obvious abnormality of thyroid function at any time in your life.

More serious eye problems may occur in patients with Graves disease and (less commonly) Hashimoto thyroiditis. The severity of these conditions is unrelated to the blood level of thyroid hormone. If the condition is mild, you may have only redness and irritation of your eyes. On the other hand, in those rare instances when the inflammation is more severe your eyes may protrude, you may have double vision, and your sight may be threatened.

It should be pointed out that the thyroid eye disease does not necessarily progress in an orderly fashion from mild to severe in any given patient. In fact, a rapid decrease in vision can occur due to pressure upon the optic nerve in a patient with only minimal swelling of the eyelids. For this reason, if you have Graves disease and begin to show signs of eye trouble, you should have a complete eye examination. If your eye involvement is severe, your physician may refer you to an ophthalmologist (eye specialist), who will have at his/her disposal all of the equipment needed to evaluate the various eye problems that may occur in Graves disease. Your vision can be accurately tested. The amount of eye protrusion can be accurately measured with an exophthalmometer. The cornea and other tissues of your eye can be examined by the use of a microscope-like instrument known as a slit lamp. Ultrasound pictures of your eye and eye socket (orbit) may be taken, using sound waves in a technique similar to radar. Alternatively, your physician may request special x-rays of your orbits done by computerized tomography (CT scan) or by a newer technique called Magnetic Resonance Imaging (MRI). These techniques will provide a clear picture of the inflamed tissues behind your eye.

Treatment of your eye condition will depend upon the kind of eye disease you have and whether it is getting worse. Mild inflammation may be treated simply by elevating the head of your bed at night and by lubricating your eyes with drops of artificial tears. On the other hand, if you have a severe and rapidly progressive inflammatory condition with double vision or decreased vision, you may require special glasses or treatment with steroids. If your eye tissues continue to swell despite the use of steroid hormones, additional therapy is available. This may include x-ray treatments to the tissues behind the eye or surgery on the bony orbit (surgical decompression) to relieve the increased pressure behind your eye.

New research suggests that cigarette smokers are at greater risk for these troubles than non-smokers, so if you smoke and have just developed Graves disease, stop smoking at once. Fortunately, serious eye problems are rare among thyroid patients. When they do occur, the treatment methods are excellent and are usually successful in improving the problem. Occasionally excessive drooping of the upper or lower eyelids may cause cosmetic problems, but plastic eye surgery can be very helpful for such patients.

Antibodies Against a Hormone Receptor for TSH Can Predict Course of Eye Disease in Common Thyroid Condition

The prevalence and levels of thyroid-stimulating hormone receptor antibodies (TSHR-AB) are significantly higher in patients with a severe course of a thyroid-associated eye disease compared to patients with a mild course, according to a study presented September 21, 2003 at the 75th Annual Meeting of the American Thyroid Association.

Based on this knowledge, physicians can predict a good or bad course of the eye disease, called thyroid-associated ophthalmopathy (TAO), at certain stages. The researchers believe that they can make an accurate prediction in about half of the patients.

TAO is an inflammatory eye disease that occurs most in cases of autoimmune hyperthyroidism, known as Graves disease, a common form of the overactive thyroid condition often characterized by goiter and a slight protrusion of the eyeballs. Half of the patients with Graves disease show signs of eye disease. Graves hyperthyroidism affects 22 out of 1000 people.

The symptoms of TAO, which is also called Graves ophthalmopathy, are lid retraction, inflammatory lid and conjunctival swellings, forward projection or displacement of the eyeball, impairment of eye motility with double vision, blurred vision due to dryness of the surface of the eye, and very rarely optic nerve compression. The severity of the eye disease goes along with the severity of thyroid disease in many cases.

To evaluate the influence of TSH-receptor antibodies on predicting the course of TAO, researchers in Germany identified 66 patients with TAO and monitored their progress over two years. Their antibodies were measured within 4, 8, 12, 16, 20, and 24 months after the onset of TAO. After two years, the patients were classified into having either a bad or good course of the disease. The classification was done with a certain severity and activity score, and the physician classifying the cases was unaware of the antibody levels. The researchers note that the newest, most sensitive assay, using the human TSH receptor, was used to measure TSHR-AB.

Anja K. Eckstein, M.D., Ph.D., of the University Eye Hospital in Essen, Germany, and lead author of the study, explained that many studies have addressed the issue of using TSHR-AB to classify TAO. However, until recently, "The overall picture has been inconclusive due to differences in the classification of the patients and low sensitivity of former assay systems," she said. "A number of recent clinical and experimental studies applying a more stringent selection criteria found evidence that TSH receptor antibodies trigger the autoimmune process in TAO. But we are the first who have shown that TSH receptor antibodies not only trigger but also constantly maintain the autoimmune process in the eye."

Dr. Eckstein advises ophthalmologists to use TSH receptor antibody prevalence and levels as an additional marker to estimate the risk for a bad or good course of TAO. "The study provides certain levels to guide physicians in predicting the course of the disease," she added.

Additional Information

American Thyroid Association
6066 Leesburg Pike, Suite 550
Falls Church, VA 22041
Toll-Free: 800-THYROID (849-7643)
Phone: 703-998-8890
Fax: 703-998-8893
Website: http://www.thyroid.org
E-mail: admin@thyroid.org

Thyroid Foundation of America
One Longfellow Place, Suite 1518
Boston, MA 02114
Toll-Free: 800-832-8321
Phone: 617-534-1500
Fax: 617-534-1515
Website: http://www.allthyroid.org
E-mail: info@allthyroid.org

Chapter 55

Thyroid Treatment and Bone Loss

Osteoporosis is a major threat to Americans. In the United States today, 10 million individuals already have osteoporosis, and 18 million more have low bone mass, placing them at increased risk for this disorder.

Osteoporosis, once thought to be a natural part of aging among women, is no longer considered age or gender dependent. It is largely preventable due to the remarkable progress in the scientific understanding of its causes, diagnosis, and treatment. Optimization of bone health is a process that must occur throughout the lifespan in both males and females. Factors that influence bone health at all ages are essential to prevent osteoporosis and its devastating consequences.

Osteoporosis and Its Consequences

Osteoporosis is defined as a skeletal disorder characterized by compromised bone strength predisposing to an increased risk of fracture. Bone strength reflects the integration of two main features: bone density and bone quality. Bone density is expressed as grams of mineral per area or volume and in any given individual is determined by peak bone mass and amount of bone loss. Bone quality refers to architecture,

Excerpts from "Osteoporosis Prevention, Diagnosis, and Therapy," NIH Consensus Statement, March 2000. National Institutes of Health (NIH). And "The Low-Down on Osteoporosis: What We Know and What We Don't," by Bobbi Bennett, *NIH Word on Health*, December 2003, National Institutes of Health (NIH).

turnover, damage accumulation (e.g., micro-fractures) and mineralization. A fracture occurs when a failure-inducing force (e.g., trauma) is applied to osteoporotic bone. Thus, osteoporosis is a significant risk factor for fracture, and a distinction between risk factors that affect bone metabolism and risk factors for fracture must be made.

It is important to acknowledge a common misperception that osteoporosis is always the result of bone loss. Bone loss commonly occurs as men and women age; however, an individual who does not reach optimal (i.e., peak) bone mass during childhood and adolescence may develop osteoporosis without the occurrence of accelerated bone loss. Hence sub-optimal bone growth in childhood and adolescence is as important as bone loss to the development of osteoporosis.

Currently there is no accurate measure of overall bone strength. Bone mineral density (BMD) is frequently used as a proxy measure and accounts for approximately 70 percent of bone strength. The World Health Organization (WHO) operationally defines osteoporosis as bone density 2.5 standard deviations below the mean for young, white, adult women. It is not clear how to apply this diagnostic criterion to men, children, and across ethnic groups. Because of the difficulty in accurate measurement and standardization between instruments and sites, controversy exists among experts regarding the continued use of this diagnostic criterion.

Osteoporosis can be further characterized as either primary or secondary. Primary osteoporosis can occur in both genders at all ages, but often follows menopause in women and occurs later in life in men. In contrast, secondary osteoporosis is a result of medications, other conditions, or diseases. Examples include glucocorticoid-induced osteoporosis, hypogonadism, and celiac disease.

The consequences of osteoporosis include the financial, physical, and psychosocial, which significantly affect the individual as well as the family and community. An osteoporotic fracture is a tragic outcome of a traumatic event in the presence of compromised bone strength, and its incidence is increased by various other risk factors. Traumatic events can range from high-impact falls to normal lifting and bending. The incidence of fracture is high in individuals with osteoporosis and increases with age. The probability that a 50-year-old will have a hip fracture during his or her lifetime is 14 percent for a white female and 5 to 6 percent for a white male. The risk for African Americans is much lower at 6 percent and 3 percent for 50-year-old women and men, respectively. Osteoporotic fractures, particularly vertebral fractures, can be associated with chronic disabling pain. Nearly one-third of patients with hip fractures are discharged to nursing homes within the year following a fracture. Notably, one in five patients is no longer living 1 year after sustaining an osteoporotic hip fracture. Hip and vertebral fractures are a problem for women in their late 70s and 80s, wrist fractures are a problem in the late 50s to early 70s, and all other fractures (e.g., pelvic and rib) are a problem throughout postmenopausal years. The impact of osteoporosis on other body systems, such as gastrointestinal, respiratory, genitourinary, and craniofacial is acknowledged, but reliable prevalence rates are unknown.

Hip fracture has a profound impact on quality of life, as evidenced by findings that 80 percent of women older than 75 years preferred death to a bad hip fracture resulting in nursing home placement. However, little data exist on the relationship between fractures and psychological and social well-being. Other quality-of-life issues include adverse effects on physical health (impact of skeletal deformity) and financial resources. An osteoporotic fracture is associated with increased difficulty in activities of daily life, as only one-third of fracture patients regain pre-fracture level of function and one-third require nursing home placement. Fear, anxiety, and depression are frequently reported in women with established osteoporosis and such consequences are likely under-addressed when considering the overall impact of this condition.

Direct financial expenditures for treatment of osteoporotic fracture are estimated at $10 to $15 billion annually. A majority of these estimated costs are due to in-patient care, but do not include the costs of treatment for individuals without a history of fractures, nor do they include the indirect costs of lost wages or productivity of either the individual or the caregiver. More needs to be learned about these indirect costs, which are considerable. Consequently, these figures significantly underestimate the true costs of osteoporosis.

Risk Factors

Gender/Ethnicity

The prevalence of osteoporosis, and incidence of fracture vary by gender and race/ethnicity. White, postmenopausal women experience almost three-quarters of hip fractures and have the highest age-adjusted fracture incidence. Most of the information regarding diagnosis and treatment is derived from research on this population. However, women of other ages, racial, and ethnic groups, and men, and children are also affected. Much of the difference in fracture rates among these groups appears to be explained by differences in peak bone mass and rate of bone loss; however, differences in bone geometry, frequency of falls, and prevalence of other risk factors appear to play a role as well.

Both men and women experience an age-related decline in BMD starting in midlife. Women experience more rapid bone loss in the early years following menopause, which places them at earlier risk for fractures. In men, hypogonadism is also an important risk factor. Men and peri-menopausal women with osteoporosis more commonly have secondary causes for the bone loss than do postmenopausal women.

African American women have higher bone mineral density than white non-Hispanic women throughout life, and experience lower hip fracture rates. Some Japanese women have lower peak BMD than white, non-Hispanic women, but have a lower hip fracture rate, the reasons for which are not fully understood. Mexican American women have bone densities intermediate between those of white, non-Hispanic women and African American women. Limited available information on Native American women suggests they have lower BMD than white non-Hispanic women.

Predictive Risk Factors

Risks associated with low bone density are supported by good evidence, including large prospective studies. Predictors of low bone mass include female gender, increased age, estrogen deficiency, white race, low weight and body mass index (BMI), family history of osteoporosis, smoking, and history of prior fracture. Use of alcohol and caffeine-containing beverages is inconsistently associated with decreased bone mass. In contrast, some measures of physical function and activity have been associated with increased bone mass, including grip strength and current exercise. Levels of exercise in childhood and adolescence have an inconsistent relationship to BMD later in life. Late menarche, early menopause, and low endogenous estrogen levels are also associated with low BMD in several studies.

Although low BMD has been established as an important predictor of future fracture risk, the results of many studies indicate that clinical risk factors related to risk of fall also serve as important predictors of fracture. Fracture risk has been consistently associated with a history of falls, low physical function such as slow gait speed and decreased quadriceps strength, impaired cognition, impaired vision, and the presence of environmental hazards (e.g., throw rugs). Increased risk of a fracture with a fall includes a fall to the side and attributes of bone geometry, such as tallness, hip axis, and femur length. Some risks for fracture, such as age, a low BMI, and low levels of physical activity, probably affect fracture incidence through their effects on both bone density and propensity to fall and inability to absorb impact.

Results of studies of persons with osteoporotic fractures have led to the development of models of risk prediction, which incorporate clinical risk factors along with BMD measurements. Results from the Study of Osteoporotic Fractures (SOF), a large longitudinal study of postmenopausal, white, non-Hispanic women, suggest that clinical risk factors can contribute greatly to fracture risk assessment. In this study, 14 clinical risk factors predictive of fracture were identified. The presence of five or more of these factors increased the rate of hip fracture for women in the highest tertile of BMD from 1.1 per 1,000 woman-years to 9.9 per 1,000 woman-years. Women in the lowest tertile of BMD with no other risk factors had a hip fracture rate of 2.6 per 1,000 woman-years as compared with 27.3 per 1,000 woman-years with five or more risk factors present. A second model, derived from the Rotterdam study, predicted hip fractures using a smaller number of variables, including gender, age, height, weight, use of a walking aid, and current smoking. However, these models have not been validated in a population different from that in which they were derived.

Secondary Osteoporosis

A large number of medical disorders are associated with osteoporosis and increased fracture risk. These can be organized into several categories: genetic disorders, hypogonadal states, endocrine disorders, gastrointestinal diseases, hematologic disorders, connective tissue disease, nutritional deficiencies, drugs, and a variety of other common serious chronic systemic disorders, such as congestive heart failure, end-stage renal disease, and alcoholism.

The distribution of the most common causes appears to differ by demographic group.

- Among men, 30 to 60 percent of osteoporosis is associated with secondary causes; with hypogonadism, glucocorticoids, and alcoholism the most common.

- In peri-menopausal women, more than 50 percent is associated with secondary causes, and the most common causes are hypo-estrogenemia, glucocorticoids, thyroid hormone excess, and anticonvulsant therapy.

- In postmenopausal women, the prevalence of secondary conditions is thought to be much lower, but the actual proportion is not known.

- In one study, hypercalciuria, hyperparathyroidism, and malabsorption were identified in a group of white, postmenopausal, osteoporotic women who had no history of conditions that cause bone loss.

These data suggest that additional testing of white postmenopausal women with osteoporosis may be indicated, but an appropriate or cost-effective evaluation strategy has not been determined.

- Glucocorticoid use is the most common form of drug-related osteoporosis, and its long-term administration for disorders such as rheumatoid arthritis and chronic obstructive pulmonary disease is associated with a high rate of fracture. For example, in one study, a group of patients treated with 10 milligrams (mg) of prednisone for 20 weeks experienced an 8 percent loss of BMD in the spine. Some experts suggest that any patient who receives orally administered glucocorticoids (such as prednisone) in a dose of 5 mg or more for longer than 2 months is at high risk for excessive bone loss.

- People who have undergone organ transplant are at high risk for osteoporosis due to a variety of factors, including pretransplant organ failure and use of glucocorticoids after transplantation.

- Hyperthyroidism is a well-described risk factor for osteoporosis. In addition, some studies have suggested that women taking thyroid replacement may also be at increased risk for excess bone loss, suggesting that careful regulation of thyroid replacement is important.

Factors Involved in Building and Maintaining Skeletal Health Throughout Life

Growth in bone size and strength occurs during childhood, but bone accumulation is not completed until the third decade of life, after the cessation of linear growth. The bone mass attained early in life is perhaps the most important determinant of lifelong skeletal health. Individuals with the highest peak bone mass after adolescence have the greatest protective advantage when the inexorable declines in bone density associated with increasing age, illness, and diminished sex-steroid production take their toll. Bone mass may be related not only to osteoporosis and fragility later in life, but also to fractures in childhood and adolescence. Genetic factors exert a strong and perhaps predominant influence on peak bone mass, but physiological, environmental, and modifiable lifestyle factors can also play a significant role. Among these are adequate nutrition and body weight, exposure to sex hormones at puberty, and physical activity. Thus, maximizing bone mass early in life presents a critical opportunity to reduce the impact of bone loss related to aging. Childhood is also a critical time for the development of lifestyle habits conducive to maintaining good bone health throughout life. Cigarette smoking, which usually starts in adolescence, may have a deleterious effect on achieving bone mass.

Nutrition

Good nutrition is essential for normal growth. A balanced diet, adequate calories, and appropriate nutrients are the foundation for development of all tissues, including bone. Adequate and appropriate nutrition is important for all individuals, but not all follow a diet that is optimal for bone health. Supplementation of calcium and vitamin D may be necessary. In particular, excessive pursuit of thinness may affect adequate nutrition and bone health.

Calcium is the specific nutrient most important for attaining peak bone mass and for preventing and treating osteoporosis. Sufficient data exist to recommend specific dietary calcium intakes at various stages of life. Although the Institute of Medicine recommends calcium intakes of 800 mg/day for children ages 3 to 8 and 1,300 mg/day for children and adolescents ages 9 to 17, only about 25 percent of boys and 10 percent of girls ages 9 to 17 are estimated to meet these recommendations. Factors contributing to low calcium intakes are restriction of dairy products, a generally low level of fruit and vegetable consumption, and a high intake of low calcium beverages such as sodas. For older adults, calcium intake should be maintained at 1,000 to 1,500 mg/day, yet only about 50 to 60 percent of this population meets this recommendation.

Vitamin D is required for optimal calcium absorption and thus is also important for bone health. Most infants and young children in the United States have adequate vitamin D intake because of supplementation and fortification of milk. During adolescence, when consumption of dairy products decreases, vitamin D intake is less likely to be adequate, and this may adversely affect calcium absorption. A recommended vitamin D intake of 400 to 600 IU/day has been established for adults.

Other nutrients have been evaluated for their relation to bone health. High dietary protein, caffeine, phosphorus, and sodium can adversely affect calcium balance, but their effects appear not to be important in individuals with adequate calcium intakes.

Exercise

Regular physical activity has numerous health benefits for individuals of all ages. The specific effects of physical activity on bone health have been investigated in randomized clinical trials and observational studies. There is strong evidence that physical activity early in life contributes to higher peak bone mass. Some evidence indicates that resistance and high impact exercise are likely the most beneficial. Exercise during the middle years of life has numerous health benefits, but there are few studies on the effects of exercise on BMD. Exercise during the later years, in the presence of adequate calcium and vitamin D intake, probably has a modest effect on slowing the decline in BMD. It is clear that exercise late in life, even beyond 90 years of age, can increase muscle mass and strength twofold or more in frail individuals. There is convincing evidence that exercise in elderly persons also improves function, delays loss of independence, and thus contributes to quality of life. Randomized clinical trials of exercise have been shown to reduce the risk of falls by approximately 25 percent, but there is no experimental evidence that exercise affects fracture rates. It also is possible that regular exercisers might fall differently and thereby reduce the risk of fracture due to falls, but this hypothesis requires testing.

Gonadal Steroids

Sex steroids secreted during puberty substantially increase BMD and peak bone mass. Gonadal steroids influence skeletal health throughout life in both women and men. In adolescents and young women, sustained production of estrogens is essential for the maintenance of bone mass. Reduction in estrogen production with menopause is the major cause of loss of BMD during later life. Timing of menarche, absent or infrequent menstrual cycles, and the timing of menopause influence both the attainment of peak bone mass and the preservation of BMD. Testosterone production in adolescent boys and

524

men is similarly important in achieving and maintaining maximal bone mass. Estrogens have also been implicated in the growth and maturation of the male skeleton. Pathologic delay in the onset of puberty is a risk factor for diminished bone mass in men. Disorders that result in hypogonadism in adult men result in osteoporosis.

Growth Hormone and Body Composition

Growth hormone and insulin-like growth factor-I, which are maximally secreted during puberty, continue to play a role in the acquisition and maintenance of bone mass and the determination of body composition into adulthood. Growth hormone deficiency is associated with a decrease in BMD. Children and youth with low BMI are likely to attain lower-than-average peak bone mass. Although there is a direct association between BMI and bone mass throughout the adult years, it is not known whether the association between body composition and bone mass is due to hormones, nutritional factors, higher impact during weight-bearing activities, or other factors. There are several observational studies of fractures in older persons that show an inverse relationship between fracture rates and BMI.

The Low-Down on Osteoporosis: What We Know and What We Don't Know

Many myths have sprung up about osteoporosis and its fractures that are not based on solid science. While scientists do not yet have all the answers about the best ways to diagnose, treat, or prevent osteoporosis, the National Institutes of Health (NIH), led by the National Institute of Arthritis and Musculoskeletal and Skin Diseases (NIAMS), is conducting and supporting research to help find those answers. Here is what we know now about some of those myths.

Myth: Our Bones Do not Change after We Have Finished Growing

We reach our peak bone mass around age 30, but our bones are changing constantly throughout our lives. This process—known as remodeling—involves two major types of bone cells: osteoclasts, which break down old or worn bone and thus create bone cavities, and osteoblasts which fill in the cavities. If the amount of new bone equals the amount being dissolved, your bones stay strong. But several things can shift the balance so that bones become weaker and more brittle.

Myth: We Know All the Risk Factors for Osteoporosis

"We don't have a complete set of risk factors that describe a person who is at very high risk for fracture," says Dr. Joan McGowan, director of NIAMS' Musculoskeletal Diseases Branch. One of the biggest risk factors, she points out, is age. "Forty to fifty percent of women over 50 will have an osteoporotic fracture sometime in their life," she says. "As you age, your bones become less dense and weaker due to an increased rate of bone loss—the osteoclasts are breaking down more bone than the osteoblasts are filling in. Younger people ice skate or ski without severe trauma when they fall, they don't break any bones. We get older, do the same activities and fall, and we do suffer a fracture."

We also know that being a woman makes a big difference, too. Women have an increase in the rate of bone loss during the first three to five years after menopause. After that, it continues at a slower but steady rate.

Myth: A DXA Scan Can Predict Whether or Not You Will Have a Fracture

A DXA scan, a special type of x-ray exam, is used to measure the bone mineral density (BMD) of the spine or hip. BMD is used as a common indicator of bone health. But BMD is just one component of bone strength and is not the perfect marker for gauging a person's risk of fracture.

"There is a lot more about the quality of bone that isn't captured by DXA," says Dr. McGowan. "Yet DXA is as good at predicting fracture as blood pressure measurement is at predicting stroke, and better than cholesterol numbers at predicting heart disease. However, just because you have normal blood pressure doesn't mean that you won't have a stroke, or just because you have normal cholesterol levels doesn't mean that you are protected from having a heart attack. There are many different risk factors involved for those diseases and the same is true for osteoporosis and for fractures."

Myth: You Can Not Get All the Calcium You Need from Food

On the contrary, Dr. McGowan says it is best to get your daily amounts of calcium from food whenever possible. "You won't have to worry about getting enough calcium, vitamin D and vitamin K," she explains, "if you eat a balanced diet of fruits, vegetables—especially leafy green ones—grains, protein, and low-fat dairy products." And with so many calcium-fortified products on the market, it's getting easier all the time to get all the calcium you need from food.

If you cannot get enough calcium from your diet, you may need a calcium supplement. They come in different forms, such as calcium carbonate and calcium citrate. Dr. McGowan says there is no significant difference among the various forms. So if one type seems to disagree with you, switch to another. Check your supplement's label to ensure that your calcium supplement meets USP standards. (USP, or the U.S. Pharmacopeia, is an organization that helps ensure consumers receive quality medicines by setting standards that drug manufacturers must meet.)

Men and women between the ages of 19 and 50 should get about 1,000 milligrams (mg) of calcium daily while those over 50 should get 1,200 mg. Dr. McGowan recommends spreading out the calcium over the day so that you get better overall absorption of the calcium, and taking it with food helps, too.

You also need enough vitamin D every day in order to absorb calcium from the diet. Vitamin D is found in food, particularly fortified food, but can also be made by your body after exposure to the sun; 15 minutes outside in the sun per day is usually sufficient for your body to make all the vitamin D you need. If you have limited sun exposure, especially during the winter, you should take vitamin pills with 200 to 400 international units (IU) of vitamin D per day if you are below age 70, or 600 IU if you are over 70. Too much vitamin D can be harmful, so do not take more than 800 IU per day without a doctor's supervision.

What You Can Do to Prevent Osteoporosis

- Get enough daily calcium:
  - Kids ages 8–18 need 1,300 mg
  - Adults 19–50 need 1,000 mg
  - Those over 50 need 1,200 mg
  - Do not exceed 2,000 mg per day

- Take calcium with meals; the body absorbs it better that way and you are more likely to remember to take it. Buy fortified orange juice and cereals, and eat lots of green leafy vegetables and low-fat dairy products like cheese, milk, ice cream, and yogurt.

- If you cannot get enough calcium through foods, take calcium supplements from well-known manufacturers. Be wary of supplements from natural sources.

- It is best to take only 500 mg of calcium at a time if you can.

- Get enough vitamin D. Spend 15 minutes outside in the sun each day or take 200 to 400 IU below age 70 and 600 over 70.

- Get out of that chair and walk or do other weight-bearing exercises like jogging, dancing, or tennis.

The U.S. Food and Drug Administration (FDA) has approved several medications for the prevention or treatment of osteoporosis. However, Dr. McGowan cautions, "None of these can completely stop fractures and may not be suitable for taking the rest of your life since we don't yet know what their long-term effects are." Millions of women were taking estrogen along with progestin—known as hormone replacement therapy or HRT—beginning at menopause, and planning to continue it for the rest of their lives. "Estrogen used to be considered a sheet of armor for your bones," Dr. McGowan says. But NIH's long-term clinical trial, the Women's Health Initiative (WHI), revealed in 2002 that, although estrogen and progestin combined to prevent fractures, the overall health risks of taking HRT outweighed the benefits.

Another part of the WHI that is not scheduled to be completed until 2005 is investigating the effect of 1,000 mg of calcium carbonate plus 400 IU of vitamin D daily on hip and other osteoporosis-related fractures and colorectal cancer. Until these studies are finished, women should consult their doctor or health care provider about the risks and benefits of the various options available for treating or preventing osteoporosis.

There are several FDA-approved medications available. Most inhibit the osteoclasts, the cells that break down bone; only one, teriparatide, actually stimulates the growth of new bone. These drugs have not been available for very long, so we do not yet know all their long-term effects. Here is a brief description of each:

- Teriparatide (brand name Forteo®) is a synthetic form of human parathyroid hormone (PTH) that FDA has approved for the treatment of osteoporosis in postmenopausal women at high risk of fracture. This drug must be injected daily for no longer than two years.

- Two drugs in a class known as bisphosphonates, alendronate (brand name Fosamax®) and risedronate (brand name Actonel®), reduce the risk of fractures in postmenopausal women with osteoporosis and now come in a once-a-week pill. Both can cause problems in your stomach and esophagus (the tube that connects the mouth with the stomach) if not taken with 6–8 ounces of water and if you do not remain upright for 30 minutes after taking it.

- Raloxifene (brand name Evista®) mimics estrogen's positive effects on bone without the negative effects on the breast or uterus. It prevents bone loss and reduces the risk of vertebral fractures. However, it could cause blood clots and hot flashes.

- Calcitonin (brand names Miacalcin® and Calcimar®) is a synthetic protein similar to a hormone made by the thyroid. It is approved for treating osteoporosis in women at least five years beyond menopause. It can be taken as a daily nasal spray or by injection under the skin. Calcitonin increases spinal bone density, but its effects on fracture risk are still unclear. The nasal form has few side effects, but may not be as effective as the injected one which may cause an allergic reaction.

NIAMS is funding trials to test various combinations of these drugs. Recently, a trial of PTH and alendronate showed that the concurrent combination provided no additional improvement in BMD than PTH alone. Ongoing studies will determine whether the sequential use of the two drugs is superior to just one of the drugs. NIAMS and several other NIH components are investigating other agents for preventing or treating osteoporosis as well. These include statins (cholesterol-lowering drugs), phytoestrogens (chemicals found in plants that can act like estrogen), and nitric oxide (a drug given to heart patients in the form of nitroglycerin).

Final Advice

Dr. McGowan has one last recommendation: Do regular weight-bearing exercise, such as walking, jogging, stair-climbing, tennis, weight-training, and dancing. These activities may not only help strengthen your bones; they can build muscle and help with your balance, reducing your risk of falling. As doctors are learning with many other functions of the body, use it or lose it—in this case, exercise or lose your bone and muscle strength.

Additional Information

Osteoporosis and Related Bone Diseases–
National Resource Center
NIH ORBD-NRC
2 AMS Circle
Washington, DC 20892-3676
Toll-Free: 800-624-BONE (2663)
Phone: 202-223-0344
TTY: 202-466-4315
Fax: 202-293-2356
Website: http://www.osteo.org
E-mail: osteoinfo@osteo.org

Chapter 56

Anemia Caused by Thyroid Disease

Anemia is a disorder characterized by a decrease in the number of red blood cells that carry oxygen to various body tissues. If you have hypothyroidism, you may also have an associated mild anemia as one manifestation of the general slowing of your body functions that occurs in your condition. The anemia usually causes no symptoms and corrects itself when your hypothyroidism is treated. It is not a separate disease, but is due instead to the low thyroid hormone level.

Pernicious Anemia

A more serious type of anemia, known as pernicious anemia, is a separate disease that tends to occur in older patients who have or have had Graves disease or Hashimoto thyroiditis, and their relatives. This kind of anemia is caused by a deficiency of vitamin B_{12}.

Under normal circumstances, cells lining your stomach make a substance known as intrinsic factor that enables your body to absorb vitamin B_{12} from food. Some individuals lose the ability to absorb vitamin B_{12} due to failure of the cells that make intrinsic factor. The damage seems to be caused by a self-destructive process involving the body's immune system, similar to what occurs in Addison's and Hashimoto diseases.

Vitamin B_{12} is an important ingredient in the manufacturing of red blood cells, and if levels of this vitamin fall, anemia may result. Vitamin

531

B_{12} is also important in nourishing your nervous system, so if you develop pernicious anemia, you also may experience numbness and tingling of your hands and feet, loss of balance, and even leg weakness. It is not clear how many patients who have thyroid functional problems also develop pernicious anemia. Some studies have suggested that as many as 5 percent of patients with Graves disease and 10 percent of those who have Hashimoto disease may develop this condition.

Since pernicious anemia tends to develop in later years, it is probably even more common in older patients with either condition. Therefore, it seems appropriate to measure the blood level of vitamin B in every patient over the age of sixty who has ever had Graves disease or Hashimoto thyroiditis. Doctors do this because pernicious anemia is both common and treatable. If your blood level of vitamin B_{12} appears low or borderline low, another test, known as a Schilling test, can be performed. This test demonstrates whether you have difficulty absorbing vitamin B_{12} from your food. If you do have pernicious anemia, it can be easily treated.

On the basis of new research, your physician may choose to treat you initially with tablets of B_{12} to see if you are able to absorb enough of the vitamin to restore your blood level to normal and thus cure the condition. However, since your body's ability to absorb B_{12} tends to decrease with time, you will probably need treatment with a monthly intramuscular injection of vitamin B_{12} as you grow older.

Platelet Disorders

Platelet disorders are also more common in this group of thyroid patients than they are in the general population. Normally you have about 2.5 million platelets in every teaspoonful of your blood. Despite their small size, they play a major role in helping your blood to clot normally. Some thyroid patients experience easy bruising due to a decrease in the number or function of their platelets. The bruising can become much worse if you take aspirin, or one of the non-steroidal anti-inflammatory drugs such as ibuprofen (Advil or Motrin) or Naprosyn. If that is your situation, your physician may choose to order a platelet count or check your platelet function with a bleeding time test, which tells how long it takes your blood to clot. He or she may also recommend that you take an alternative pain medication such as acetaminophen (Tylenol) which will not worsen your bleeding tendency.

Very rarely, immune processes may destroy large numbers of platelets producing thrombocytopenic purpura. The word purpura refers to red or blue bruises which appear on the skin in this condition, especially on the legs. Tiny purplish-red spots known as petechiae that represent smaller areas of bleeding within the skin are also commonly present in this condition. If you develop this type of rash, your physician is likely consider it an emergency and order an immediate platelet count because of the risk of more serious bleeding elsewhere. If thrombocytopenic purpura proves to be your problem, treatment is usually helpful, and often includes steroid medication.

Additional Information

Thyroid Foundation of America
One Longfellow Place, Suite 1518
Boston, MA 02114
Toll-Free: 800-832-8321
Phone: 617-534-1500
Fax: 617-534-1515
Website: http://www.allthyroid.org
E-mail: info@allthyroid.org

Chapter 57

Low Neonatal Thyroid Function Linked to Cerebral Palsy

Scientists have linked low levels of a thyroid hormone in premature infants to the development of disabling cerebral palsy. They examined more than 400 premature infants screened for blood levels of the hormone thyroxine during the first week of life. They found that infants with low levels of thyroxine at birth had a 3- to 4-fold increase in the incidence of disabling cerebral palsy at age 2.

The study is the most comprehensive to date that explores the relationship between low levels of thyroid hormone (called hypothyroxinemia) at birth and neurodevelopment in preterm infants. The work was funded by the National Institute of Neurological Disorders and Stroke (NINDS) and the National Institute of Child Health and Human Development. It appeared in the March 28, 1996 issue of the *New England Journal of Medicine.* Investigators also found lowered mental development scores at age 2 in the affected children, who had a gestational age of 33 weeks or less.

Cerebral palsy is a group of chronic disorders characterized by impaired body movement. Faulty development or damage to motor areas in the brain disrupts the brain's ability to adequately control movement and posture. Over 500,000 Americans have the disorder, and 4,500 American infants are diagnosed each year.

"Our data gives strong support to the concept that a low level of thyroid hormone around the time of birth is an important cause of

"Study Links Neonatal Thyroid Function to Cerebral Palsy," National Institute of Neurological Disorders and Stroke (NINDS), March 27, 1996, reviewed July 1, 2001.

motor and cognitive problems in preterm infants," said Nigel Paneth, M.D., M.P.H., professor of epidemiology and pediatrics at Michigan State University and one of the authors of the paper. "We will not know, however, whether treatment with thyroid hormone will improve neurodevelopmental outcome until a suitable randomized trial of thyroid supplementation is completed."

- Thyroid hormone is indispensable to cerebral development.

- Babies in the United States are routinely screened for abnormal thyroid function.

- Premature infants often go through a period of transient hypothyroxinemia. They are already at risk for cerebral palsy and account for approximately one-third of cerebral palsy cases.

- In most cases, thyroid function returns to normal within a period of months.

- Rarely, a premature child will have permanently low thyroid hormone levels.

Reference

Reuss, Mary Lynne; Paneth, Nigel; Pinto-Martin, Jennifer A.; Lorenz, John M.; Susser, Mervyn. "The Relation of Transient Hypothyroxinemia in Preterm Infants to Neurologic Development at Two Years of Age." *New England Journal of Medicine*, Vol. 334, No. 13, (pp. 821-827).

Part Ten

Additional Help
and Information

Chapter 58

Glossary of Thyroid Terms

Anaplasia: Loss of structural differentiation, especially as seen in most, but not all, malignant neoplasms.

Addison's disease: Permanent loss of function of the adrenal glands, which make essential steroid hormones for the body. [1]

Anemia: Too few of the red blood cells that deliver essential oxygen to the body's cells. [1]

Antibodies: Proteins that the body's immune system makes to attack invaders like bacteria and viruses. [1]

Antigen: Any substance that, as a result of coming in contact with appropriate cells, induces a state of sensitivity and/or immune responsiveness after a latent period (days to weeks) and that reacts in a demonstrable way with antibodies and/or immune cells of the sensitized subject in vivo or in vitro.

Antithyroid: Relating to an agent that suppresses thyroid function (e.g., propylthiouracil).

Unmarked definitions in this chapter are reprinted with permission from *Stedman's Medical Dictionary, 27th Edition*, Copyright © 2000 Lippincott Williams & Wilkins. All rights reserved. Terms marked [1] are reprinted with permission from the *ATA Hypothyroidism Booklet*, Copyright © 2003 The American Thyroid Association. All rights reserved.

Anti-TPO antibodies: In autoimmune thyroid disease, proteins that mistakenly try to attack the thyroid peroxidase (TPO) enzymes that help the thyroid gland make hormone. [1]

Autoantibody: Antibody occurring in response to antigenic constituents of the host's tissue against self antigen, and which reacts with the inciting tissue component.

Autoimmune disease: Any disease in which the body's immune system, designed to protect the body from outside invaders like viruses and bacteria, mistakes a normal part of the body for an invader and tries to destroy it. [1]

Autoimmune thyroiditis: Inflammation of the thyroid, caused by autoimmune disease. [1]

Atrophic thyroiditis: A form of autoimmune thyroiditis in which the immune system's attack on the thyroid causes it to shrink and stop making thyroid hormone. [1]

Beta-blocker: A compound that selectively blocks or inhibits responses to sympathetic adrenergic nerve activity (sympatholytic agent) and to epinephrine, norepinephrine, and other adrenergic amines (adrenolytic agent).

Biopsy: Process of removing tissue from patients for diagnostic examination.

C cell: Calcitonin-secreting round or spindle shaped follicular thyroid cell.

Calcitonin: A peptide hormone, of which eight forms in five species are known; composed of 32 amino acids and produced by the parathyroid, thyroid, and thymus glands; its action is opposite to that of parathyroid hormone in that calcitonin increases deposition of calcium and phosphate in bone and lowers the level of calcium in the blood.

Cancer: General term frequently used to indicate any of various types of malignant neoplasms, most of which invade surrounding tissues, may metastasize to several sites.

Coma: Unconsciousness from which a person cannot be awakened. [1]

Congenital hypothyroidism: Hypothyroidism in a newborn baby. [1]

Cretinism: Mental and physical retardation caused by severe congenital hypothyroidism. [1]

Deficiency: A lack, too little. [1]

Ectopic: In the wrong place; an ectopic thyroid gland is usually in the tongue and/or upper neck. [1]

Endocrine gland: Any gland that produces and releases hormones directly into the blood, for example, the thyroid, pituitary, adrenals, and pancreas. [1]

Endocrinologist: A medical doctor who specializes in endocrinology, the treatment of endocrine gland diseases like thyroid disease and diabetes. [1]

Enzyme: Protein that helps chemical processes take place within the body but does not get used up in the process; the major enzymes in the thyroid gland are peroxidases. [1]

Exophthalmos: Protrusion of one or both eyeballs; can be congenital and familial, or due to pathology, such as a retroorbital tumor (usually unilateral) or thyroid disease (usually bilateral).

Feedback loop: A system in which A affects B, which in turn affects A again. [1]

Fetus: A developing baby inside the mother. [1]

Fine needle biopsy: The aspiration and removal of tissue or suspensions of cells through a small needle.

Follicular carcinoma: Carcinoma of the thyroid composed of well or poorly differentiated epithelial follicles without papillary formation, which is difficult to distinguish from adenoma; the criteria include blood vessel invasion and the finding of metastases of follicular thyroid tissue in other structures such as cervical lymph nodes and bone; follicular carcinoma may take up radioactive iodine.

Free T4: The thyroid hormone T4 that circulates in the blood unattached to a protein, and that can be taken up by cells in tissues. [1]

Free T4 index: An estimate of the amount of free T4 in the blood. [1]

Gland: An organ or tissue that makes and sends out a hormone or other substance. [1]

541

Goiter: An enlarged thyroid gland, which can cause swelling in the front of the neck. [1]

Graves disease: Autoimmune hyperthyroidism, usually with goiter and eye symptoms. [1]

Hashimoto thyroiditis: Autoimmune thyroiditis in which the immune system's attack on the thyroid causes a goiter (swelling), and sometimes, hypothyroidism. [1]

Hormone: Substance made by an organ or tissue that affects the function of one or more other organs. [1]

Hot nodule: A thyroid nodule with a much higher uptake of radioactive iodine than the surrounding cells; usually benign but sometimes causing hyperthyroidism.

Hürthle cell: A large, granular eosinophilic cell derived from thyroid follicular layer by accumulation of mitochondria, e.g., in Hashimoto disease.

Hyperparathyroidism: A condition due to an increase in the secretion of the parathyroids, causing elevated serum calcium, decreased serum phosphorus, and increased excretion of both calcium and phosphorus, calcium stones, and sometimes generalized osteitis fibrosa cystica.

Hypoparathyroidism: A condition due to diminution or absence of the secretion of the parathyroid hormones, with low serum calcium and tetany, and sometimes with increased bone density.

Hyperthyroidism: An overactive thyroid gland. [1]

Hypothyroidism: An underactive thyroid gland. [1]

I-131: One of several forms of radioactive iodine; low-dose I-131 is used for medical testing and to destroy an overactive thyroid gland. [1]

Infiltrate: To deposit an abnormal substance in a tissue. [1]

Immune response: Any response of the immune system to an antigen including antibody production and/or cell-mediated immunity.

Immune system: The body's way of protecting itself from invaders like bacteria and viruses. [1]

Immunosuppressant: An agent that induces immunosuppression (e.g., cyclosporine, corticosteroids).

Infection: Invasion of the body with organisms that have the potential to cause disease.

Inflammation: The body's response to injured cells. [1]

Iodine: Chemical element that is an essential ingredient of thyroid hormone. [1]

Lymph node: One of numerous round, oval, or bean-shaped bodies located along the course of lymphatic vessels, varying greatly in size (1–25 mm in diameter) and usually presenting a depressed area, the hilum, on one side through which blood vessels enter and efferent lymphatic vessels emerge.

Malignant: In reference to a neoplasm, having the property of locally invasive and destructive growth and metastasis.

mcg: Unit of measure, abbreviation for micrograms; thyroxine doses may be measured in mcg (also written as μg); 50 mcg = .05 mg (milligrams). [1]

Medullary thyroid cancer: A malignant thyroid neoplasm composed of calcitonin producing C-cells and amyloid rich stroma; it may be sporadic or familial; the familial form may be part of the multiple endocrine neoplasia syndrome, type 2A and 2B.

Metabolism: All the processes by which the body makes and uses energy and builds tissues. [1]

Metastases: The spread of a disease process from one part of the body to another, as in the appearance of neoplasms in parts of the body remote from the site of the primary tumor.

Mild hypothyroidism: Subclinical hypothyroidism. [1]

Multiple endocrine neoplasia 3: Characterized by tumors found in MEN2; tall, thin, physical appearance; prominent lips, and neuromas of the tongue and eyelids; autosomal dominant inheritance, caused by mutation in the *RET* oncogene on 10q.

Multiple endocrine neoplasia syndrome, type 1: An autosomal-dominant predisposition to tumors of parathyroid glands, anterior pituitary, endocrine pancreas, and less commonly, other organs.

Multiple endocrine neoplasia syndrome, type 2A: An autosomal-dominant predisposition to tumors of thyroid C cells (medullary carcinoma), adrenal medulla (pheochromocytoma), and nodular hyperplasia of parathyroid glands.

Multiple endocrine neoplasia syndrome, type 2B: An autosomal-dominant predisposition to tumors of thyroid C cells (medullary carcinoma), adrenal medulla (pheochromocytoma), peripheral nerves (mucosal neurinoma), and intestinal ganglioneuromatosis; associated with a tall, thin physical appearance.

mU/L: Unit of measure, abbreviation for milliunits per liter; TSH levels are measured in mU/L. [1]

Myxedema: Severe hypothyroidism; the brain, heart, lungs, kidneys, and other organs slow to the point that they cannot keep up critical functions like maintaining temperature, heart rate, blood pressure, and breathing. [1]

Myxedema coma: Often-fatal unconsciousness resulting from severe hypothyroidism. [1]

Nodule: Small abnormal mass or lump; nodules in the thyroid are very common, but few are cancerous. [1]

Papillary carcinoma: A malignant neoplasm characterized by the formation of numerous, irregular, finger-like projections of fibrous stroma that is covered with a surface layer of neoplastic epithelial cells.

Parathyroid gland: One of two small paired endocrine glands, superior and inferior, usually found embedded in the connective tissue capsule on the posterior surface of the thyroid gland; they secrete parathyroid hormone that regulates the metabolism of calcium and phosphorus.

Parathyroid hormone: A peptide hormone formed by the parathyroid glands; it raises the serum calcium levels when injected by causing bone resorption, reducing renal clearance of calcium and increasing efficiency of calcium absorption in the intestine. It acts in conjunction with calcitonin and other hormones.

Paresthesia: Feeling of pins and needles in the hands and feet. [1]

Pernicious anemia: Chronic progressive anemia of older adults (occurring more frequently during the fifth and later decades, rarely prior to 30 years of age), due to failure of absorption of vitamin B_{12}, usually resulting from a defect of the stomach.

Pituitary (master) gland: From its position in the base of the brain, the pituitary monitors most basic body functions and sends out hormones that control those functions, for example, the rate at which the thyroid gland makes hormone. [1]

Polyglandular autoimmune syndromes: Combinations of autoimmune diseases affecting both endocrine and non-endocrine organs and usually involving the thyroid.

Postpartum: After giving birth. [1]

Premature ovarian failure: Before the normal age for menopause, the ovaries' loss of ability to produce estrogen and release eggs, leaving a woman unable to become pregnant. [1]

Radioactive iodine, radioiodine: Iodine that has naturally or artificially been made radioactive. [1]

Secondary hypothyroidism: Hypothyroidism caused not by damage to the thyroid gland, but by damage to the pituitary gland, preventing it from being able to tell the thyroid to make hormone. [1]

Set point: The body's preferred level or range for a function; for example, the pituitary gland knows the body's normal T4 range (set point) and works to keep the T4 within that range. [1]

Silent: Not causing symptoms. [1]

Subclinical (mild) hypothyroidism: A T4 in the normal range, but a slightly high TSH of 4.0 to 10.0 mU/L, causing few or no symptoms. [1]

Supportive care: General medical care, such as nutrition and fluids, to help a patient recover when no targeted treatment can improve the person's condition. [1]

Suppressive treatment: Thyroxine dose high enough to keep the TSH below normal. [1]

Syndrome: A combination of symptoms. [1]

Synthetic: Made in a laboratory. [1]

T3: Triiodothyronine, a hormone with 3 iodine molecules, made in small amounts by the thyroid gland and in larger amounts from T4 in other body tissues. [1]

T4: Thyroxine, the main hormone made by the thyroid gland, containing 4 iodine molecules. [1]

Thyroglobulin:

1. A protein that contains precursors of thyroid hormone usually stored in the colloid within the thyroid follicles; a defect in thyroglobulin metabolism will lead to hypothyroidism.

2. A substance obtained by the fractionation of thyroid glands from the hog containing not less than 0.7% of total iodine; used as a thyroid hormone in the treatment of hypothyroidism.

Thyroid gland: An endocrine gland, normally in the lower front of the neck, that makes and sends out the hormones T4 and T3, which regulate the metabolism of every cell in the body. [1]

Thyroid hormone: T4 and T3, the products of the thyroid gland. [1]

Thyroid insufficiency: Subnormal secretion of hormones by the thyroid gland.

Thyroiditis: Inflammation of the thyroid gland. [1]

Thyroidectomy: Removal of the thyroid gland.

Thyroidologist: A medical doctor who specializes in the diagnosis and treatment of thyroid diseases. [1]

Thyroid peroxidase (TPO) enzymes: Enzymes within the thyroid gland that help thyroid cells make hormone. [1]

Thyroid-stimulating hormone (TSH): Hormone that the pituitary gland makes and sends into the blood to tell the thyroid gland how much T4 and T3 to make. [1]

Thyroxine: T4, the main hormone made by the thyroid gland; also pills used to treat hypothyroidism by replacing the missing T4. [1]

Toxic goiter: A goiter that forms an excessive secretion, causing signs and symptoms of hyperthyroidism.

Trimester: Three months; the nine months of a pregnancy are broken into three trimesters. [1]

TPO: Thyroid peroxidase. [1]

Trigger: Term describing a system in which a relatively small input turns on a relatively large output, the magnitude of which is unrelated to the magnitude of the input.

TSH: Thyroid-stimulating hormone. [1]

Chapter 59

Directory of Organizations for Thyroid Information

Agency for Toxic Substances and Disease Registry (ATSDR)
Division of Toxicology
Information Center
1600 Clifton Road N.E.
Mail Stop F-32
Atlanta, GA 30333
Toll-Free: 888-422-8737
Phone: 404-498-0110
Fax: 404-498-0093
Website: http://www.atsdr.cdc.gov
E-mail: ATSDRIC@cdc.gov

Alliance of Genetic Support Groups
4301 Connecticut Ave., N.W., Suite 404
Washington, DC 20008-2304
Toll-Free Help Line: 800-336-GENE (4363)
Phone: 202-966-5557
Fax: 202-966-8553
Website: http://www.geneticalliance.org
E-mail: info@geneticalliance.org

American Academy of Otolaryngology–Head and Neck Surgery
One Prince Street
Alexandria, VA 22314-3357
Phone: 703-836-4444
Website: http://www.entnet.org
E-mail: info@entnet.org

Resources in this chapter were compiled from several sources deemed reliable; all contact information was verified and updated in December 2004.

American Association of Clinical Endocrinologists

1000 Riverside Ave., Suite 205
Jacksonville, FL 32204
Phone: 904-353-7878
Fax: 904-353-8185
Website: http://www.aace.com
E-mail: info@aace.com

American Autoimmune Related Diseases Association

22100 Gratiot Avenue
East Detroit, MI 48201-2227
Toll-Free Literature Requests:
800-598-4668
Phone: 586-776-3900
Fax: 586-776-3903
Website: http://www.aarda.org
E-mail: aarda@aarda.org

American Cancer Society

Thyroid Cancer Resource Center
P.O. Box 102454
Atlanta, GA 30368-2425
Toll-Free: 800-ACS-2345 (227-2345)
Website: http://www.cancer.org/docroot/home/index.asp

American Foundation of Thyroid Patients

4322 Douglas Ave.
Midland, TX 79703
Phone: 915-694-9966
Website: http://www.thyroidfoundation.org
E-mail: thyroid@flash.net

American Thyroid Association

6066 Leesburg Pike, Suite 550
Falls Church, VA 22041
Toll-Free: 800-THYROID (849-7643)
Phone: 703-998-8890
Fax: 703-998-8893
Website: http://www.thyroid.org
Thyroid Specialist Locator:
http://www.thyroid.org/patients/specialists.php3
E-mail: admin@thyroid.org

Dana-Farber Cancer Institute

44 Binney Street
Boston, MA 02115
Toll-Free: 866-408-3324
Website: http://www.dana-farber.org

Endocrine Society

8401 Connecticut Ave., Suite 900
Chevy Chase, MD 20815-5817
Phone: 301-941-0200
Website: http://www.endo-society.org
E-mail: societyservices@endo-society.org

Hormone Foundation

8401 Connecticut Ave., Suite 900
Chevy Chase, MD 20815-5817
Toll-Free: 800-HORMONE (467-6663)
Website: http://www.hormone.org

Hypoparathyroidism Association, Inc.
2835 Salmon
Idaho Falls, ID 83406
Phone: 208-524-3857
Website: http://www
.hypoparathyroidism.org
E-mail: hpth@
hypoparathyroidism.org

Johns Hopkins Thyroid Tumor Center
Website: http://www.thyroid-cancer.net
Thyroid Specialist Locator:
http://www.thyroid-cancer.net/resources/findaspec.php3

Light of Life Foundation
Thyroid Cancer Information
P.O. Box 163
Manalapan, NJ 07726
Toll-Free: 877-565-6325
Website: http://
www.checkyourneck.com
E-mail: info@checkyourneck.com

Magic Foundation
6645 W. North Ave.
Oak Park, IL 60302
Phone: 708-383-0808
Fax: 708-383-0899
Website: http://
www.magicfoundation.org

March of Dimes/Birth Defects Foundation
1275 Mamaroneck Avenue
White Plains, NY 10605
Phone: 914-428-7100
Website: http://
www.modimes.org

National Cancer Institute
6116 Executive Blvd., MSC 8322
Bethesda, MD 20892-8322
Toll-Free: 800-4-CANCER (800-422-6237)
Toll-Free TTY: 800-332-8615
Website: http://www.cancer.gov
E-mail: cancergovstaff@mail
.nih.gov.

National Coalition for Cancer Survivorship
1010 Wayne Ave., Suite 770
Silver Spring, MD 20910
Toll-Free: 877-622-7937
Phone: 301-650-9127
Fax: 301-565-9670
Website: http://
www.canceradvocacy.org
E-mail: info@canceradvocacy.org

National Graves' Disease Foundation
P.O. Box 8387
Fleming Island, FL 32006
Phone: 904-278-9488
Website: http://www.ngdf.org

National Health Information Center
P.O. Box 1133
Washington, DC 20013-1133
Toll-Free: 800-336-4797
Phone: 301-565-4167
Website: http://
www.healthfinder.gov
E-mail: healthfinder@nhic.org

National Institute of Diabetes and Digestive and Kidney Diseases (NIDDK)
NIH Building 31, Room 9A04
Center Drive, MSC 2560
Bethesda, MD 20892-2560
Phone: 301-496-3583
Website: http://
www.niddk.nih.gov

National Pesticides Information Center (NPIC)
Oregon State University
333 Weniger Hall
Corvallis, OR 97331-6502
Toll-Free: 800-858-7378 (7 days/
week, except holidays, 6:30 a.m.
to 4:30 p.m. Pacific Time)
Website: http://npic.orst.edu
E-mail: npic@ace.orst.edu

National Service Center for Environmental Publications (NSCEP)
P.O. Box 42419
Cincinnati, OH 45242-2419
Toll-Free: 800-490-9198
Phone: 513-489-8190
Fax: 513-489-8695
Website: http://www.epa.gov/
ncepihom

National Women's Health Information Center
8550 Arlington Blvd.
Suite 300
Fairfax, VA 22031
Toll-Free: 800-994-9662
Website: http://
www.4woman.gov

Norman Endocrine Surgery Clinic
505 South Boulevard
Tampa, FL 33606
Phone: 813-991-6922
Fax: 813-991-6918
Website: http://
www.endocrineweb.com

Osteoporosis and Related Bone Diseases–National Resource Center
2 AMS Circle
Washington, DC 20892-3676
Toll-Free: 800-624-BONE (2663)
Phone: 202-223-0344
TTY: 202-466-4315
Fax: 202-293-2356
Website: http://www.osteo.org
E-mail: osteoinfo@osteo.org

Patient Recruitment and Public Liaison Office
10 Cloister Ct., Bldg. 61
Bethesda, MD 20892-4754
Toll Free: 800-411-1222
Toll-Free TTY: 866-411-1010
Fax: 301-480-9793
Website: http://
clinicalstudies.info.nih.gov
E-mail: prpl@mail.cc.nih.gov

Pituitary Network Association
P.O. Box 1958
Thousand Oaks, CA 91358
Phone: 805-499-9973
Fax: 805-480-0633
Website: http://
www.pituitary.org

Santa Monica Thyroid Diagnostic Center

1328 16th Street
Santa Monica, CA 90404
Toll-Free (outside CA): 800-408-4909
Phone: 310-393-8860
Fax: 310-395-8147
Website: http://www.thyroid.com
E-mail: Dr.Guttler@thyroid.com

ThyCa: Thyroid Cancer Survivors' Association, Inc.

P.O. Box 1545
New York, NY 10159-1545
Toll-Free: 877-588-7904
Fax: 630-604-6078
Website: http://www.thyca.org
E-mail: thyca@thyca.org

Thyroid Federation International

797 Princess St., Suite 304
Kingston, ON K7L 1G1
Canada
Phone: 613-544-8364
Fax: 613-544-9731
Website: http://www.thyroid-fed.org
E-mail: tfi@on.aibn.com

Thyroid Foundation of America, Inc.

One Longfellow Place, Suite 1518
Boston, MA 02114
Toll-Free: 800-832-8321
Phone: 617-534-1500
Fax: 617-534-1515
Website: http://www.allthyroid.org
E-mail: info@allthyroid.org

Thyroid Today

ACCESS Medical Group
Department of Continuing
Medical Education
8420 W. Bryn Mawr Ave.
Suite 800
Chicago, IL 60631
Phone: 847-392-2227
Fax: 847-392-2257
Website: http://www.thyroidtoday.com
E-mail: access@access-medical.com

University of Texas M. D. Anderson Cancer Center

1515 Holcombe Blvd.
Houston, TX 77030
Toll-Free: 800-392-1611
Phone: 713-792-6161
Website: http://www.mdanderson.org

U.S. Preventive Services Task Force

Project Director, USPSTF
Agency for Healthcare Research
and Quality
540 Gaither Road
Rockville, MD 20850
Toll-Free: 800-358-9295
Website: http://www.ahrq.gov/clinic/uspstfix.htm
E-mail: uspstf@ahrq.gov

Index

Index

Page numbers followed by 'n' indicate a footnote. Page numbers in *italics* indicate a table or illustration.

heredity
  goiter 67
  hyperparathyroidism 310
  hypothyroidism 203
  medullary thyroid cancer 401, 402–3
  multiple endocrine neoplasia type 1
    320
  multiple endocrine neoplasia type 2
    330
  Pendred syndrome 251–55
  pseudohypoparathyroidism 337–38
  thyroid cancer 347
  thyroid disorders 9, 10
  thyrotoxic periodic paralysis 294
Hirschsprung disease 409
Hollowell, Joe 140n
"Home Preparation Procedure for
  Emergency Administration of Potassium Iodide Tablets to Infants and
  Small Children" (FDA) 116n
Hormone Foundation
  contact information 53, 455, 548
  endocrinologists publication 47n
hormones
  defined 223, 542
  endocrine system 24–25
  sexual characteristics 24
  see also thyroid hormones
hormone treatment, thyroid cancer
  356–57
hot nodules
  defined 542
  described 74, 350
Howdeshell, Kembra L. 99, 104
"How to Take the Thyroid 'Neck
  Check'" (AACE) 153n
human chorionic gonadotropin (hCG),
  pregnancy 226, 266
Hürthle cell, defined 542
hyperparathyroidism
  defined 542
  overview 309–17
  treatment 321, 491–93
hypertension, endocrinologists 52
hyperthyroidism
  defined 223, 542
  described 4, 6, 27, 58, 482–83
  iodine 143
  medications 449–55

hyperthyroidism, continued
  osteoporosis 522
  overview 260–66
  pregnancy 266–70
  symptoms 62–65
  see also Graves disease
"Hyperthyroidism: Information for
  Patients" (AACE) 260n
hypocalcemia 339
hypoglycemia, growth hormone 27
hypomagnesemia 335
hypoparathyroidism
  defined 542
  overview 333–36
"Hypoparathyroidism" (Norman) 333n
Hypoparathyroidism Association,
  Inc., contact information 549
hypothalamus, described 22
hypothyroidism
  defined 223, 542
  described 5, 6, 27, 58
  iodine 144–45
  medications 437–48
  overview 198–225
  pregnancy 226–33
  symptoms 59–62
  treatment 10–11
  see also congenital hypothyroidism;
    myxedema; subclinical hypo-
    thyroidism

I

I-131
  defined 223, 542
  thyroid cancer 356–57, 376–85
  thyroid disorders 101–3
Idaho, thyroid cancer mortality *367*
"If a genetic disorder runs in my family,
  what are the chances that my children will have the condition?"
  (NLM) 251n
Illinois, thyroid cancer mortality *367*
immune response, defined 34, 542
immune system
  defined 34, 223, 542
  Hashimoto thyroiditis 236
  pregnancy 230–31

563

liver disorders, antithyroid medications 453–54
"Living with Graves' Disease" (Patterson) 283n
Long Island Breast Cancer Study 125
Lopressor (metoprolol) 272
Louisiana, thyroid cancer mortality *367*
"The Low-Down on Osteoporosis: What We Know and What We Don't" (Bennett) 517n
LT4 *see* levothyroxine sodium
L-thyroxine 248
luteinizing hormone (LH), hyperparathyroidism 322
lymph nodes, defined 543

M

Magic Foundation, contact information 250, 549
magnetic resonance imaging (MRI), thyroid cancer 350
Maine, thyroid cancer mortality *367*
major depression, described 84
"Making Choices: Screening for Thyroid Disease" (NCI) 376n, 382n, 385n
malignant, defined 543
malignant nodules, described 345
mania, symptoms 95
March of Dimes/Birth Defects Foundation, contact information 329, 549
Maryland, thyroid cancer mortality *367*
Massachusetts, thyroid cancer mortality *368*
master gland, defined 224
McClain, R. Michael 99
mcg, defined 223, 543
McGowan, Joan 526–29
medications
combinations 214
factitious hyperthyroidism 303–4
Graves disease 283–84
hyperthyroidism 265
hypothyroidism 202
thyroxine 211–12

Medmaster, thyroid medication publication 437n
MedPointe, Inc., contact information 121
medullary thyroid cancer
defined 543
described 346, 393–94
overview 399–430
treatment 396–97
"Medullary Thyroid Cancer Overview" (Norman) 399n
melatonin, described 24
Memorial Sloan-Kettering Cancer Center, TSH-producing tumors publication 297n
MEN-1 *see* multiple endocrine neoplasia type 1
MEN-2 *see* multiple endocrine neoplasia type 2
metabolism, defined 223, 543
metastases, defined 543
methimazole (MMI) 263, 268, 272, 450–54
metoprolol 272
Miacalcin (calcitonin) 529
Michigan
thyroid cancer diagnoses *371*
thyroid cancer mortality *368*
microbial inflammatory thyroiditis *458*, 462–63, *463*
mild hypothyroidism, defined 224
see also subclinical hypothyroidism
minimally invasive parathyroidectomy 315
minimally invasive radioguided parathyroid (MIRP) 187, 493
Minnesota, thyroid cancer mortality *368*
MIRP *see* minimally invasive radioguided parathyroid
Mississippi, thyroid cancer mortality *368*
Missouri, thyroid cancer mortality *368*
MMI *see* methimazole
Montana, thyroid cancer mortality *368*
Morreale de Escobar, Gabriella 98
mU/L, defined 223, 544
"Multiple Endocrine Neoplasia (MEN) II" (A.D.A.M., Inc.) 330n

Health Reference Series
COMPLETE CATALOG

Adolescent Health Sourcebook

Basic Consumer Health Information about Common Medical, Mental, and Emotional Concerns in Adolescents, Including Facts about Acne, Body Piercing, Mononucleosis, Nutrition, Eating Disorders, Stress, Depression, Behavior Problems, Peer Pressure, Violence, Gangs, Drug Use, Puberty, Sexuality, Pregnancy, Learning Disabilities, and More

Along with a Glossary of Terms and Other Resources for Further Help and Information

Edited by Chad T. Kimball. 658 pages. 2002. 0-7808-0248-9. $78.

"It is written in clear, nontechnical language aimed at general readers. . . . Recommended for public libraries, community colleges, and other agencies serving health care consumers."
— American Reference Books Annual, 2003

"Recommended for school and public libraries. Parents and professionals dealing with teens will appreciate the easy-to-follow format and the clearly written text. This could become a 'must have' for every high school teacher." — E-Streams, Jan '03

"A good starting point for information related to common medical, mental, and emotional concerns of adolescents." — School Library Journal, Nov '02

"This book provides accurate information in an easy to access format. It addresses topics that parents and caregivers might not be aware of and provides practical, useable information." — Doody's Health Sciences Book Review Journal, Sep-Oct '02

"Recommended reference source."
— Booklist, American Library Association, Sep '02

■

AIDS Sourcebook, 3rd Edition

Basic Consumer Health Information about Acquired Immune Deficiency Syndrome (AIDS) and Human Immunodeficiency Virus (HIV) Infection, Including Facts about Transmission, Prevention, Diagnosis, Treatment, Opportunistic Infections, and Other Complications, with a Section for Women and Children, Including Details about Associated Gynecological Concerns, Pregnancy, and Pediatric Care

Along with Updated Statistical Information, Reports on Current Research Initiatives, a Glossary, and Directories of Internet, Hotline, and Other Resources

Edited by Dawn D. Matthews. 664 pages. 2003. 0-7808-0631-X. $78.

ALSO AVAILABLE: AIDS Sourcebook, 1st Edition. Edited by Karen Bellenir and Peter D. Dresser. 831 pages. 1995. 0-7808-0031-1. $78.

AIDS Sourcebook, 2nd Edition. Edited by Karen Bellenir. 751 pages. 1999. 0-7808-0225-X. $78.

"The 3rd edition of the *AIDS Sourcebook*, part of Omnigraphics' *Health Reference Series*, is a welcome update. . . . This resource is highly recommended for academic and public libraries."
—American Reference Books Annual, 2004

"Excellent sourcebook. This continues to be a highly recommended book. There is no other book that provides as much information as this book provides."
— AIDS Book Review Journal, Dec-Jan 2000

"Recommended reference source."
—Booklist, American Library Association, Dec '99

"A solid text for college-level health libraries."
—The Bookwatch, Aug '99

Cited in Reference Sources for Small and Medium-Sized Libraries, American Library Association, 1999

■

Alcoholism Sourcebook

Basic Consumer Health Information about the Physical and Mental Consequences of Alcohol Abuse, Including Liver Disease, Pancreatitis, Wernicke-Korsakoff Syndrome (Alcoholic Dementia), Fetal Alcohol Syndrome, Heart Disease, Kidney Disorders, Gastrointestinal Problems, and Immune System Compromise and Featuring Facts about Addiction, Detoxification, Alcohol Withdrawal, Recovery, and the Maintenance of Sobriety

Along with a Glossary and Directories of Resources for Further Help and Information

Edited by Karen Bellenir. 613 pages. 2000. 0-7808-0325-6. $78.

"This title is one of the few reference works on alcoholism for general readers. For some readers this will be a welcome complement to the many self-help books on the market. Recommended for collections serving general readers and consumer health collections."
— E-Streams, Mar '01

"This book is an excellent choice for public and academic libraries."
— American Reference Books Annual, 2001

"Recommended reference source."
—Booklist, American Library Association, Dec '00

"Presents a wealth of information on alcohol use and abuse and its effects on the body and mind, treatment, and prevention." — SciTech Book News, Dec '00

"Important new health guide which packs in the latest consumer information about the problems of alcoholism." — Reviewer's Bookwatch, Nov '00

SEE ALSO Drug Abuse Sourcebook, Substance Abuse Sourcebook

575

Allergies Sourcebook, 2nd Edition

Basic Consumer Health Information about Allergic Disorders, Triggers, Reactions, and Related Symptoms, Including Anaphylaxis, Rhinitis, Sinusitis, Asthma, Dermatitis, Conjunctivitis, and Multiple Chemical Sensitivity

Along with Tips on Diagnosis, Prevention, and Treatment, Statistical Data, a Glossary, and a Directory of Sources for Further Help and Information

Edited by Annemarie S. Muth. 598 pages. 2002. 0-7808-0376-0. $78.

ALSO AVAILABLE: Allergies Sourcebook, 1st Edition. Edited by Allan R. Cook. 611 pages. 1997. 0-7808-0036-2. $78.

"This book brings a great deal of useful material together. . . . This is an excellent addition to public and consumer health library collections."
— *American Reference Books Annual, 2003*

"This second edition would be useful to laypersons with little or advanced knowledge of the subject matter. This book would also serve as a resource for nursing and other health care professions students. It would be useful in public, academic, and hospital libraries with consumer health collections." — *E-Streams, Jul '02*

■

Alternative Medicine Sourcebook, 2nd Edition

Basic Consumer Health Information about Alternative and Complementary Medical Practices, Including Acupuncture, Chiropractic, Herbal Medicine, Homeopathy, Naturopathic Medicine, Mind-Body Interventions, Ayurveda, and Other Non-Western Medical Traditions

Along with Facts about such Specific Therapies as Massage Therapy, Aromatherapy, Qigong, Hypnosis, Prayer, Dance, and Art Therapies, a Glossary, and Resources for Further Information

Edited by Dawn D. Matthews. 618 pages. 2002. 0-7808-0605-0. $78.

ALSO AVAILABLE: Alternative Medicine Sourcebook, 1st Edition. Edited by Allan R. Cook. 737 pages. 1999. 0-7808-0200-4. $78.

"Recommended for public, high school, and academic libraries that have consumer health collections. Hospital libraries that also serve the public will find this to be a useful resource." — *E-Streams, Feb '03*

"Recommended reference source."
— *Booklist, American Library Association, Jan '03*

"An important alternate health reference."
— *MBR Bookwatch, Oct '02*

"A great addition to the reference collection of every type of library." — *American Reference Books Annual, 2000*

Alzheimer's Disease Sourcebook, 3rd Edition

Basic Consumer Health Information about Alzheimer's Disease, Other Dementias, and Related Disorders, Including Multi-Infarct Dementia, AIDS Dementia Complex, Dementia with Lewy Bodies, Huntington's Disease, Wernicke-Korsakoff Syndrome (Alcohol-Reated Dementia), Delirium, and Confusional States

Along with Information for People Newly Diagnosed with Alzheimer's Disease and Caregivers, Reports Detailing Current Research Efforts in Prevention, Diagnosis, and Treatment, Facts about Long-Term Care Issues, and Listings of Sources for Additional Information

Edited by Karen Bellenir. 645 pages. 2003. 0-7808-0666-2. $78.

ALSO AVAILABLE: Alzheimer's, Stroke & 29 Other Neurological Disorders Sourcebook, 1st Edition. Edited by Frank E. Bair. 579 pages. 1993. 1-55888-748-2. $78.

ALSO AVAILABLE: Alzheimer's Disease Sourcebook, 2nd Edition. Edited by Karen Bellenir. 524 pages. 1999. 0-7808-0223-3. $78.

"This very informative and valuable tool will be a great addition to any library serving consumers, students and health care workers."
— *American Reference Books Annual, 2004*

"This is a valuable resource for people affected by dementias such as Alzheimer's. It is easy to navigate and includes important information and resources."
— *Doody's Review Service, Feb. 2004*

"Recommended reference source."
— *Booklist, American Library Association, Oct '99*

SEE ALSO Brain Disorders Sourcebook

■

Arthritis Sourcebook, 2nd Edition

Basic Consumer Health Information about Osteoarthritis, Rheumatoid Arthritis, Other Rheumatic Disorders, Infectious Forms of Arthritis, and Diseases with Symptoms Linked to Arthritis, Featuring Facts about Diagnosis, Pain Management, and Surgical Therapies

Along with Coping Strategies, Research Updates, a Glossary, and Resources for Additional Help and Information

Edited by Amy L. Sutton. 593 pages. 2004. 0-7808-0667-0. $78.

ALSO AVAILABLE: Arthritis Sourcebook, 1st Edition. Edited by Allan R. Cook. 550 pages. 1998. 0-7808-0201-2. $78.

". . . accessible to the layperson."
— *Reference and Research Book News, Feb '99*

Asthma Sourcebook

Basic Consumer Health Information about Asthma, Including Symptoms, Traditional and Nontraditional Remedies, Treatment Advances, Quality-of-Life Aids, Medical Research Updates, and the Role of Allergies, Exercise, Age, the Environment, and Genetics in the Development of Asthma

Along with Statistical Data, a Glossary, and Directories of Support Groups, and Other Resources for Further Information

Edited by Annemarie S. Muth. 628 pages. 2000. 0-7808-0381-7. $78.

"A worthwhile reference acquisition for public libraries and academic medical libraries whose readers desire a quick introduction to the wide range of asthma information." —Choice, Association of College & Research Libraries, Jun '01

"Recommended reference source." —Booklist, American Library Association, Feb '01

"Highly recommended." —The Bookwatch, Jan '01

"There is much good information for patients and their families who deal with asthma daily." —American Medical Writers Association Journal, Winter '01

"This informative text is recommended for consumer health collections in public, secondary school, and community college libraries and the libraries of universities with a large undergraduate population." —American Reference Books Annual, 2001

Attention Deficit Disorder Sourcebook

Basic Consumer Health Information about Attention Deficit/Hyperactivity Disorder in Children and Adults, Including Facts about Causes, Symptoms, Diagnostic Criteria, and Treatment Options Such as Medications, Behavior Therapy, Coaching, and Homeopathy

Along with Reports on Current Research Initiatives, Legal Issues, and Government Regulations, and Featuring a Glossary of Related Terms, Internet Resources, and a List of Additional Reading Material

Edited by Dawn D. Matthews. 470 pages. 2002. 0-7808-0624-7. $78.

"Recommended reference source." —Booklist, American Library Association, Jan '03

"This book is recommended for all school libraries and the reference or consumer health sections of public libraries." —American Reference Books Annual, 2003

Back & Neck Sourcebook, 2nd Edition

Basic Consumer Health Information about Spinal Pain, Spinal Cord Injuries, and Related Disorders, Such as Degenerative Disk Disease, Osteoarthritis, Scoliosis, Sciatica, Spina Bifida, and Spinal Stenosis, and Featuring Facts about Maintaining Spinal Health, Self-Care, Pain Management, Rehabilitative Care, Chiro-

practic Care, Spinal Surgeries, and Complementary Therapies

Along with Suggestions for Preventing Back and Neck Pain, a Glossary of Related Terms, and a Directory of Resources

Edited by Amy L. Sutton. 633 pages. 2004. 0-7808-0738-3 $78.

ALSO AVAILABLE: Back & Neck Disorders Sourcebook, 1st Edition. Edited by Karen Bellenir. 548 pages. 1997. 0-7808-0202-0. $78.

"The strength of this work is its basic, easy-to-read format. Recommended." —Reference and User Services Quarterly, American Library Association, Winter '97

Blood & Circulatory Disorders Sourcebook, 2nd Edition

Basic Consumer Health Information about the Blood and Circulatory System and Related Disorders, Such as Anemia and Other Hemoglobin Diseases, Cancer of the Blood and Associated Bone Marrow Disorders, Clotting and Bleeding Problems, and Conditions That Affect the Veins, Blood Vessels, and Arteries, Including Facts about the Donation and Transplantation of Bone Marrow, Stem Cells, and Blood and Tips for Keeping the Blood and Circulatory System Healthy

Along with a Glossary of Related Terms and Resources for Additional Help and Information

Edited by Amy L. Sutton. 650 pages. 2005. 0-7808-0746-4. $78.

ALSO AVAILABLE: Blood and Circulatory Disorders Sourcebook, 1st Edition. Edited by Karen Bellenir and Linda M. Shin. 554 pages. 1998. 0-7808-0203-9. $78.

"Recommended reference source." —Booklist, American Library Association, Feb '99

"An important reference sourcebook written in simple language for everyday, non-technical users. " —Reviewer's Bookwatch, Jan '99

Brain Disorders Sourcebook, 2nd Edition

Basic Consumer Health Information about Acquired and Traumatic Brain Injuries, Infections of the Brain, Epilepsy and Seizure Disorders, Cerebral Palsy, and Degenerative Neurological Disorders, Including Amyotrophic Lateral Sclerosis (ALS), Dementias, Multiple Sclerosis, and More

Along with Information on the Brain's Structure and Function, Treatment and Rehabilitation Options, Reports on Current Research Initiatives, a Glossary of Terms Related to Brain Disorders and Injuries, and a Directory of Sources for Further Help and Information

Edited by Sandra J. Judd. 625 pages. 2005. 0-7808-0744-8. $78.

ALSO AVAILABLE: Brain Disorders Sourcebook, 1st Edition. Edited by Karen Bellenir. 481 pages. 1999. 0-7808-0229-2. $78.

SEE ALSO *Alzheimer's Disease Sourcebook*

Breast Cancer Sourcebook, 2nd Edition

Basic Consumer Health Information about Breast Cancer, Including Facts about Risk Factors, Prevention, Screening and Diagnostic Methods, Treatment Options, Complementary and Alternative Therapies, Post-Treatment Concerns, Clinical Trials, Special Risk Populations, and New Developments in Breast Cancer Research

Along with Breast Cancer Statistics, a Glossary of Related Terms, and a Directory of Resources for Additional Help and Information

Edited by Sandra J. Judd. 595 pages. 2004. 0-7808-0668-9. $78.

ALSO AVAILABLE: Breast Cancer Sourcebook, 1st Edition. Edited by Edward J. Prucha and Karen Bellenir. 580 pages. 2001. 0-7808-0244-6. $78.

SEE ALSO *Cancer Sourcebook for Women, Women's Health Concerns Sourcebook*

Breastfeeding Sourcebook

Basic Consumer Health Information about the Benefits of Breastmilk, Preparing to Breastfeed, Breastfeeding as a Baby Grows, Nutrition, and More, Including Information on Special Situations and Concerns Such as Mastitis, Illness, Medications, Allergies, Multiple Births, Prematurity, Special Needs, and Adoption

Along with a Glossary and Resources for Additional Help and Information

Edited by Jenni Lynn Colson. 388 pages. 2002. 0-7808-0332-9. $78.

SEE ALSO *Pregnancy & Birth Sourcebook*

Burns Sourcebook

Basic Consumer Health Information about Various Types of Burns and Scalds, Including Flame, Heat, Cold, Electrical, Chemical, and Sun Burns

Along with Information on Short-Term and Long-Term Treatments, Tissue Reconstruction, Plastic Surgery, Prevention Suggestions, and First Aid

Edited by Allan R. Cook. 604 pages. 1999. 0-7808-0204-7. $78.

SEE ALSO *Skin Disorders Sourcebook*

Cancer Sourcebook, 4th Edition

Basic Consumer Health Information about Major Forms and Stages of Cancer, Featuring Facts about Head and Neck Cancers, Lung Cancers, Gastrointestinal Cancers, Genitourinary Cancers, Lymphomas, Blood Cell Cancers, Endocrine Cancers, Skin Cancers, Bone Cancers, Sarcomas, and Others, and Including Information about Cancer Treatments and Therapies, Identifying and Reducing Cancer Risks, and Strategies for Coping with Cancer and the Side Effects of Treatment

Along with a Cancer Glossary, Statistical and Demographic Data, and a Directory of Sources for Additional Help and Information

Edited by Karen Bellenir. 1,119 pages. 2003. 0-7808-0633-6. $78.

ALSO AVAILABLE: Cancer Sourcebook, 1st Edition. Edited by Frank E. Bair. 932 pages. 1990. 1-55888-888-8. $78.

New Cancer Sourcebook, 2nd Edition. Edited by Allan R. Cook. 1,313 pages. 1996. 0-7808-0041-9. $78.

Cancer Sourcebook, 3rd Edition. Edited by Edward J. Prucha. 1,069 pages. 2000. 0-7808-0227-6. $78.

"With cancer being the second leading cause of death for Americans, a prodigious work such as this one, which locates centrally so much cancer-related information, is clearly an asset to this nation's citizens and others." —*Journal of the National Medical Association, 2004*

"This title is recommended for health sciences and public libraries with consumer health collections." —*E-Streams, Feb '01*

". . . can be effectively used by cancer patients and their families who are looking for answers in a language they can understand. Public and hospital libraries should have it on their shelves." —*American Reference Books Annual, 2001*

"Recommended reference source." —*Booklist, American Library Association, Dec '00*

Cited in *Reference Sources for Small and Medium-Sized Libraries, American Library Association, 1999*

"The amount of factual and useful information is extensive. The writing is very clear, geared to general readers. Recommended for all levels." —*Choice, Association of College & Research Libraries, Jan '97*

SEE ALSO *Breast Cancer Sourcebook, Cancer Sourcebook for Women, Pediatric Cancer Sourcebook, Prostate Cancer Sourcebook*

∎

Cancer Sourcebook for Women, 2nd Edition

Basic Consumer Health Information about Gynecologic Cancers and Related Concerns, Including Cervical Cancer, Endometrial Cancer, Gestational Trophoblastic Tumor, Ovarian Cancer, Uterine Cancer, Vaginal Cancer, Vulvar Cancer, Breast Cancer, and Common Non-Cancerous Uterine Conditions, with Facts about Cancer Risk Factors, Screening and Prevention, Treatment Options, and Reports on Current Research Initiatives

Along with a Glossary of Cancer Terms and a Directory of Resources for Additional Help and Information

Edited by Karen Bellenir. 604 pages. 2002. 0-7808-0226-8. $78.

ALSO AVAILABLE: *Cancer Sourcebook for Women, 1st Edition.* Edited by Allan R. Cook and Peter D. Dresser. 524 pages. 1996. 0-7808-0076-1. $78.

"An excellent addition to collections in public, consumer health, and women's health libraries." —*American Reference Books Annual, 2003*

"Overall, the information is excellent, and complex topics are clearly explained. As a reference book for the consumer it is a valuable resource to assist them to make informed decisions about cancer and its treatments." —*Cancer Forum, Nov '02*

"Highly recommended for academic and medical reference collections." —*Library Bookwatch, Sep '02*

"This is a highly recommended book for any public or consumer library, being reader friendly and containing accurate and helpful information." —*E-Streams, Aug '02*

"Recommended reference source." —*Booklist, American Library Association, Jul '02*

SEE ALSO *Breast Cancer Sourcebook, Women's Health Concerns Sourcebook*

∎

Cardiovascular Diseases & Disorders Sourcebook, 3rd Edition

Basic Consumer Health Information about Heart and Vascular Diseases and Disorders, Such as Angina, Heart Attacks, Arrhythmias, Cardiomyopathy, Valve Disease, Atherosclerosis, and Aneurysms, with Information about Managing Cardiovascular Risk Factors and Maintaining Heart Health, Medications and Procedures Used to Treat Cardiovascular Disorders, and Concerns of Special Significance to Women

long with Reports on Current Research Initiatives, a Glossary of Related Medical Terms, and a Directory of Sources for Further Help and Information

Edited by Sandra J. Judd. 713 pages. 2005. 0-7808-0739-1. $78.

ALSO AVAILABLE: *Heart Diseases & Disorders Sourcebook, 2nd Edition.* Edited by Karen Bellenir. 612 pages. 2000. 0-7808-0238-1. $78.

Cardiovascular Diseases & Disorders Sourcebook, 1st Edition. Edited by Karen Bellenir and Peter D. Dresser. 683 pages. 1995. 0-7808-0032-X. $78.

"This work stands out as an imminently accessible resource for the general public. It is recommended for the reference and circulating shelves of school, public, and academic libraries." —*American Reference Books Annual, 2001*

"Recommended reference source." —*Booklist, American Library Association, Dec '00*

"Provides comprehensive coverage of matters related to the heart. This title is recommended for health sciences and public libraries with consumer health collections." —*E-Streams, Oct '00*

SEE ALSO *Healthy Heart Sourcebook for Women*

∎

Caregiving Sourcebook

Basic Consumer Health Information for Caregivers, Including a Profile of Caregivers, Caregiving Responsibilities and Concerns, Tips for Specific Conditions, Care Environments, and the Effects of Caregiving

Along with Facts about Legal Issues, Financial Information, and Future Planning, a Glossary, and a Listing of Additional Resources

Edited by Joyce Brennfleck Shannon. 600 pages. 2001. 0-7808-0331-0. $78.

Child Abuse Sourcebook

Basic Consumer Health Information about the Physical, Sexual, and Emotional Abuse of Children, with Additional Facts about Neglect, Munchausen Syndrome by Proxy (MSBP), Shaken Baby Syndrome, and Controversial Issues Related to Child Abuse, Such as Withholding Medical Care, Corporal Punishment, and Child Maltreatment in Youth Sports, and Featuring Facts about Child Protective Services, Foster Care, Adoption, Parenting Challenges, and Other Abuse Prevention Efforts

Along with a Glossary of Related Terms and Resources for Additional Help and Information

Edited by Dawn D. Matthews. 620 pages. 2004. 0-7808-0705-7. $78.

Childhood Diseases & Disorders Sourcebook

Basic Consumer Health Information about Medical Problems Often Encountered in Pre-Adolescent Children, Including Respiratory Tract Ailments, Ear Infections, Sore Throats, Disorders of the Skin and Scalp, Digestive and Genitourinary Diseases, Infectious Diseases, Inflammatory Disorders, Chronic Physical and Developmental Disorders, Allergies, and More

Along with Information about Diagnostic Tests, Common Childhood Surgeries, and Frequently Used Medications, with a Glossary of Important Terms and Resource Directory

Edited by Chad T. Kimball. 662 pages. 2003. 0-7808-0458-9. $78.

Colds, Flu & Other Common Ailments Sourcebook

Basic Consumer Health Information about Common Ailments and Injuries, Including Colds, Coughs, the Flu, Sinus Problems, Headaches, Fever, Nausea and Vomiting, Menstrual Cramps, Diarrhea, Constipation, Hemorrhoids, Back Pain, Dandruff, Dry and Itchy Skin, Cuts, Scrapes, Sprains, Bruises, and More

Along with Information about Prevention, Self-Care, Choosing a Doctor, Over-the-Counter Medications, Folk

Remedies, and Alternative Therapies, and Including a Glossary of Important Terms and a Directory of Resources for Further Help and Information

Edited by Chad T. Kimball. 638 pages. 2001. 0-7808-0435-X. $78.

Communication Disorders Sourcebook

Basic Information about Deafness and Hearing Loss, Speech and Language Disorders, Voice Disorders, Balance and Vestibular Disorders, and Disorders of Smell, Taste, and Touch

Edited by Linda M. Ross. 533 pages. 1996. 0-7808-0077-X. $78.

Congenital Disorders Sourcebook

Basic Information about Disorders Acquired during Gestation, Including Spina Bifida, Hydrocephalus, Cerebral Palsy, Heart Defects, Craniofacial Abnormalities, Fetal Alcohol Syndrome, and More

Along with Current Treatment Options and Statistical Data

Edited by Karen Bellenir. 607 pages. 1997. 0-7808-0205-5. $78.

SEE ALSO Pregnancy & Birth Sourcebook

Consumer Issues in Health Care Sourcebook

Basic Information about Health Care Fundamentals and Related Consumer Issues, Including Exams and Screening Tests, Physician Specialties, Choosing a Doctor, Using Prescription and Over-the-Counter Medications Safely, Avoiding Health Scams, Managing Common Health Risks in the Home, Care Options for Chronically or Terminally Ill Patients, and a List of Resources for Obtaining Help and Further Information

Edited by Karen Bellenir. 618 pages. 1998. 0-7808-0221-7. $78.

Contagious Diseases Sourcebook

Basic Consumer Health Information about Infectious Diseases Spread by Person-to-Person Contact through Direct Touch, Airborne Transmission, Sexual Contact, or Contact with Blood or Other Body Fluids, Including Hepatitis, Herpes, Influenza, Lice, Measles, Mumps, Pinworm, Ringworm, Severe Acute Respiratory Syndrome (SARS), Streptococcal Infections, Tuberculosis, and Others

Along with Facts about Disease Transmission, Antimicrobial Resistance, and Vaccines, with a Glossary and Directories of Resources for More Information

Edited by Karen Bellenir. 643 pages. 2004. 0-7808-0736-7. $78.

Contagious & Non-Contagious Infectious Diseases Sourcebook

Basic Information about Contagious Diseases like Measles, Polio, Hepatitis B, and Infectious Mononucleosis, and Non-Contagious Infectious Diseases like Tetanus and Toxic Shock Syndrome, and Diseases Occurring as Secondary Infections Such as Shingles and Reye Syndrome

Along with Vaccination, Prevention, and Treatment Information, and a Section Describing Emerging Infectious Disease Threats

Edited by Karen Bellenir and Peter D. Dresser. 566 pages. 1996. 0-7808-0075-3. $78.

Death & Dying Sourcebook

Basic Consumer Health Information for the Layperson about End-of-Life Care and Related Ethical and Legal Issues, Including Chief Causes of Death, Autopsies, Pain Management for the Terminally Ill, Life Support Systems, Insurance, Euthanasia, Assisted Suicide, Hospice Programs, Living Wills, Funeral Planning, Counseling, Mourning, Organ Donation, and Physician Training

Along with Statistical Data, a Glossary, and Listings of Sources for Further Help and Information

Edited by Annemarie S. Muth. 641 pages. 1999. 0-7808-0230-6. $78.

Dental Care & Oral Health Sourcebook, 2nd Edition

Basic Consumer Health Information about Dental Care, Including Oral Hygiene, Dental Visits, Pain Management, Cavities, Crowns, Bridges, Dental Implants, and Fillings, and Other Oral Health Concerns, Such as Gum Disease, Bad Breath, Dry Mouth, Genetic and Developmental Abnormalities, Oral Cancers, Orthodontics, and Temporomandibular Disorders

Along with Updates on Current Research in Oral Health, a Glossary, a Directory of Dental and Oral Health Organizations, and Resources for People with Dental and Oral Health Disorders

Edited by Amy L. Sutton. 609 pages. 2003. 0-7808-0634-4. $78.

ALSO AVAILABLE: Oral Health Sourcebook, 1st Edition. Edited by Allan R. Cook. 558 pages. 1997. 0-7808-0082-6. $78.

Depression Sourcebook

Basic Consumer Health Information about Unipolar Depression, Bipolar Disorder, Postpartum Depression, Seasonal Affective Disorder, and Other Types of Depression in Children, Adolescents, Women, Men, the Elderly, and Other Selected Populations

Along with Facts about Causes, Risk Factors, Diagnostic Criteria, Treatment Options, Coping Strategies, Suicide Prevention, a Glossary, and a Directory of Sources for Additional Help and Information

Edited by Karen Belleni. 602 pages. 2002. 0-7808-0611-5. $78.

"*Depression Sourcebook* is of a very high standard. Its purpose, which is to serve as a reference source to the lay reader, is very well served."
— *Journal of the National Medical Association, 2004*

"Invaluable reference for public and school library collections alike." — *Library Bookwatch, Apr '03*

"Recommended for purchase."
— *American Reference Books Annual, 2003*

■

Diabetes Sourcebook, 3rd Edition

Basic Consumer Health Information about Type 1 Diabetes (Insulin-Dependent or Juvenile-Onset Diabetes), Type 2 Diabetes (Noninsulin-Dependent or Adult-Onset Diabetes), Gestational Diabetes, Impaired Glucose Tolerance (IGT), and Related Complications, Such as Amputation, Eye Disease, Gum Disease, Nerve Damage, and End-Stage Renal Disease, Including Facts about Insulin, Oral Diabetes Medications, Blood Sugar Testing, and the Role of Exercise and Nutrition in the Control of Diabetes

Along with a Glossary and Resources for Further Help and Information

Edited by Dawn D. Matthews. 622 pages. 2003. 0-7808-0629-8. $78.

ALSO AVAILABLE: Diabetes Sourcebook, 1st Edition. Edited by Karen Bellenir and Peter D. Dresser. 827 pages. 1994. 1-55888-751-2. $78.

Diabetes Sourcebook, 2nd Edition. Edited by Karen Bellenir. 688 pages. 1998. 0-7808-0224-1. $78.

"This edition is even more helpful than earlier versions. . . . It is a truly valuable tool for anyone seeking readable and authoritative information on diabetes."
— *American Reference Books Annual, 2004*

"An invaluable reference." — *Library Journal, May '00*

Selected as one of the 250 "Best Health Sciences Books of 1999." — *Doody's Rating Service, Mar-Apr 2000*

"Provides useful information for the general public."
— *Healthlines, University of Michigan Health Management Research Center, Sep/Oct '99*

". . . provides reliable mainstream medical information . . . belongs on the shelves of any library with a consumer health collection." — *E-Streams, Sep '99*

"Recommended reference source."
— *Booklist, American Library Association, Feb '99*

■

Diet & Nutrition Sourcebook, 2nd Edition

Basic Consumer Health Information about Dietary Guidelines, Recommended Daily Intake Values, Vitamins, Minerals, Fiber, Fat, Weight Control, Dietary Supplements, and Food Additives

Along with Special Sections on Nutrition Needs throughout Life and Nutrition for People with Such Specific Medical Concerns as Allergies, High Blood Cholesterol, Hypertension, Diabetes, Celiac Disease, Seizure Disorders, Phenylketonuria (PKU), Cancer, and

Eating Disorders, and Including Reports on Current Nutrition Research and Source Listings for Additional Help and Information

Edited by Karen Bellenir. 650 pages. 1999. 0-7808-0228-4. $78.

ALSO AVAILABLE: Diet & Nutrition Sourcebook, 1st Edition. Edited by Dan R. Harris. 662 pages. 1996. 0-7808-0084-2. $78.

"This book is an excellent source of basic diet and nutrition information." — *Booklist Health Sciences Supplement, American Library Association, Dec '00*

"This reference document should be in any public library, but it would be a very good guide for beginning students in the health sciences. If the other books in this publisher's series are as good as this, they should all be in the health sciences collections."
— *American Reference Books Annual, 2000*

"This book is an excellent general nutrition reference for consumers who desire to take an active role in their health care for prevention. Consumers of all ages who select this book can feel confident they are receiving current and accurate information." — *Journal of Nutrition for the Elderly, Vol. 19, No. 4, '00*

"Recommended reference source."
— *Booklist, American Library Association, Dec '99*

SEE ALSO Digestive Diseases & Disorders Sourcebook, Eating Disorders Sourcebook, Gastrointestinal Diseases & Disorders Sourcebook, Vegetarian Sourcebook

■

Digestive Diseases & Disorders Sourcebook

Basic Consumer Health Information about Diseases and Disorders that Impact the Upper and Lower Digestive System, Including Celiac Disease, Constipation, Crohn's Disease, Cyclic Vomiting Syndrome, Diarrhea, Diverticulosis and Diverticulitis, Gallstones, Heartburn, Hemorrhoids, Hernias, Indigestion (Dyspepsia), Irritable Bowel Syndrome, Lactose Intolerance, Ulcers, and More

Along with Information about Medications and Other Treatments, Tips for Maintaining a Healthy Digestive Tract, a Glossary, and Directory of Digestive Diseases Organizations

Edited by Karen Bellenir. 335 pages. 2000. 0-7808-0327-2. $78.

"This title would be an excellent addition to all public or patient-research libraries."
— *American Reference Books Annual, 2001*

"This title is recommended for public, hospital, and health sciences libraries with consumer health collections." — *E-Streams, Jul-Aug '00*

"Recommended reference source."
— *Booklist, American Library Association, May '00*

SEE ALSO Diet & Nutrition Sourcebook, Eating Disorders Sourcebook, Gastrointestinal Diseases & Disorders Sourcebook

Disabilities Sourcebook

Basic Consumer Health Information about Physical and Psychiatric Disabilities, Including Descriptions of Major Causes of Disability, Assistive and Adaptive Aids, Workplace Issues, and Accessibility Concerns

Along with Information about the Americans with Disabilities Act, a Glossary, and Resources for Additional Help and Information

Edited by Dawn D. Matthews. 616 pages. 2000. 0-7808-0389-2. $78.

"It is a must for libraries with a consumer health section." — *American Reference Books Annual 2002*

"A much needed addition to the Omnigraphics *Health Reference Series*. A current reference work to provide people with disabilities, their families, caregivers or those who work with them, a broad range of information in one volume, has not been available until now. . . . It is recommended for all public and academic library reference collections." — *E-Streams, May '01*

"An excellent source book in easy-to-read format covering many current topics; highly recommended for all libraries." — *Choice, Association of College and Research Libraries, Jan '01*

"Recommended reference source." —*Booklist, American Library Association, Jul '00*

∎

Domestic Violence Sourcebook, 2nd Edition

Basic Consumer Health Information about the Causes and Consequences of Abusive Relationships, Including Physical Violence, Sexual Assault, Battery, Stalking, and Emotional Abuse, and Facts about the Effects of Violence on Women, Men, Young Adults, and the Elderly, with Reports about Domestic Violence in Selected Populations, and Featuring Facts about Medical Care, Victim Assistance and Protection, Prevention Strategies, Mental Health Services, and Legal Issues

Along with a Glossary of Related Terms and Resources for Additional Help and Information

Edited by Dawn D. Matthews. 628 pages. 2004. 0-7808-0669-7. $78.

ALSO AVAILABLE: Domestic Violence & Child Abuse Sourcebook, 1st Edition. Edited by Helene Henderson. 1,064 pages. 2001. 0-7808-0235-7. $78.

"Interested lay persons should find the book extremely beneficial. . . . A copy of *Domestic Violence and Child Abuse Sourcebook* should be in every public library in the United States." — *Social Science & Medicine, No. 56, 2003*

"This is important information. The Web has many resources but this sourcebook fills an important societal need. I am not aware of any other resources of this type." — *Doody's Review Service, Sep '01*

"Recommended for all libraries, scholars, and practitioners." — *Choice, Association of College & Research Libraries, Jul '01*

"Recommended reference source." — *Booklist, American Library Association, Apr '01*

"Important pick for college-level health reference libraries." — *The Bookwatch, Mar '01*

"Because this problem is so widespread and because this book includes a lot of issues within one volume, this work is recommended for all public libraries." — *American Reference Books Annual, 2001*

∎

Drug Abuse Sourcebook, 2nd Edition

Basic Consumer Health Information about Illicit Substances of Abuse and the Misuse of Prescription and Over-the-Counter Medications, Including Depressants, Hallucinogens, Inhalants, Marijuana, Stimulants, and Anabolic Steroids

Along with Facts about Related Health Risks, Treatment Programs, Prevention Programs, a Glossary of Abuse and Addiction Terms, a Glossary of Drug-Related Street Terms, and a Directory of Resources for More Information

Edited by Catherine Ginther. 607 pages. 2004. 0-7808-0740-5. $78.

ALSO AVAILABLE: Drug Abuse Sourcebook, 1st Edition. Edited by Karen Bellenir. 629 pages. 2000. 0-7808-0242-X. $78.

"Containing a wealth of information . . . . This resource belongs in libraries that serve a lower-division undergraduate or community college clientele as well as the general public." — *Choice, Association of College and Research Libraries, Jun '01*

"Recommended reference source." — *Booklist, American Library Association, Feb '01*

"Highly recommended." — *The Bookwatch, Jan '01*

"Even though there is a plethora of books on drug abuse, this volume is recommended for school, public, and college libraries." —*American Reference Books Annual, 2001*

SEE ALSO Alcoholism Sourcebook, Substance Abuse Sourcebook

∎

Ear, Nose & Throat Disorders Sourcebook

Basic Information about Disorders of the Ears, Nose, Sinus Cavities, Pharynx, and Larynx, Including Ear Infections, Tinnitus, Vestibular Disorders, Allergic and Non-Allergic Rhinitis, Sore Throats, Tonsillitis, and Cancers That Affect the Ears, Nose, Sinuses, and Throat

Along with Reports on Current Research Initiatives, a Glossary of Related Medical Terms, and a Directory of Sources for Further Help and Information

Edited by Karen Bellenir and Linda M. Shin. 576 pages. 1998. 0-7808-0206-3. $78.

■

Eating Disorders Sourcebook

Basic Consumer Health Information about Eating Disorders, Including Information about Anorexia Nervosa, Bulimia Nervosa, Binge Eating, Body Dysmorphic Disorder, Pica, Laxative Abuse, and Night Eating Syndrome

Along with Information about Causes, Adverse Effects, and Treatment and Prevention Issues, and Featuring a Section on Concerns Specific to Children and Adolescents, a Glossary, and Resources for Further Help and Information

Edited by Dawn D. Matthews. 322 pages. 2001. 0-7808-0335-3. $78.

SEE ALSO *Diet & Nutrition Sourcebook, Digestive Diseases & Disorders Sourcebook, Gastrointestinal Diseases & Disorders Sourcebook*

■

Emergency Medical Services Sourcebook

Basic Consumer Health Information about Preventing, Preparing for, and Managing Emergency Situations, When and Who to Call for Help, What to Expect in the Emergency Room, the Emergency Medical Team, Patient Issues, and Current Topics in Emergency Medicine

Along with Statistical Data, a Glossary, and Sources of Additional Help and Information

Edited by Jenni Lynn Colson. 494 pages. 2002. 0-7808-0420-1. $78.

Endocrine & Metabolic Disorders Sourcebook

Basic Information for the Layperson about Pancreatic and Insulin-Related Disorders Such as Pancreatitis, Diabetes, and Hypoglycemia; Adrenal Gland Disorders Such as Cushing's Syndrome, Addison's Disease, and Congenital Adrenal Hyperplasia; Pituitary Gland Disorders Such as Growth Hormone Deficiency, Acromegaly, and Pituitary Tumors; Thyroid Disorders Such as Hypothyroidism, Graves' Disease, Hashimoto's Disease, and Goiter; Hyperparathyroidism; and Other Diseases and Syndromes of Hormone Imbalance or Metabolic Dysfunction

Along with Reports on Current Research Initiatives

Edited by Linda M. Shin. 574 pages. 1998. 0-7808-0207-1. $78.

■

Environmental Health Sourcebook, 2nd Edition

Basic Consumer Health Information about the Environment and Its Effect on Human Health, Including the Effects of Air Pollution, Water Pollution, Hazardous Chemicals, Food Hazards, Radiation Hazards, Biological Agents, Household Hazards, Such as Radon, Asbestos, Carbon Monoxide, and Mold, and Information about Associated Diseases and Disorders, Including Cancer, Allergies, Respiratory Problems, and Skin Disorders

Along with Information about Environmental Concerns for Specific Populations, a Glossary of Related Terms, and Resources for Further Help and Information

Edited by Dawn D. Matthews. 673 pages. 2003. 0-7808-0632-8. $78.

ALSO AVAILABLE: *Environmentally Induced Disorders Sourcebook, 1st Edition.* Edited by Allan R. Cook. 620 pages. 1997. 0-7808-0083-4. $78.

Environmentally Induced Disorders Sourcebook, 1st Edition

SEE Environmental Health Sourcebook, 2nd Edition

Ethnic Diseases Sourcebook

Basic Consumer Health Information for Ethnic and Racial Minority Groups in the United States, Including General Health Indicators and Behaviors, Ethnic Diseases, Genetic Testing, the Impact of Chronic Diseases, Women's Health, Mental Health Issues, and Preventive Health Care Services

Along with a Glossary and a Listing of Additional Resources

Edited by Joyce Brennfleck Shannon. 664 pages. 2001. 0-7808-0336-1. $78.

"Recommended for health sciences libraries where public health programs are a priority."
—E-Streams, Jan '02

"Not many books have been written on this topic to date, and the Ethnic Diseases Sourcebook is a strong addition to the list. It will be an important introductory resource for health consumers, students, health care personnel, and social scientists. It is recommended for public, academic, and large hospital libraries."
—American Reference Books Annual 2002

"Recommended reference source."
—Booklist, American Library Association, Oct '01

"Will prove valuable to any library seeking to maintain a current, comprehensive reference collection of health resources. . . . An excellent source of health information about genetic disorders which affect particular ethnic and racial minorities in the U.S."
—The Bookwatch, Aug '01

Eye Care Sourcebook, 2nd Edition

Basic Consumer Health Information about Eye Care and Eye Disorders, Including Facts about the Diagnosis, Prevention, and Treatment of Common Refractive Problems Such as Myopia, Hyperopia, Astigmatism, and Presbyopia, and Eye Diseases, Including Glaucoma, Cataract, Age-Related Macular Degeneration, and Diabetic Retinopathy

Along with a Section on Vision Correction and Refractive Surgeries, Including LASIK and LASEK, a Glossary, and Directories of Resources for Additional Help and Information

Edited by Amy L. Sutton. 543 pages. 2003. 0-7808-0635-2. $78.

ALSO AVAILABLE: Ophthalmic Disorders Sourcebook, 1st Edition. Edited by Linda M. Ross. 631 pages. 1996. 0-7808-0081-8. $78.

". . . a solid reference tool for eye care and a valuable addition to a collection."
—American Reference Books Annual, 2004

Family Planning Sourcebook

Basic Consumer Health Information about Planning for Pregnancy and Contraception, Including Traditional Methods, Barrier Methods, Hormonal Methods, Permanent Methods, Future Methods, Emergency Contraception, and Birth Control Choices for Women at Each Stage of Life

Along with Statistics, a Glossary, and Sources of Additional Information

Edited by Amy Marcaccio Keyzer. 520 pages. 2001. 0-7808-0379-5. $78.

"Recommended for public, health, and undergraduate libraries as part of the circulating collection."
—E-Streams, Mar '02

"Information is presented in an unbiased, readable manner, and the sourcebook will certainly be a necessary addition to those public and high school libraries where Internet access is restricted or otherwise problematic." —American Reference Books Annual 2002

"Recommended reference source."
—Booklist, American Library Association, Oct '01

"Will prove valuable to any library seeking to maintain a current, comprehensive reference collection of health resources. . . . Excellent reference."
—The Bookwatch, Aug '01

SEE ALSO Pregnancy & Birth Sourcebook

Fitness & Exercise Sourcebook, 2nd Edition

Basic Consumer Health Information about the Fundamentals of Fitness and Exercise, Including How to Begin and Maintain a Fitness Program, Fitness as a Lifestyle, the Link between Fitness and Diet, Advice for Specific Groups of People, Exercise as It Relates to Specific Medical Conditions, and Recent Research in Fitness and Exercise

Along with a Glossary of Important Terms and Resources for Additional Help and Information

Edited by Kristen M. Gledhill. 646 pages. 2001. 0-7808-0334-5. $78.

ALSO AVAILABLE: Fitness & Exercise Sourcebook, 1st Edition. Edited by Dan R. Harris. 663 pages. 1996. 0-7808-0186-5. $78.

"This work is recommended for all general reference collections."
—American Reference Books Annual 2002

"Highly recommended for public, consumer, and school grades fourth through college."
—E-Streams, Nov '01

"Recommended reference source." — Booklist, American Library Association, Oct '01

"The information appears quite comprehensive and is considered reliable. . . . This second edition is a welcomed addition to the series."
—Doody's Review Service, Sep '01

585

"This reference is a valuable choice for those who desire a broad source of information on exercise, fitness, and chronic-disease prevention through a healthy lifestyle." —*American Medical Writers Association Journal, Fall '01*

"Will prove valuable to any library seeking to maintain a current, comprehensive reference collection of health resources. . . . Excellent reference." —*The Bookwatch, Aug '01*

■

Food & Animal Borne Diseases Sourcebook

Basic Information about Diseases That Can Be Spread to Humans through the Ingestion of Contaminated Food or Water or by Contact with Infected Animals and Insects, Such as Botulism, E. Coli, Hepatitis A, Trichinosis, Lyme Disease, and Rabies

Along with Information Regarding Prevention and Treatment Methods, and Including a Special Section for International Travelers Describing Diseases Such as Cholera, Malaria, Travelers' Diarrhea, and Yellow Fever, and Offering Recommendations for Avoiding Illness

Edited by Karen Bellenir and Peter D. Dresser. 535 pages. 1995. 0-7808-0033-8. $78.

"Targeting general readers and providing them with a single, comprehensive source of information on selected topics, this book continues, with the excellent caliber of its predecessors, to catalog topical information on health matters of general interest. Readable and thorough, this valuable resource is highly recommended for all libraries." —*Academic Library Book Review, Summer '96*

"A comprehensive collection of authoritative information." —*Emergency Medical Services, Oct '95*

■

Food Safety Sourcebook

Basic Consumer Health Information about the Safe Handling of Meat, Poultry, Seafood, Eggs, Fruit Juices, and Other Food Items, and Facts about Pesticides, Drinking Water, Food Safety Overseas, and the Onset, Duration, and Symptoms of Foodborne Illnesses, Including Types of Pathogenic Bacteria, Parasitic Protozoa, Worms, Viruses, and Natural Toxins

Along with the Role of the Consumer, the Food Handler, and the Government in Food Safety; a Glossary, and Resources for Additional Help and Information

Edited by Dawn D. Matthews. 339 pages. 1999. 0-7808-0326-4. $78.

"This book is recommended for public libraries and universities with home economic and food science programs." —*E-Streams, Nov '00*

"Recommended reference source." —*Booklist, American Library Association, May '00*

"This book takes the complex issues of food safety and foodborne pathogens and presents them in an easily understood manner. [It does] an excellent job of covering a large and often confusing topic." —*American Reference Books Annual, 2000*

Forensic Medicine Sourcebook

Basic Consumer Information for the Layperson about Forensic Medicine, Including Crime Scene Investigation, Evidence Collection and Analysis, Expert Testimony, Computer-Aided Criminal Identification, Digital Imaging in the Courtroom, DNA Profiling, Accident Reconstruction, Autopsies, Ballistics, Drugs and Explosives Detection, Latent Fingerprints, Product Tampering, and Questioned Document Examination

Along with Statistical Data, a Glossary of Forensics Terminology, and Listings of Sources for Further Help and Information

Edited by Annemarie S. Muth. 574 pages. 1999. 0-7808-0232-2. $78.

"Given the expected widespread interest in its content and its easy to read style, this book is recommended for most public and all college and university libraries." —*E-Streams, Feb '01*

"Recommended for public libraries." —*Reference & User Services Quarterly, American Library Association, Spring 2000*

"Recommended reference source." —*Booklist, American Library Association, Feb '00*

"A wealth of information, useful statistics, references are up-to-date and extremely complete. This wonderful collection of data will help students who are interested in a career in any type of forensic field. It is a great resource for attorneys who need information about types of expert witnesses needed in a particular case. It also offers useful information for fiction and nonfiction writers whose work involves a crime. A fascinating compilation. All levels." —*Choice, Association of College and Research Libraries, Jan 2000*

"There are several items that make this book attractive to consumers who are seeking certain forensic data. . . . This is a useful current source for those seeking general forensic medical answers." —*American Reference Books Annual, 2000*

■

Gastrointestinal Diseases & Disorders Sourcebook

Basic Information about Gastroesophageal Reflux Disease (Heartburn), Ulcers, Diverticulosis, Irritable Bowel Syndrome, Crohn's Disease, Ulcerative Colitis, Diarrhea, Constipation, Lactose Intolerance, Hemorrhoids, Hepatitis, Cirrhosis, and Other Digestive Problems, Featuring Statistics, Descriptions of Symptoms, and Current Treatment Methods of Interest for Persons Living with Upper and Lower Gastrointestinal Maladies

Edited by Linda M. Ross. 413 pages. 1996. 0-7808-0078-8. $78.

". . . very readable form. The successful editorial work that brought this material together into a useful and understandable reference makes accessible to all readers information that can help them more effectively understand and obtain help for digestive tract problems." —*Choice, Association of College & Research Libraries, Feb '97*

SEE ALSO *Diet & Nutrition Sourcebook, Digestive Diseases & Disorders, Eating Disorders Sourcebook*

■

Genetic Disorders Sourcebook, 3rd Edition

Basic Consumer Health Information about Hereditary Diseases and Disorders, Including Facts about the Human Genome, Genetic Inheritance Patterns, Disorders Associated with Specific Genes, Such as Sickle Cell Disease, Hemophilia, and Cystic Fibrosis, Chromosome Disorders, Such as Down Syndrome, Fragile X Syndrome, and Turner Syndrome, and Complex Diseases and Disorders Resulting from the Interaction of Environmental and Genetic Factors, Such as Allergies, Cancer, and Obesity

Along with Facts about Genetic Testing, Suggestions for Parents of Children with Special Needs, Reports on Current Research Initiatives, a Glossary of Genetic Terminology, and Resources for Additional Help and Information

Edited by Karen Bellenir. 777 pages. 2004. 0-7808-0742-1. $78.

ALSO AVAILABLE: Genetic Disorders Sourcebook, 1st Edition. Edited by Karen Bellenir. 642 pages. 1996. 0-7808-0034-6. $78.

Genetic Disorders Sourcebook, 2nd Edition. Edited by Kathy Massimini. 768 pages. 2001. 0-7808-0241-1. $78.

"Recommended for public libraries and medical and hospital libraries with consumer health collections."
— *E-Streams, May '01*

"Recommended reference source."
— *Booklist, American Library Association, Apr '01*

"Important pick for college-level health reference libraries." — *The Bookwatch, Mar '01*

"Provides essential medical information to both the general public and those diagnosed with a serious or fatal genetic disease or disorder." —*Choice, Association of College and Research Libraries, Jan '97*

■

Head Trauma Sourcebook

Basic Information for the Layperson about Open-Head and Closed-Head Injuries, Treatment Advances, Recovery, and Rehabilitation

Along with Reports on Current Research Initiatives

Edited by Karen Bellenir. 414 pages. 1997. 0-7808-0208-X. $78.

■

Headache Sourcebook

Basic Consumer Health Information about Migraine, Tension, Cluster, Rebound and Other Types of Headaches, with Facts about the Cause and Prevention of Headaches, the Effects of Stress and the Environment, Headaches during Pregnancy and Menopause, and Childhood Headaches

Along with a Glossary and Other Resources for Additional Help and Information

Edited by Dawn D. Matthews. 362 pages. 2002. 0-7808-0337-X. $78.

"Highly recommended for academic and medical reference collections." — *Library Bookwatch, Sep '02*

■

Health Insurance Sourcebook

Basic Information about Managed Care Organizations, Traditional Fee-for-Service Insurance, Insurance Portability and Pre-Existing Conditions Clauses, Medicare, Medicaid, Social Security, and Military Health Care

Along with Information about Insurance Fraud

Edited by Wendy Wilcox. 530 pages. 1997. 0-7808-0222-5. $78.

"Particularly useful because it brings much of this information together in one volume. This book will be a handy reference source in the health sciences library, hospital library, college and university library, and medium to large public library."
— *Medical Reference Services Quarterly, Fall '98*

Awarded "Books of the Year Award"
— *American Journal of Nursing, 1997*

"The layout of the book is particularly helpful as it provides easy access to reference material. A most useful addition to the vast amount of information about health insurance. The use of data from U.S. government agencies is most commendable. Useful in a library or learning center for healthcare professional students."
— *Doody's Health Sciences Book Reviews, Nov '97*

■

Health Reference Series Cumulative Index 1999

A Comprehensive Index to the Individual Volumes of the Health Reference Series, Including a Subject Index, Name Index, Organization Index, and Publication Index

Along with a Master List of Acronyms and Abbreviations

Edited by Edward J. Prucha, Anne Holmes, and Robert Rudnick. 990 pages. 2000. 0-7808-0382-5. $78.

"This volume will be most helpful in libraries that have a relatively complete collection of the Health Reference Series." — *American Reference Books Annual, 2001*

"Essential for collections that hold any of the numerous *Health Reference Series* titles."
— *Choice, Association of College and Research Libraries, Nov '00*

■

Healthy Aging Sourcebook

Basic Consumer Health Information about Maintaining Health through the Aging Process, Including Advice on Nutrition, Exercise, and Sleep, Help in Making Decisions about Midlife Issues and Retirement, and

Guidance Concerning Practical and Informed Choices in Health Consumerism

Along with Data Concerning the Theories of Aging, Different Experiences in Aging by Minority Groups, and Facts about Aging Now and Aging in the Future; and Featuring a Glossary, a Guide to Consumer Help, Additional Suggested Reading, and Practical Resource Directory

Edited by Jenifer Swanson. 536 pages. 1999. 0-7808-0390-6. $78.

"Recommended reference source."
— Booklist, American Library Association, Feb '00

SEE ALSO *Physical & Mental Issues in Aging Sourcebook*

■

Healthy Children Sourcebook

Basic Consumer Health Information about the Physical and Mental Development of Children between the Ages of 3 and 12, Including Routine Health Care, Preventative Health Services, Safety and First Aid, Healthy Sleep, Dental Care, Nutrition, and Fitness, and Featuring Parenting Tips on Such Topics as Bedwetting, Choosing Day Care, Monitoring TV and Other Media, and Establishing a Foundation for Substance Abuse Prevention

Along with a Glossary of Commonly Used Pediatric Terms and Resources for Additional Help and Information.

Edited by Chad T. Kimball. 647 pages. 2003. 0-7808-0247-0. $78.

"It is hard to imagine that any other single resource exists that would provide such a comprehensive guide of timely information on health promotion and disease prevention for children aged 3 to 12."
— American Reference Books Annual, 2004

"The strengths of this book are many. It is clearly written, presented and structured."
— Journal of the National Medical Association, 2004

■

Healthy Heart Sourcebook for Women

Basic Consumer Health Information about Cardiac Issues Specific to Women, Including Facts about Major Risk Factors and Prevention, Treatment and Control Strategies, and Important Dietary Issues

Along with a Special Section Regarding the Pros and Cons of Hormone Replacement Therapy and Its Impact on Heart Health, and Additional Help, Including Recipes, a Glossary, and a Directory of Resources

Edited by Dawn D. Matthews. 336 pages. 2000. 0-7808-0329-9. $78.

"A good reference source and recommended for all public, academic, medical, and hospital libraries."
— Medical Reference Services Quarterly, Summer '01

"Because of the lack of information specific to women on this topic, this book is recommended for public libraries and consumer libraries."
— American Reference Books Annual, 2001

"Contains very important information about coronary artery disease that all women should know. The information is current and presented in an easy-to-read format. The book will make a good addition to any library."
— American Medical Writers Association Journal, Summer '00

"Important, basic reference."
— Reviewer's Bookwatch, Jul '00

SEE ALSO *Heart Diseases & Disorders Sourcebook, Women's Health Concerns Sourcebook*

■

Heart Diseases & Disorders Sourcebook, 2nd Edition

SEE *Cardiovascular Diseases & Disorders Sourcebook, 3rd Edition*

■

Household Safety Sourcebook

Basic Consumer Health Information about Household Safety, Including Information about Poisons, Chemicals, Fire, and Water Hazards in the Home

Along with Advice about the Safe Use of Home Maintenance Equipment, Choosing Toys and Nursery Furniture, Holiday and Recreation Safety, a Glossary, and Resources for Further Help and Information

Edited by Dawn D. Matthews. 606 pages. 2002. 0-7808-0338-8. $78.

"This work will be useful in public libraries with large consumer health and wellness departments."
— American Reference Books Annual, 2003

"As a sourcebook on household safety this book meets its mark. It is encyclopedic in scope and covers a wide range of safety issues that are commonly seen in the home."
— E-Streams, Jul '02

■

Hypertension Sourcebook

Basic Consumer Health Information about the Causes, Diagnosis, and Treatment of High Blood Pressure, with Facts about Consequences, Complications, and Co-Occurring Disorders, Such as Coronary Heart Disease, Diabetes, Stroke, Kidney Disease, and Hypertensive Retinopathy, and Issues in Blood Pressure Control, Including Dietary Choices, Stress Management, and Medications

Along with Reports on Current Research Initiatives and Clinical Trials, a Glossary, and Resources for Additional Help and Information

Edited by Dawn D. Matthews and Karen Bellenir. 613 pages. 2004. 0-7808-0674-3. $78.

Immune System Disorders Sourcebook

Basic Information about Lupus, Multiple Sclerosis, Guillain-Barré Syndrome, Chronic Granulomatous Disease, and More

Along with Statistical and Demographic Data and Reports on Current Research Initiatives

Edited by Allan R. Cook. 608 pages. 1997. 0-7808-0209-8. $78.

Infant & Toddler Health Sourcebook

Basic Consumer Health Information about the Physical and Mental Development of Newborns, Infants, and Toddlers, Including Neonatal Concerns, Nutrition Recommendations, Immunization Schedules, Common Pediatric Disorders, Assessments and Milestones, Safety Tips, and Advice for Parents and Other Caregivers

Along with a Glossary of Terms and Resource Listings for Additional Help

Edited by Jenifer Swanson. 585 pages. 2000. 0-7808-0246-2. $78.

"As a reference for the general public, this would be useful in any library." — *E-Streams, May '01*

"Recommended reference source."
— *Booklist, American Library Association, Feb '01*

"This is a good source for general use."
— *American Reference Books Annual, 2001*

Infectious Diseases Sourcebook

Basic Consumer Health Information about Non-Contagious Bacterial, Viral, Prion, Fungal, and Parasitic Diseases Spread by Food and Water, Insects and Animals, or Environmental Contact, Including Botulism, E. Coli, Encephalitis, Legionnaires' Disease, Lyme Disease, Malaria, Plague, Rabies, Salmonella, Tetanus, and Others, and Facts about Newly Emerging Diseases, Such as Hantavirus, Mad Cow Disease, Monkeypox, and West Nile Virus

Along with Information about Preventing Disease Transmission, the Threat of Bioterrorism, and Current Research Initiatives, with a Glossary and Directory of Resources for More Information

Edited by Karen Bellenir. 634 pages. 2004. 0-7808-0675-1. $78.

Injury & Trauma Sourcebook

Basic Consumer Health Information about the Impact of Injury, the Diagnosis and Treatment of Common and Traumatic Injuries, Emergency Care, and Specific Injuries Related to Home, Community, Workplace, Transportation, and Recreation

Along with Guidelines for Injury Prevention, a Glossary, and a Directory of Additional Resources

Edited by Joyce Brennfleck Shannon. 696 pages. 2002. 0-7808-0421-X. $78.

"This publication is the most comprehensive work of its kind about injury and trauma."
— *American Reference Books Annual, 2003*

"This sourcebook provides concise, easily readable, basic health information about injuries. . . . This book is well organized and an easy to use reference resource suitable for hospital, health sciences and public libraries with consumer health collections."
— *E-Streams, Nov '02*

"Practitioners should be aware of guides such as this in order to facilitate their use by patients and their families." — *Doody's Health Sciences Book Review Journal, Sep-Oct '02*

"Recommended reference source."
— *Booklist, American Library Association, Sep '02*

"Highly recommended for academic and medical reference collections." — *Library Bookwatch, Sep '02*

Kidney & Urinary Tract Diseases & Disorders Sourcebook

Basic Information about Kidney Stones, Urinary Incontinence, Bladder Disease, End Stage Renal Disease, Dialysis, and More

Along with Statistical and Demographic Data and Reports on Current Research Initiatives

Edited by Linda M. Ross. 602 pages. 1997. 0-7808-0079-6. $78.

Learning Disabilities Sourcebook, 2nd Edition

Basic Consumer Health Information about Learning Disabilities, Including Dyslexia, Developmental Speech and Language Disabilities, Non-Verbal Learning Disorders, Developmental Arithmetic Disorder, Developmental Writing Disorder, and Other Conditions That Impede Learning Such as Attention Deficit/ Hyperactivity Disorder, Brain Injury, Hearing Impairment, Klinefelter Syndrome, Dyspraxia, and Tourette Syndrome

Along with Facts about Educational Issues and Assistive Technology, Coping Strategies, a Glossary of Related Terms, and Resources for Further Help and Information

Edited by Dawn D. Matthews. 621 pages. 2003. 0-7808-0626-3. $78.

ALSO AVAILABLE: Learning Disabilities Sourcebook, 1st Edition. Edited by Linda M. Shin. 579 pages. 1998. 0-7808-0210-1. $78.

"The second edition of *Learning Disabilities Sourcebook* far surpasses the earlier edition in that it is more focused on information that will be useful as a consumer health resource."
— *American Reference Books Annual, 2004*

589

"Teachers as well as consumers will find this an essential guide to understanding various syndromes and their latest treatments. [An] invaluable reference for public and school library collections alike."
— *Library Bookwatch, Apr '03*

Named *"Outstanding Reference Book of 1999."*
— *New York Public Library, Feb 2000*

"An excellent candidate for inclusion in a public library reference section. It's a great source of information. Teachers will also find the book useful. Definitely worth reading."
— *Journal of Adolescent & Adult Literacy, Feb 2000*

"Readable . . . provides a solid base of information regarding successful techniques used with individuals who have learning disabilities, as well as practical suggestions for educators and family members. Clear language, concise descriptions, and pertinent information for contacting multiple resources add to the strength of this book as a useful tool." — *Choice, Association of College and Research Libraries, Feb '99*

"Recommended reference source."
— *Booklist, American Library Association, Sep '98*

"A useful resource for libraries and for those who don't have the time to identify and locate the individual publications." — *Disability Resources Monthly, Sep '98*

■

Leukemia Sourcebook

Basic Consumer Health Information about Adult and Childhood Leukemias, Including Acute Lymphocytic Leukemia (ALL), Chronic Lymphocytic Leukemia (CLL), Acute Myelogenous Leukemia (AML), Chronic Myelogenous Leukemia (CML), and Hairy Cell Leukemia, and Treatments Such as Chemotherapy, Radiation Therapy, Peripheral Blood Stem Cell and Marrow Transplantation, and Immunotherapy

Along with Tips for Life During and After Treatment, a Glossary, and Directories of Additional Resources

Edited by Joyce Brennfleck Shannon. 587 pages. 2003. 0-7808-0627-1. $78.

"Unlike other medical books for the layperson, . . . the language does not talk down to the reader. . . . This volume is highly recommended for all libraries."
— *American Reference Books Annual, 2004*

■

Liver Disorders Sourcebook

Basic Consumer Health Information about the Liver and How It Works; Liver Diseases, Including Cancer, Cirrhosis, Hepatitis, and Toxic and Drug Related Diseases; Tips for Maintaining a Healthy Liver; Laboratory Tests, Radiology Tests, and Facts about Liver Transplantation

Along with a Section on Support Groups, a Glossary, and Resource Listings

Edited by Joyce Brennfleck Shannon. 591 pages. 2000. 0-7808-0383-3. $78.

"A valuable resource."
— *American Reference Books Annual, 2001*

"This title is recommended for health sciences and public libraries with consumer health collections."
— *E-Streams, Oct '00*

"Recommended reference source."
— *Booklist, American Library Association, Jun '00*

■

Lung Disorders Sourcebook

Basic Consumer Health Information about Emphysema, Pneumonia, Tuberculosis, Asthma, Cystic Fibrosis, and Other Lung Disorders, Including Facts about Diagnostic Procedures, Treatment Strategies, Disease Prevention Efforts, and Such Risk Factors as Smoking, Air Pollution, and Exposure to Asbestos, Radon, and Other Agents

Along with a Glossary and Resources for Additional Help and Information

Edited by Dawn D. Matthews. 678 pages. 2002. 0-7808-0339-6. $78.

"This title is a great addition for public and school libraries because it provides concise health information on the lungs."
— *American Reference Books Annual, 2003*

"Highly recommended for academic and medical reference collections." — *Library Bookwatch, Sep '02*

■

Medical Tests Sourcebook, 2nd Edition

Basic Consumer Health Information about Medical Tests, Including Age-Specific Health Tests, Important Health Screenings and Exams, Home-Use Tests, Blood and Specimen Tests, Electrical Tests, Scope Tests, Genetic Testing, and Imaging Tests, Such as X-Rays, Ultrasound, Computed Tomography, Magnetic Resonance Imaging, Angiography, and Nuclear Medicine

Along with a Glossary and Directory of Additional Resources

Edited by Joyce Brennfleck Shannon. 654 pages. 2004. 0-7808-0670-0. $78.

ALSO AVAILABLE: Medical Tests, 1st Edition. Edited by Joyce Brennfleck Shannon. 691 pages. 1999. 0-7808-0243-8. $78.

"Recommended for hospital and health sciences libraries with consumer health collections."
— *E-Streams, Mar '00*

"This is an overall excellent reference with a wealth of general knowledge that may aid those who are reluctant to get vital tests performed."
— *Today's Librarian, Jan 2000*

"A valuable reference guide."
— *American Reference Books Annual, 2000*

Men's Health Concerns Sourcebook, 2nd Edition

Basic Consumer Health Information about the Medical and Mental Concerns of Men, Including Theories about the Shorter Male Lifespan, the Leading Causes of Death and Disability, Physical Concerns of Special Significance to Men, Reproductive and Sexual Concerns, Sexually Transmitted Diseases, Men's Mental and Emotional Health, and Lifestyle Choices That Affect Wellness, Such as Nutrition, Fitness, and Substance Use

Along with a Glossary of Related Terms and a Directory of Organizational Resources in Men's Health

Edited by Robert Aquinas McNally. 644 pages. 2004. 0-7808-0671-9. $78.

ALSO AVAILABLE: Men's Health Concerns Sourcebook, 1st Edition. Edited by Allan R. Cook. 738 pages. 1998. 0-7808-0212-8. $78.

"This comprehensive resource and the series are highly recommended."
—*American Reference Books Annual, 2000*

"Recommended reference source."
—*Booklist, American Library Association, Dec '98*

∎

Mental Health Disorders Sourcebook, 2nd Edition

Basic Consumer Health Information about Anxiety Disorders, Depression and Other Mood Disorders, Eating Disorders, Personality Disorders, Schizophrenia, and More, Including Disease Descriptions, Treatment Options, and Reports on Current Research Initiatives

Along with Statistical Data, Tips for Maintaining Mental Health, a Glossary, and Directory of Sources for Additional Help and Information

Edited by Karen Bellenir. 605 pages. 2000. 0-7808-0240-3. $78.

ALSO AVAILABLE: Mental Health Disorders Sourcebook, 1st Edition. Edited by Karen Bellenir. 548 pages. 1995. 0-7808-0040-0. $78.

"Well organized and well written."
—*American Reference Books Annual, 2001*

"Recommended reference source."
—*Booklist, American Library Association, Jun '00*

∎

Mental Retardation Sourcebook

Basic Consumer Health Information about Mental Retardation and Its Causes, Including Down Syndrome, Fetal Alcohol Syndrome, Fragile X Syndrome, Genetic Conditions, Injury, and Environmental Sources

Along with Preventive Strategies, Parenting Issues, Educational Implications, Health Care Needs, Employment and Economic Matters, Legal Issues, a Glossary, and a Resource Listing for Additional Help and Information

Edited by Joyce Brennfleck Shannon. 642 pages. 2000. 0-7808-0377-9. $78.

"Public libraries will find the book useful for reference and as a beginning research point for students, parents, and caregivers."
—*American Reference Books Annual, 2001*

"The strength of this work is that it compiles many basic fact sheets and addresses for further information in one volume. It is intended and suitable for the general public. This sourcebook is relevant to any collection providing health information to the general public."
—*E-Streams, Nov '00*

"From preventing retardation to parenting and family challenges, this covers health, social and legal issues and will prove an invaluable overview."
—*Reviewer's Bookwatch, Jul '00*

∎

Movement Disorders Sourcebook

Basic Consumer Health Information about Neurological Movement Disorders, Including Essential Tremor, Parkinson's Disease, Dystonia, Cerebral Palsy, Huntington's Disease, Myasthenia Gravis, Multiple Sclerosis, and Other Early-Onset and Adult-Onset Movement Disorders, Their Symptoms and Causes, Diagnostic Tests, and Treatments

Along with Mobility and Assistive Technology Information, a Glossary, and a Directory of Additional Resources

Edited by Joyce Brennfleck Shannon. 655 pages. 2003. 0-7808-0628-X. $78.

". . . a good resource for consumers and recommended for public, community college and undergraduate libraries."
—*American Reference Books Annual, 2004*

∎

Muscular Dystrophy Sourcebook

Basic Consumer Health Information about Congenital, Childhood-Onset, and Adult-Onset Forms of Muscular Dystrophy, Such as Duchenne, Becker, Emery-Dreifuss, Distal, Limb-Girdle, Facioscapulohumeral (FSHD), Myotonic, and Ophthalmoplegic Muscular Dystrophies, Including Facts about Diagnostic Tests, Medical and Physical Therapies, Management of Co-Occurring Conditions, and Parenting Guidelines

Along with Practical Tips for Home Care, a Glossary, and Directories of Additional Resources

Edited by Joyce Brennfleck Shannon. 577 pages. 2004. 0-7808-0676-X. $78.

∎

Obesity Sourcebook

Basic Consumer Health Information about Diseases and Other Problems Associated with Obesity, and Including Facts about Risk Factors, Prevention Issues, and Management Approaches

Along with Statistical and Demographic Data, Information about Special Populations, Research Updates, a Glossary, and Source Listings for Further Help and Information

Edited by Wilma Caldwell and Chad T. Kimball. 376 pages. 2001. 0-7808-0333-7. $78.

"The book synthesizes the reliable medical literature on obesity into one easy-to-read and useful resource for the general public."
— *American Reference Books Annual 2002*

"This is a very useful resource book for the lay public."
— *Doody's Review Service, Nov '01*

"Well suited for the health reference collection of a public library or an academic health science library that serves the general population." — *E-Streams, Sep '01*

"Recommended reference source."
— *Booklist, American Library Association, Apr '01*

" Recommended pick both for specialty health library collections and any general consumer health reference collection." — *The Bookwatch, Apr '01*

Ophthalmic Disorders Sourcebook, 1st Edition

SEE Eye Care Sourcebook, 2nd Edition

Oral Health Sourcebook

SEE Dental Care & Oral Health Sourcebook, 2nd Ed.

Osteoporosis Sourcebook

Basic Consumer Health Information about Primary and Secondary Osteoporosis and Juvenile Osteoporosis and Related Conditions, Including Fibrous Dysplasia, Gaucher Disease, Hyperthyroidism, Hypophosphatasia, Myeloma, Osteopetrosis, Osteogenesis Imperfecta, and Paget's Disease

Along with Information about Risk Factors, Treatments, Traditional and Non-Traditional Pain Management, a Glossary of Related Terms, and a Directory of Resources

Edited by Allan R. Cook. 584 pages. 2001. 0-7808-0239-X. $78.

"This would be a book to be kept in a staff or patient library. The targeted audience is the layperson, but the therapist who needs a quick bit of information on a particular topic will also find the book useful."
— *Physical Therapy, Jan '02*

"This resource is recommended as a great reference source for public, health, and academic libraries, and is another triumph for the editors of Omnigraphics."
— *American Reference Books Annual 2002*

"Recommended for all public libraries and general health collections, especially those supporting patient education or consumer health programs."
— *E-Streams, Nov '01*

"Will prove valuable to any library seeking to maintain a current, comprehensive reference collection of health resources. . . . From prevention to treatment and associated conditions, this provides an excellent survey."
— *The Bookwatch, Aug '01*

"Recommended reference source."
— *Booklist, American Library Association, July '01*

SEE ALSO Women's Health Concerns Sourcebook

Pain Sourcebook, 2nd Edition

Basic Consumer Health Information about Specific Forms of Acute and Chronic Pain, Including Muscle and Skeletal Pain, Nerve Pain, Cancer Pain, and Disorders Characterized by Pain, Such as Fibromyalgia, Shingles, Angina, Arthritis, and Headaches

Along with Information about Pain Medications and Management Techniques, Complementary and Alternative Pain Relief Options, Tips for People Living with Chronic Pain, a Glossary, and a Directory of Sources for Further Information

Edited by Karen Bellenir. 670 pages. 2002. 0-7808-0612-3. $78.

ALSO AVAILABLE: Pain Sourcebook, 1st Edition. Edited by Allan R. Cook. 667 pages. 1997. 0-7808-0213-6. $78.

"A source of valuable information. . . . This book offers help to nonmedical people who need information about pain and pain management. It is also an excellent reference for those who participate in patient education."
— *Doody's Review Service, Sep '02*

"The text is readable, easily understood, and well indexed. This excellent volume belongs in all patient education libraries, consumer health sections of public libraries, and many personal collections."
— *American Reference Books Annual, 1999*

"A beneficial reference." — *Booklist Health Sciences Supplement, American Library Association, Oct '98*

"The information is basic in terms of scholarship and is appropriate for general readers. Written in journalistic style . . . intended for non-professionals. Quite thorough in its coverage of different pain conditions and summarizes the latest clinical information regarding pain treatment." — *Choice, Association of College and Research Libraries, Jun '98*

"Recommended reference source."
— *Booklist, American Library Association, Mar '98*

Pediatric Cancer Sourcebook

Basic Consumer Health Information about Leukemias, Brain Tumors, Sarcomas, Lymphomas, and Other Cancers in Infants, Children, and Adolescents, Including Descriptions of Cancers, Treatments, and Coping Strategies

Along with Suggestions for Parents, Caregivers, and Concerned Relatives, a Glossary of Cancer Terms, and Resource Listings

Edited by Edward J. Prucha. 587 pages. 1999. 0-7808-0245-4. $78.

"An excellent source of information. Recommended for public, hospital, and health science libraries with consumer health collections." — *E-Streams, Jun '00*

"Recommended reference source."
— *Booklist, American Library Association, Feb '00*

Physical & Mental Issues in Aging Sourcebook

Basic Consumer Health Information on Physical and Mental Disorders Associated with the Aging Process, Including Concerns about Cardiovascular Disease, Pulmonary Disease, Oral Health, Digestive Disorders, Musculoskeletal and Skin Disorders, Metabolic Changes, Sexual and Reproductive Issues, and Changes in Vision, Hearing, and Other Senses

Along with Data about Longevity and Causes of Death, Information on Acute and Chronic Pain, Descriptions of Mental Concerns, a Glossary of Terms, and Resource Listings for Additional Help

Edited by Jenifer Swanson. 660 pages. 1999. 0-7808-0233-0. $78.

SEE ALSO Healthy Aging Sourcebook

Podiatry Sourcebook

Basic Consumer Health Information about Foot Conditions, Diseases, and Injuries, Including Bunions, Corns, Calluses, Athlete's Foot, Plantar Warts, Hammertoes and Clawtoes, Clubfoot, Heel Pain, Gout, and More

Along with Facts about Foot Care, Disease Prevention, Foot Safety, Choosing a Foot Care Specialist, a Glossary of Terms, and Resource Listings for Additional Information

Edited by M. Lisa Weatherford. 380 pages. 2001. 0-7808-0215-2. $78.

Pregnancy & Birth Sourcebook, 2nd Edition

Basic Consumer Health Information about Conception and Pregnancy, Including Facts about Fertility, Infertility, Pregnancy Symptoms and Complications, Fetal Growth and Development, Labor, Delivery, and the Postpartum Period, as Well as Information about Maintaining Health and Wellness during Pregnancy and Caring for a Newborn

Along with Information about Public Health Assistance for Low-Income Pregnant Women, a Glossary, and Directories of Agencies and Organizations Providing Help and Support

Edited by Amy L. Sutton. 626 pages. 2004. 0-7808-0672-7. $78.

ALSO AVAILABLE: Pregnancy & Birth Sourcebook, 1st Edition. Edited by Heather E. Aldred. 737 pages. 1997. 0-7808-0216-0. $78.

SEE ALSO Congenital Disorders Sourcebook, Family Planning Sourcebook

---

Prostate Cancer Sourcebook

Basic Consumer Health Information about Prostate Cancer, Including Information about the Associated Risk Factors, Detection, Diagnosis, and Treatment of Prostate Cancer

Along with Information on Non-Malignant Prostate Conditions, and Featuring a Section Listing Support and Treatment Centers and a Glossary of Related Terms

Edited by Dawn D. Matthews. 358 pages. 2001. 0-7808-0324-8. $78.

Public Health Sourcebook

Basic Information about Government Health Agencies, Including National Health Statistics and Trends, Healthy People 2000 Program Goals and Objectives, the Centers for Disease Control and Prevention, the Food and Drug Administration, and the National Institutes of Health

Along with Full Contact Information for Each Agency

Edited by Wendy Wilcox. 698 pages. 1998. 0-7808-0220-9. $78.

Reconstructive & Cosmetic Surgery Sourcebook

Basic Consumer Health Information on Cosmetic and Reconstructive Plastic Surgery, Including Statistical Information about Different Surgical Procedures, Things to Consider Prior to Surgery, Plastic Surgery Techniques and Tools, Emotional and Psychological Considerations, and Procedure-Specific Information

Along with a Glossary of Terms and a Listing of Resources for Additional Help and Information

Edited by M. Lisa Weatherford. 374 pages. 2001. 0-7808-0214-4. $78.

"An excellent reference that addresses cosmetic and medically necessary reconstructive surgeries. . . . The style of the prose is calm and reassuring, discussing the many positive outcomes now available due to advances in surgical techniques."
— *American Reference Books Annual 2002*

"Recommended for health science libraries that are open to the public, as well as hospital libraries that are open to the patients. This book is a good resource for the consumer interested in plastic surgery."
— *E-Streams, Dec '01*

"Recommended reference source."
— *Booklist, American Library Association, July '01*

Rehabilitation Sourcebook

Basic Consumer Health Information about Rehabilitation for People Recovering from Heart Surgery, Spinal Cord Injury, Stroke, Orthopedic Impairments, Amputation, Pulmonary Impairments, Traumatic Injury, and More, Including Physical Therapy, Occupational Therapy, Speech/ Language Therapy, Massage Therapy, Dance Therapy, Art Therapy, and Recreational Therapy

Along with Information on Assistive and Adaptive Devices, a Glossary, and Resources for Additional Help and Information

Edited by Dawn D. Matthews. 531 pages. 1999. 0-7808-0236-5. $78.

"This is an excellent resource for public library reference and health collections."
— *American Reference Books Annual, 2001*

"Recommended reference source."
— *Booklist, American Library Association, May '00*

Respiratory Diseases & Disorders Sourcebook

Basic Information about Respiratory Diseases and Disorders, Including Asthma, Cystic Fibrosis, Pneumonia, the Common Cold, Influenza, and Others, Featuring Facts about the Respiratory System, Statistical and Demographic Data, Treatments, Self-Help Management Suggestions, and Current Research Initiatives

Edited by Allan R. Cook and Peter D. Dresser. 771 pages. 1995. 0-7808-0037-0. $78.

"Designed for the layperson and for patients and their families coping with respiratory illness. . . . an extensive array of information on diagnosis, treatment, management, and prevention of respiratory illnesses for the general reader." — *Choice, Association of College and Research Libraries, Jun '96*

"A highly recommended text for all collections. It is a comforting reminder of the power of knowledge that good books carry between their covers."
— *Academic Library Book Review, Spring '96*

"A comprehensive collection of authoritative information presented in a nontechnical, humanitarian style for patients, families, and caregivers." — *Association of Operating Room Nurses, Sep/Oct '95*

SEE ALSO Lung Disorders Sourcebook

Sexually Transmitted Diseases Sourcebook, 2nd Edition

Basic Consumer Health Information about Sexually Transmitted Diseases, Including Information on the Diagnosis and Treatment of Chlamydia, Gonorrhea, Hepatitis, Herpes, HIV, Mononucleosis, Syphilis, and Others

Along with Information on Prevention, Such as Condom Use, Vaccines, and STD Education; And Featuring a Section on Issues Related to Youth and Adolescents, a Glossary, and Resources for Additional Help and Information

Edited by Dawn D. Matthews. 538 pages. 2001. 0-7808-0249-7. $78.

ALSO AVAILABLE: Sexually Transmitted Diseases Sourcebook, 1st Edition. Edited by Linda M. Ross. 550 pages. 1997. 0-7808-0217-9. $78.

"Recommended for consumer health collections in public libraries, and secondary school and community college libraries."
— *American Reference Books Annual 2002*

"Every school and public library should have a copy of this comprehensive and user-friendly reference book."
— *Choice, Association of College & Research Libraries, Sep '01*

"This is a highly recommended book. This is an especially important book for all school and public libraries." — *AIDS Book Review Journal, Jul-Aug '01*

"Recommended reference source."
— *Booklist, American Library Association, Apr '01*

"Recommended pick both for specialty health library collections and any general consumer health reference collection." — *The Bookwatch, Apr '01*

Skin Disorders Sourcebook

Basic Information about Common Skin and Scalp Conditions Caused by Aging, Allergies, Immune Reactions, Sun Exposure, Infectious Organisms, Parasites, Cosmetics, and Skin Traumas, Including Abrasions, Cuts, and Pressure Sores

Along with Information on Prevention and Treatment

Edited by Allan R. Cook. 647 pages. 1997. 0-7808-0080-X. $78.

"... comprehensive, easily read reference book."
—*Doody's Health Sciences Book Reviews, Oct '97*

SEE ALSO Burns Sourcebook

■

Sleep Disorders Sourcebook, 2nd Edition

Basic Consumer Health Information about Sleep and Sleep Disorders, Including Insomnia, Sleep Apnea, Restless Legs Syndrome, Narcolepsy, Parasomnias, and Other Health Problems That Affect Sleep, Plus Facts about Diagnostic Procedures, Treatment Strategies, Sleep Medications, and Tips for Improving Sleep Quality

Along with a Glossary of Related Terms and Resources for Additional Help and Information

Edited by Amy L. Sutton. 567 pages. 2005. 0-7808-0745-6. $78.

ALSO AVAILABLE: Sleep Disorders Sourcebook, 1st Edition. Edited by Jenifer Swanson. 439 pages. 1998. 0-7808-0234-9. $78.

"This text will complement any home or medical library. It is user-friendly and ideal for the adult reader."
—*American Reference Books Annual, 2000*

"A useful resource that provides accurate, relevant, and accessible information on sleep to the general public. Health care providers who deal with sleep disorders patients may also find it helpful in being prepared to answer some of the questions patients ask."
—*Respiratory Care, Jul '99*

"Recommended reference source."
—*Booklist, American Library Association, Feb '99*

■

Smoking Concerns Sourcebook

Basic Consumer Health Information about Nicotine Addiction and Smoking Cessation, Featuring Facts about the Health Effects of Tobacco Use, Including Lung and Other Cancers, Heart Disease, Stroke, and Respiratory Disorders, Such as Emphysema and Chronic Bronchitis

Along with Information about Smoking Prevention Programs, Suggestions for Achieving and Maintaining a Smoke-Free Lifestyle, Statistics about Tobacco Use, Reports on Current Research Initiatives, a Glossary of Related Terms, and Directories of Resources for Additional Help and Information

Edited by Karen Bellenir. 621 pages. 2004. 0-7808-0323-X. $78.

■

Sports Injuries Sourcebook, 2nd Edition

Basic Consumer Health Information about the Diagnosis, Treatment, and Rehabilitation of Common Sports-Related Injuries in Children and Adults

Along with Suggestions for Conditioning and Training, Information and Prevention Tips for Injuries Frequently Associated with Specific Sports and Special Populations, a Glossary, and a Directory of Additional Resources

Edited by Joyce Brennfleck Shannon. 614 pages. 2002. 0-7808-0604-2. $78.

ALSO AVAILABLE: Sports Injuries Sourcebook, 1st Edition. Edited by Heather E. Aldred. 624 pages. 1999. 0-7808-0218-7. $78.

"This is an excellent reference for consumers and it is recommended for public, community college, and undergraduate libraries."
—*American Reference Books Annual, 2003*

"Recommended reference source."
—*Booklist, American Library Association, Feb '03*

■

Stress-Related Disorders Sourcebook

Basic Consumer Health Information about Stress and Stress-Related Disorders, Including Stress Origins and Signals, Environmental Stress at Work and Home, Mental and Emotional Stress Associated with Depression, Post-Traumatic Stress Disorder, Panic Disorder, Suicide, and the Physical Effects of Stress on the Cardiovascular, Immune, and Nervous Systems

Along with Stress Management Techniques, a Glossary, and a Listing of Additional Resources

Edited by Joyce Brennfleck Shannon. 610 pages. 2002. 0-7808-0560-7. $78.

"Well written for a general readership, the *Stress-Related Disorders Sourcebook* is a useful addition to the health reference literature."
—*American Reference Books Annual, 2003*

"I am impressed by the amount of information. It offers a thorough overview of the causes and consequences of stress for the layperson. ... A well-done and thorough reference guide for professionals and nonprofessionals alike."
—*Doody's Review Service, Dec '02*

■

Stroke Sourcebook

Basic Consumer Health Information about Stroke, Including Ischemic, Hemorrhagic, Transient Ischemic Attack (TIA), and Pediatric Stroke, Stroke Triggers and Risks, Diagnostic Tests, Treatments, and Rehabilitation Information

Along with Stroke Prevention Guidelines, Legal and Financial Information, a Glossary, and a Directory of Additional Resources

Edited by Joyce Brennfleck Shannon. 606 pages. 2003. 0-7808-0630-1. $78.

"This volume is highly recommended and should be in every medical, hospital, and public library."
—*American Reference Books Annual, 2004*

Substance Abuse Sourcebook

Basic Health-Related Information about the Abuse of Legal and Illegal Substances Such as Alcohol, Tobacco, Prescription Drugs, Marijuana, Cocaine, and Heroin; and Including Facts about Substance Abuse Prevention Strategies, Intervention Methods, Treatment and Recovery Programs, and a Section Addressing the Special Problems Related to Substance Abuse during Pregnancy

Edited by Karen Bellenir. 573 pages. 1996. 0-7808-0038-9. $78.

"A valuable addition to any health reference section. Highly recommended."
— *The Book Report, Mar/Apr '97*

". . . a comprehensive collection of substance abuse information that's both highly readable and compact. Families and caregivers of substance abusers will find the information enlightening and helpful, while teachers, social workers and journalists should benefit from the concise format. Recommended."
— *Drug Abuse Update, Winter '96/'97*

SEE ALSO Alcoholism Sourcebook, Drug Abuse Sourcebook

■

Surgery Sourcebook

Basic Consumer Health Information about Inpatient and Outpatient Surgeries, Including Cardiac, Vascular, Orthopedic, Ocular, Reconstructive, Cosmetic, Gynecologic, and Ear, Nose, and Throat Procedures and More

Along with Information about Operating Room Policies and Instruments, Laser Surgery Techniques, Hospital Errors, Statistical Data, a Glossary, and Listings of Sources for Further Help and Information

Edited by Annemarie S. Muth and Karen Bellenir. 596 pages. 2002. 0-7808-0380-9. $78.

"Large public libraries and medical libraries would benefit from this material in their reference collections."
— *American Reference Books Annual, 2004*

"Invaluable reference for public and school library collections alike." — *Library Bookwatch, Apr '03*

■

Thyroid Disorders Sourcebook

Basic Consumer Health Information about Disorders of the Thyroid and Parathyroid Glands, Including Hypothyroidism, Hyperthyroidism, Graves Disease, Hashimoto Thyroiditis, Thyroid Cancer, and Parathyroid Disorders, Featuring Facts about Symptoms, Risk Factors, Tests, and Treatments

Along with Information about the Effects of Thyroid Imbalance on Other Body Systems, Environmental Factors That Affect the Thyroid Gland, a Glossary, and a Directory of Additional Resources

Edited by Joyce Brennfleck Shannon. 599 pages. 2005. 0-7808-0745-6. $78.

Transplantation Sourcebook

Basic Consumer Health Information about Organ and Tissue Transplantation, Including Physical and Financial Preparations, Procedures and Issues Relating to Specific Solid Organ and Tissue Transplants, Rehabilitation, Pediatric Transplant Information, the Future of Transplantation, and Organ and Tissue Donation

Along with a Glossary and Listings of Additional Resources

Edited by Joyce Brennfleck Shannon. 628 pages. 2002. 0-7808-0322-1. $78.

"Along with these advances [in transplantation technology] have come a number of daunting questions for potential transplant patients, their families, and their health care providers. This reference text is the best single tool to address many of these questions. . . . It will be a much-needed addition to the reference collections in health care, academic, and large public libraries."
— *American Reference Books Annual, 2003*

"Recommended for libraries with an interest in offering consumer health information." — *E-Streams, Jul '02*

"This is a unique and valuable resource for patients facing transplantation and their families."
— *Doody's Review Service, Jun '02*

■

Traveler's Health Sourcebook

Basic Consumer Health Information for Travelers, Including Physical and Medical Preparations, Transportation Health and Safety, Essential Information about Food and Water, Sun Exposure, Insect and Snake Bites, Camping and Wilderness Medicine, and Travel with Physical or Medical Disabilities

Along with International Travel Tips, Vaccination Recommendations, Geographical Health Issues, Disease Risks, a Glossary, and a Listing of Additional Resources

Edited by Joyce Brennfleck Shannon. 613 pages. 2000. 0-7808-0384-1. $78.

"Recommended reference source."
— *Booklist, American Library Association, Feb '01*

"This book is recommended for any public library, any travel collection, and especially any collection for the physically disabled."
— *American Reference Books Annual, 2001*

■

Vegetarian Sourcebook

Basic Consumer Health Information about Vegetarian Diets, Lifestyle, and Philosophy, Including Definitions of Vegetarianism and Veganism, Tips about Adopting Vegetarianism, Creating a Vegetarian Pantry, and Meeting Nutritional Needs of Vegetarians, with Facts Regarding Vegetarianism's Effect on Pregnant and Lactating Women, Children, Athletes, and Senior Citizens

Along with a Glossary of Commonly Used Vegetarian Terms and Resources for Additional Help and Information

Edited by Chad T. Kimball. 360 pages. 2002. 0-7808-0439-2. $78.

"Organizes into one concise volume the answers to the most common questions concerning vegetarian diets and lifestyles. This title is recommended for public and secondary school libraries." —*E-Streams, Apr '03*

"Invaluable reference for public and school library collections alike." — *Library Bookwatch, Apr '03*

"The articles in this volume are easy to read and come from authoritative sources. The book does not necessarily support the vegetarian diet but instead provides the pros and cons of this important decision. The *Vegetarian Sourcebook* is recommended for public libraries and consumer health libraries."
—*American Reference Books Annual, 2003*

∎

Women's Health Concerns Sourcebook, 2nd Edition

Basic Consumer Health Information about the Medical and Mental Concerns of Women, Including Maintaining Health and Wellness, Gynecological Concerns, Breast Health, Sexuality and Reproductive Issues, Menopause, Cancer in Women, the Leading Causes of Death and Disability among Women, Physical Concerns of Special Significance to Women, and Women's Mental and Emotional Health

Along with a Glossary of Related Terms and Directories of Resources for Additional Help and Information

Edited by Amy L. Sutton. 748 pages. 2004. 0-7808-0673-5. $78.

ALSO AVAILABLE: Women's Health Concerns Sourcebook, 1st Edition. Edited by Heather E. Aldred. 567 pages. 1997. 0-7808-0219-5. $78.

"Handy compilation. There is an impressive range of diseases, devices, disorders, procedures, and other physical and emotional issues covered . . . well organized, illustrated, and indexed." — *Choice, Association of College and Research Libraries, Jan '98*

SEE ALSO Breast Cancer Sourcebook, Cancer Sourcebook for Women, Healthy Heart Sourcebook for Women, Osteoporosis Sourcebook

∎

Workplace Health & Safety Sourcebook

Basic Consumer Health Information about Workplace Health and Safety, Including the Effect of Workplace Hazards on the Lungs, Skin, Heart, Ears, Eyes, Brain, Reproductive Organs, Musculoskeletal System, and Other Organs and Body Parts

Along with Information about Occupational Cancer, Personal Protective Equipment, Toxic and Hazardous Chemicals, Child Labor, Stress, and Workplace Violence

Edited by Chad T. Kimball. 626 pages. 2000. 0-7808-0231-4. $78.

"As a reference for the general public, this would be useful in any library." —*E-Streams, Jun '01*

"Provides helpful information for primary care physicians and other caregivers interested in occupational medicine. . . . General readers; professionals."
— *Choice, Association of College & Research Libraries, May '01*

"Recommended reference source."
—*Booklist, American Library Association, Feb '01*

"Highly recommended." — *The Bookwatch, Jan '01*

∎

Worldwide Health Sourcebook

Basic Information about Global Health Issues, Including Malnutrition, Reproductive Health, Disease Dispersion and Prevention, Emerging Diseases, Risky Health Behaviors, and the Leading Causes of Death

Along with Global Health Concerns for Children, Women, and the Elderly, Mental Health Issues, Research and Technology Advancements, and Economic, Environmental, and Political Health Implications, a Glossary, and a Resource Listing for Additional Help and Information

Edited by Joyce Brennfleck Shannon. 614 pages. 2001. 0-7808-0330-2. $78.

"Named an Outstanding Academic Title."
—*Choice, Association of College & Research Libraries, Jan '02*

"Yet another handy but also unique compilation in the extensive Health Reference Series, this is a useful work because many of the international publications reprinted or excerpted are not readily available. Highly recommended." —*Choice, Association of College & Research Libraries, Nov '01*

"Recommended reference source."
—*Booklist, American Library Association, Oct '01*

Teen Health Series

Helping Young Adults Understand, Manage, and Avoid Serious Illness

Alcohol Information For Teens

Health Tips About Alcohol And Alcoholism

Including Facts about Underage Drinking, Preventing Teen Alcohol Use, Alcohol's Effects on the Brain and the Body, Alcohol Abuse Treatment, Help for Children of Alcoholics, and More

Edited by Joyce Brennfleck Shannon. 370 pages. 2005. 0-7808-0741-3. $58.

■

Asthma Information for Teens

Health Tips about Managing Asthma and Related Concerns

Including Facts about Asthma Causes, Triggers, Symptoms, Diagnosis, and Treatment

Edited by Karen Bellenir. 375 pages. 2005. 0-7808-0770-7. $58.

■

Cancer Information for Teens

Health Tips about Cancer Awareness, Prevention, Diagnosis, and Treatment

Including Facts about Frequently Occurring Cancers, Cancer Risk Factors, and Coping Strategies for Teens Fighting Cancer or Dealing with Cancer in Friends or Family Members

Edited by Wilma R. Caldwell. 428 pages. 2004. 0-7808-0678-6. $58.

■

Diet Information for Teens

Health Tips about Diet and Nutrition

Including Facts about Nutrients, Dietary Guidelines, Breakfasts, School Lunches, Snacks, Party Food, Weight Control, Eating Disorders, and More

Edited by Karen Bellenir. 399 pages. 2001. 0-7808-0441-4. $58.

"Full of helpful insights and facts throughout the book. . . . An excellent resource to be placed in public libraries or even in personal collections."
—*American Reference Books Annual 2002*

"Recommended for middle and high school libraries and media centers as well as academic libraries that educate future teachers of teenagers. It is also a suitable addition to health science libraries that serve patrons who are interested in teen health promotion and education." —*E-Streams, Oct '01*

"This comprehensive book would be beneficial to collections that need information about nutrition, dietary guidelines, meal planning, and weight control. . . . This reference is so easy to use that its purchase is recommended." —*The Book Report, Sep-Oct '01*

"This book is written in an easy to understand format describing issues that many teens face every day, and then provides thoughtful explanations so that teens can make informed decisions. This is an interesting book that provides important facts and information for today's teens." —*Doody's Health Sciences Book Review Journal, Jul-Aug '01*

"A comprehensive compendium of diet and nutrition. The information is presented in a straightforward, plain-spoken manner. This title will be useful to those working on reports on a variety of topics, as well as to general readers concerned about their dietary health." —*School Library Journal, Jun '01*

■

Drug Information for Teens

Health Tips about the Physical and Mental Effects of Substance Abuse

Including Facts about Alcohol, Anabolic Steroids, Club Drugs, Cocaine, Depressants, Hallucinogens, Herbal Products, Inhalants, Marijuana, Narcotics, Stimulants, Tobacco, and More

Edited by Karen Bellenir. 452 pages. 2002. 0-7808-0444-9. $58.

"A clearly written resource for general readers and researchers alike." —*School Library Journal*

"The chapters are quick to make a connection to their teenage reading audience. The prose is straightforward and the book lends itself to spot reading. It should be useful both for practical information and for research, and it is suitable for public and school libraries." —*American Reference Books Annual, 2003*

"Recommended reference source." —*Booklist, American Library Association, Feb '03*

"This is an excellent resource for teens and their parents. Education about drugs and substances is key to discouraging teen drug abuse and this book provides this much needed information in a way that is interesting and factual." —*Doody's Review Service, Dec '02*

■

Fitness Information for Teens

Health Tips about Exercise, Physical Well-Being, and Health Maintenance

Including Facts about Aerobic and Anaerobic Conditioning, Stretching, Body Shape and Body Image, Sports Training, Nutrition, and Activities for Non-Athletes

Edited by Karen Bellenir. 425 pages. 2004. 0-7808-0679-4. $58.

Mental Health Information for Teens

Health Tips about Mental Health and Mental Illness

Including Facts about Anxiety, Depression, Suicide, Eating Disorders, Obsessive-Compulsive Disorders, Panic Attacks, Phobias, Schizophrenia, and More

Edited by Karen Bellenir. 406 pages. 2001. 0-7808-0442-2. $58.

"In both language and approach, this user-friendly entry in the *Teen Health Series* is on target for teens needing information on mental health concerns." *—Booklist, American Library Association, Jan '02*

"Readers will find the material accessible and informative, with the shaded notes, facts, and embedded glossary insets adding appropriately to the already interesting and succinct presentation." *—School Library Journal, Jan '02*

"This title is highly recommended for any library that serves adolescents and parents/caregivers of adolescents." *—E-Streams, Jan '02*

"Recommended for high school libraries and young adult collections in public libraries. Both health professionals and teenagers will find this book useful." *— American Reference Books Annual 2002*

"This is a nice book written to enlighten the society, primarily teenagers, about common teen mental health issues. It is highly recommended to teachers and parents as well as adolescents." *— Doody's Review Service, Dec '01*

Sexual Health Information for Teens

Health Tips about Sexual Development, Human Reproduction, and Sexually Transmitted Diseases

Including Facts about Puberty, Reproductive Health, Chlamydia, Human Papillomavirus, Pelvic Inflammatory Disease, Herpes, AIDS, Contraception, Pregnancy, and More

Edited by Deborah A. Stanley. 391 pages. 2003. 0-7808-0445-7. $58.

"This work should be included in all high school libraries and many larger public libraries. . . . highly recommended." *— American Reference Books Annual 2004*

"Sexual Health approaches its subject with appropriate seriousness and offers easily accessible advice and information." *— School Library Journal, Feb. 2004*

Skin Health Information For Teens

Health Tips about Dermatological Concerns and Skin Cancer Risks

Including Facts about Acne, Warts, Hives, and Other Conditions and Lifestyle Choices, Such as Tanning, Tattooing, and Piercing, That Affect the Skin, Nails, Scalp, and Hair

Edited by Robert Aquinas McNally. 429 pages. 2003. 0-7808-0446-5. $58.

"This volume, as with others in the series, will be a useful addition to school and public library collections." *—American Reference Books Annual 2004*

"This volume serves as a one-stop source and should be a necessity for any health collection." *— Library Media Connection*

Sports Injuries Information For Teens

Health Tips about Sports Injuries and Injury Protection

Including Facts about Specific Injuries, Emergency Treatment, Rehabilitation, Sports Safety, Competition Stress, Fitness, Sports Nutrition, Steroid Risks, and More

Edited by Joyce Brennfleck Shannon. 405 pages. 2003. 0-7808-0447-3. $58.

"This work will be useful in the young adult collections of public libraries as well as high school libraries." *— American Reference Books Annual 2004*

Suicide Information for Teens

Health Tips about Suicide Causes and Prevention

Including Facts about Depression, Risk Factors, Getting Help, Survivor Support, and More

Edited by Joyce Brennfleck Shannon. 368 pages. 2005. 0-7808-0737-5. $58.

Health Reference Series